Human Hybridomas

IMMUNOLOGY SERIES

1. Mechanisms in Allergy: Reagin-Mediated Hypersensitivity
   Edited by Lawrence Goodfriend, Alec Sehon and Robert P. Orange
2. Immunopathology: Methods and Techniques
   Edited by Theodore P. Zacharia and Sidney S. Breese, Jr.
3. Immunity and Cancer in Man: An Introduction
   Edited by Arnold E. Reif
4. *Bordetella pertussis:* Immunological and Other Biological Activities
   J.J. Munoz and R.K. Bergman
5. The Lymphocyte: Structure and Function (in two parts)
   Edited by John J. Marchalonis
6. Immunology of Receptors
   Edited by B. Cinader
7. Immediate Hypersensitivity: Modern Concepts and Development
   Edited by Michael K. Bach
8. Theoretical Immunology
   Edited by George I. Bell, Alan S. Perelson, and George H. Pimbley, Jr.
9. Immunodiagnosis of Cancer (in two parts)
   Edited by Ronald B. Herberman and K. Robert McIntire
10. Immunologically Mediated Renal Diseases: Criteria for Diagnosis and Treatment
    Edited by Robert T. McCluskey and Giuseppe A. Andres
11. Clinical Immunotherapy
    Edited by Albert F. LoBuglio
12. Mechanisms of Immunity to Virus-Induced Tumors
    Edited by John W. Blasecki
13. Manual of Macrophage Methodology: Collection, Characterization, and Function
    Edited by Herbert B. Herscowitz, Howard T. Holden, Joseph A. Bellanti, and Abdul Ghaffar
14. Suppressor Cells in Human Disease
    Edited by James S. Goodwin
15. Immunological Aspects of Aging
    Edited by Diego Segre and Lester Smith

16. Cellular and Molecular Mechanisms of Immunologic Tolerance
Edited by Tomáš Hraba and Milan Hašek

17. Immune Regulation: Evolution and Biological Significance
Edited by Laurens N. Ruben and M. Eric Gershwin

18. Tumor Immunity in Prognosis: The Role of Mononuclear Cell Infiltration
Edited by Stephen Haskill

19. Immunopharmacology and the Regulation of Leukocyte Function
Edited by David R. Webb

20. Pathogenesis and Immunology of Treponemal Infection
Edited by Ronald F. Schell and Daniel M. Musher

21. Macrophage-Mediated Antibody-Dependent Cellular Cytotoxicity
Edited by Hillel S. Koren

22. Molecular Immunology: A Textbook
Edited by M. Zouhair Atassi, Carel J. van Oss, and Darryl R. Absolom

23. Monoclonal Antibodies and Cancer
Edited by George L. Wright, Jr.

24. Stress, Immunity, and Aging
Edited by Edwin L. Cooper

25. Immune Modulation Agents and Their Mechanisms
Edited by Richard L. Fenichel and Michael A. Chirigos

26. Mononuclear Phagocyte Biology
Edited by Alvin Volkman

27. The Lactoperoxidase System: Chemistry and Biological Significance
Edited by Kenneth M. Pruitt and Jorma O. Tenovuo

28. Introduction to Medical Immunology
Edited by Gabriel Virella, Jean-Michel Goust, H. Hugh Fudenberg, and Christian C. Patrick

29. Handbook of Food Allergies
Edited by James C. Breneman

30. Human Hybridomas: Diagnostic and Therapeutic Applications
Edited by Anthony J. Strelkauskas

31. Aging and the Immune Response: Cellular and Humoral Aspects
Edited by Edmond A. Goidl

32. Complications of Organ Transplantation
Edited by Luis H. Toledo-Pereyra

33. Monoclonal Antibodies: Hybridoma Techniques
Edited by Lawrence B. Schook

Additional Volumes in Preparation

Human Hybridomas

Diagnostic and Therapeutic Applications

edited by

ANTHONY J. STRELKAUSKAS
Department of Pediatrics
Medical University of South Carolina
Charleston, South Carolina

MARCEL DEKKER, INC. New York and Basel

Library of Congress Cataloging-in-Publication Data

Human hybridomas.

(Immunology series ; 30)
Includes bibliographies and index.
1. Antibodies, Monoclonal--Diagnostic use.
2. Antibodies, Monoclonal--Therapeutic use. 3. Hybridomas.
I. Strelkauskas, Anthony J. II. Series:
Immunology series ; v. 30. [DNLM: 1. Antibodies,
Monoclonal. 2. Hybridomas. W1 IM53K v. 30 / QW 575 H9185]
ISBN 0-8247-7521-X

MARCEL DEKKER, INC.
270 Madison Avenue, New York, New York 10016

Current printing (last digit):
10 9 8 7 6 5 4 3 2 1

PRINTED IN THE UNITED STATES OF AMERICA

For

Dad, Jenky, Jennifer, and Dan

Preface

There have been several biological revolutions, perhaps the last being the elucidation of DNA structure and function and the beginnings of molecular biology. A more recent would-be revolution took place in 1976 when Köhler and Milstein reported the successful fusion of murine cells to construct a hybrid antibody-producing clone. Since that report, there has been an explosion in the area of hybridoma research and development which has resulted not only in the development of a tremendous number of clones, but also in the establishment of a growing multimillion-dollar commercial industry predicated on the construction of hybrid clones and the marketing of resultant antibodies. Together with the strides made in genetic engineering, hybridoma technology must without question be considered one of the cornerstones of biotechnology.

Several excellent books on murine monoclonals have been published, and no doubt future months will see several other equally fine volumes on the subject. This work is an attempt to describe some of the work currently being done exclusively with human hybrid cells. Although they are essentially identical to murine clones, several differences exist, perhaps the most obvious being the possibility of using these antibodies more effectively *in vivo*. Whether this proves to be the case remains to be seen, but the potential is certainly there. In compiling this book I have chosen a diverse array of work which focuses on areas of clonal construction and on the impact of human monoclonal antibodies on infectious diseases and cancer research. Also included is a chapter on the regulatory impact of the Food and Drug Administration on these antibodies. The potential for greater sensitivity, specificity, therapeutic effect, and safety of antibodies produced by human clones has made them extremely important. Many laboratories in the world are concentrating on their construction, and it is becoming obvious that, as with many other biological systems, there are many inherent problems which were not completely foreseen by those who imagined that human monoclonals could be easily constructed by following in the footsteps of our murine system predecessors.

Perhaps the current state of human monoclonal development is best described by paraphrasing the late Dr. Jacques Monod, one of the fathers of molecular biology: "We are still trying to understand."

Anthony J. Strelkauskas

Contents

Contributors

Paul H. Aldenderfer, Ph.D. Senior Scientist, Department of Pediatrics, Medical University of South Carolina, Charleston, South Carolina

Rinette B. Andreasen, M.D. Medical Department A, State University Hospital, Rigshospitalet, Copenhagen, Denmark

Tsehay Atlaw* Graduate Student, Department of Microbiology and Immunology, Queen's University, Kingston, Ontario, Canada

Phyllis D. Bear, Ph.D. Professor of Molecular Biology, Division of Microbiology and Biochemistry, University of Wyoming, Laramie, Wyoming

Marcia Bieber, M.D. Department of Radiology, Cancer Biology Research Laboratory, Stanford, California

Karen G. Burnett, Ph.D. Section Manager, Human Antibody Development, Hybritech Incorporated, San Diego, California

---

Present affiliation:

*Research Fellow, Armauer Hansen Research Institute, Addis Ababa, Ethiopia

Barbara G. Campling, M.D. Ontario Cancer Treatment and Research Foundation, and Assistant Professor, Department of Radiation Oncology, Queen's University, Kingston, Ontario, Canada

Susan P. C. Cole, Ph.D. Career Scientist, Kingston Regional Cancer Centre, Ontario Cancer Treatment and Research Foundation, and Assistant Professor, Departments of Radiation Oncology and Microbiology and Immunology, Queen's University, Kingston, Ontario, Canada

Paul A. W. Edwards, Ph.D.* Ludwig Institute for Cancer Research (London Branch), Sutton, Surrey, England

Bruce D. Freimark, Ph.D. Research Associate, Scripps Clinic and Research Foundation, La Jolla, California

Shaik A. Gaffar, Ph.D. Postgraduate Researcher, University of California-San Diego Cancer Center, San Diego, California

Mark C Glassy, Ph.D. Assistant Research Immunologist, University of California-San Diego Cancer Center, San Diego, California

Michael Glembourtt Research Associate, Cetus Immune Corporation, Palo Alto, California

Sarah Hart† Research Laboratories, Cetus Immune Corporation, Palo Alto, California

Joan M. Hayden Senior Research Assistant, Cell Biology-Human Antibody Development, Hybritech Incorporated, San Diego, California

Rachel Hernandez, Ph.D. Senior Research Associate, Hybritech Incorporated, San Diego, California

May-Kin Ho, Ph.D. Supervisor, Immunology Research, Biomedical Products Department, E. I. Du Pont de Nemours & Company, North Billerica, Massachusetts

Yao-Pi Hsu Research Assistant, Department of Pediatrics, Stanford University School of Medicine, Palo Alto, California

---

Present affiliations:
*Department of Pathology, University of Cambridge, Cambridge, England
†Biotherapy Systems, Inc., Mountain View, California

Danuta Kozbor, Ph.D. Associate Scientist, The Wistar Institute, Philadelphia, Pennsylvania

James W. Larrick, M.D., Ph.D. Director, Research Laboratories, Cetus Immune Corporation, Palo Alto, California

David S. Lippman* Laboratory Associate II, Research Laboratories, Cetus Immune Corporation, Palo Alto, California

Nicki J. McRoberts, Ph.D. Senior Research Assistant, Hybritech Incorporated, San Diego, California

Richard B. Moss, M.D. Assistant Professor, Department of Pediatrics, Stanford University School of Medicine, Stanford, California

Esther H. Oh Research Scientist, Hybritech Incorporated, San Diego, California

Michael J. O'Hare, Ph.D. Research Scientist, Ludwig Institute for Cancer Research (London Branch), Sutton, Surrey, England

Lennart Olsson, M.D., Dsc. Cancer Biology Laboratory, State University Hospital, Rigshospitalet, Copenhagen, Denmark

Howard Ozer, M.D., Ph.D. Professor and Chief, Division of Oncology, University of North Carolina at Chapel Hill, and Associate Director for Clinical Affairs, Lineberger Cancer Research Center, Chapel Hill, North Carolina

Robert E. Peters, Ph.D.[†] Postdoctoral Fellow, University of California-San Diego Cancer Center, San Diego, California

John C. Roder, Ph.D.[‡] Department of Microbiology and Immunology, Queen's University, Kingston, Ontario, Canada

Ivor Royston, M.D. Associate Professor, Department of Medicine, University of California-San Diego Cancer Center, San Diego, California

---

Present affiliations:
*Biotherapy Systems, Inc., Mountain View, California
†Research Scientist, Cytotech, Inc., San Diego, California
‡Mount Sinai Research Institute, Toronto, Ontario, Canada

Victoria Schauf, M.D.* Professor and Chairman, Department of Pediatrics, Nassau County Medical Center, East Meadow, New York

Karol Sikora, M.D., Ph.D., F.R.C.R., F.R.C.P. Professor, Department of Clinical Oncology, Royal Postgraduate Medical School, London, England

Lloyd H. Smith, M.D., Ph.D. Fellow, Division of Gynecologic Oncology, Department of Gynecology and Obstetrics, Stanford University School of Medicine, Stanford, California

Matthew R. Smith† Student, Summer Undergraduate Research Program, Department of Pediatrics, Medical University of South Carolina, Charleston, South Carolina

Anthony J. Strelkauskas, Ph.D. Associate Professor, Department of Pediatrics, Medical University of South Carolina, Charleston, South Carolina

Catherine L. Taylor Graduate Student, Department of Molecular and Cellular Biology and Pathobiology, Medical University of South Carolina, Charleston, South Carolina

Nelson N. H. Teng, M.D., Ph.D. Assistant Professor, Section of Gynecologic Oncology, Department of Gynecology and Obstetrics, and Cancer Biology Research Laboratories, Stanford University School of Medicine, Stanford, California

Kathleen M. Waldron Senior Research Assistant, Cell Biology-Human Antibody Development, Hybritech Incorporated, San Diego, California

Glenn A. Warner, M.D. Director, Northwest Oncology Clinics, Seattle, Washington

---

**Previous affiliation*: Center for Drugs and Biologics, Division of Anti-infective Drug Products and Division of Bacterial Products, Food and Drug Administration, Bethesda, Maryland

†*Present affiliation*: Student, Medical Scientist Training Program, Biochemistry Department, Duke University Medical Center, Durham, North Carolina

Human Hybridomas

I

GENERAL AND TECHNICAL CONSIDERATIONS

1

The EBV Hybridoma Technique and Its Applications

BARBARA G. CAMPLING and SUSAN P. C. COLE
Ontario Cancer Treatment and Research Foundation and Queen's University, Kingston, Ontario, Canada

TSEHAY ATLAW* and JOHN C. RODER†
Queen's University, Kingston, Ontario, Canada

DANUTA KOZBOR
The Wistar Institute, Philadelphia, Pennsylvania

The development of *in vitro* methods for the production of human antibodies of desired specificity has long been an elusive goal. The first successful attempts at achieving this involved the immortalization of human B lymphocytes with Epstein-Barr virus (EBV). Epstein-Barr virus is a B-lymphotropic herpes virus that causes polyclonal activation and immortalization of antibody-producing human B cells (1). Steinitz *et al.* (2) were the first to recognize that this capability could be used to establish permanent cell lines to produce human antibodies of predetermined specificity. By using lymphocytes from subjects with high natural antibody titers to the synthetic hapten NNP (4-hydroxy-3,5-dinitrophenacetic acid), they preselected antigen-binding lymphocytes and then established permanent lines by infection with EBV. Others (3-18) subsequently applied this technique to produce antibodies that react with a variety of specific antigens.

It soon became apparent that there were major limitations with the EBV method. Although specific antibodies could be produced, the levels of immunoglobulin production were low (<1 μg/ml), and antibody production declined rapidly with time (3). Furthermore, the lines were very difficult to clone (19).

When the use of the murine hybridoma technology of Kohler and Milstein (20) became widespread, it was felt that the same techniques could be easily applied

---

Present affiliations:
*Armauer Hansen Research Institute, Addis Ababa, Ethiopia
†Mount Sinai Research Institute, Toronto, Ontario, Canada

to the production of human monoclonal antibodies (MAbs). The first reports (21,22) of successful human-human hybridomas appeared in 1980. Since then, one of the major problems has been the lack of an ideal human myeloma fusion partner.

We have developed a human hybridoma system that combines many of the advantages of the EBV technique and the human hybridoma technique, while avoiding some of the pitfalls. In this chapter, we will describe:

I. the development of the EBV hybridoma technique,
II. methods,
III. advantages and disadvantages of this technique,
IV. attempts currently underway to improve this technology, and
V. applications of this method to produce specific monoclonal antibodies.

I. THE DEVELOPMENT OF THE EBV HYBRIDOMA TECHNIQUE

Our initial efforts to produce human monoclonal antibodies began before any human fusion partners were available. Tetanus toxoid (TT) was selected as a "model antigen," since it was ethically possible to immunize human subjects with this antigen, and the antibody screening assays were well established. Zurawski *et al.* (3) had already been successful in establishing lymphoblastoid lines that secreted antibody to TT, but levels of antibody production were low (0.1-0.3 μg/ml) and declined rapidly with time. We set out to optimize the conditions for production of human MAbs by the EBV technique (17).

B lymphocytes from a multiply immunized donor, obtained 2 to 3 weeks after the last injection of TT, were found to produce the greatest amount of specific antibody after transformation with EBV. The first step was to enrich the donor's peripheral blood lymphocytes for B cells by removal of T cells and adherent macrophages. Different methods for preselection of antigen-specific B cells were then investigated. A negative preselection method that involved removal of cells not binding TT proved to be the most successful technique, and resulted in a sixfold increase in TT-binding B cells and a threefold increase in anti-TT antibody production. Positive selection by rosetting with TT-coupled sheep red blood cells (SRBC) or by sorting strongly binding cells on a fluorescence activated cell sorter, was unsuccessful.

Even when antigen-specific preselected B cells were transformed with EBV, only a minority (2%) of the resultant lymphoblastoid cells secreted specific antibody, as detected in a plaque-forming cell assay. If unselected cells had been used, antigen-specific cells would have been undetectable. Early cloning of the EBV-transformed cells was essential if antibody production was to be maintained because specific antibody production quickly declined to undetectable levels in bulk cultures.

Using this method, three clonal cell lines producing anti-TT antibody of the IgM-kappa class were obtained. The levels of antibody produced were in the range of 1 μg/ml, which was much higher than in those in previous reports. One of these clones, B6, which produced the highest levels of antibody, was subcloned, and was stable in culture for up to 8 months, but then shut off production of light chains.

After the report of Levy and Dilley (23), showing that it was possible to "rescue" human immunoglobulin production by fusion of human antibody producing cells with mouse myeloma cells, it seemed appropriate to fuse the anti-TT-specific clone, B6, with a nonsecreting variant of the mouse myeloma line, P3x63Ag8 (24). Others (25-33) have also found that human X mouse fusion is a useful technique for the production of human MAbs. Fused cells were selected in medium containing hypoxanthine/aminopterin/thymidine (HAT) and ouabain. Because of the natural resistance to ouabain of mouse compared with human cell lines, only mouse-human hybrids were able to grow. Of 100 hybridoma clones screened, 70 secreted anti-TT antibody, though only 15 of these had sustained production. Levels of antibody production were improved by fusion; thus, the human parent B6 produced up to 0.95 μg/ml, whereas the B6 X P3x63Ag8 hybrids produced up to 2 μg/ml of specific antibody. Because the mouse fusion partner was a nonsecreting line, there was no contamination or dilution of specific antibody with irrelevant immunoglobulins. Another advantage of this method was that the hybridomas were able to grow in very low levels (1%) of serum.

The first reports (21,22) of human-human hybridomas appeared in 1980. Human hybrids were expected to be more stable than interspecies hybrids because of the tendency of human-mouse somatic cell hybrids to lose human chromosomes. A major limitation of human hybridoma technology at the present time continues to be the lack of an ideal human fusion partner. Human myeloma lines have been exceptionally difficult to establish in culture, and only two true myeloma lines are readily available for distribution (33,34). Both of these have been shown to be less than ideal as human fusion partners (29,30).

As a result, a number of laboratories, including our own, have used the more readily available lymphoblastoid cell lines as fusion partners for human hybridomas (22,29,30,35-44). The GM-1500 cell line, available from the American Type Culture Collection (ATCC), was rendered resistant to 6-thioguanine by Croce *et al.* (22). This line was established from a patient with myeloma and, thus, was originally believed to be a plasmacytoma cell line. However, it has now been shown to be a lymphoblastoid line by its morphology and its expression of Epstein-Barr nuclear antigen (EBNA) (35,45). It secretes small amounts of gamma heavy chains and kappa light chains.

Because both the HAT-sensitive fusion partner GM-1500 and our TT-specific lymphoblastoid line B6 were immortal cell lines, it was necessary to introduce another selection marker into the fusion partner before hybridization. Thus, we developed a ouabain-resistant variant of the 6-thioguanine-resistant GM-1500 cell line by mutagenizing with low-level gamma irradiation, and then growing the cells in gradually increasing concentrations of ouabain. One resulting line, called KR-4, was found to be resistant to a remarkably high level (0.5 mM) of ouabain, 5 months after mutagenesis.

II. METHODS

The fusion protocol for producing human MAbs is essentially the same as that for producing mouse MAbs. Some 10^7 B6 cells were fused with 10^7 KR-4 cells using 45% (wt/vol) polyethylene glycol (MW 4000). Fused cells were plated in microtiter wells at 2×10^5 cells/well, using irradiated mouse spleen cells (2×10^5 cells/well) and mouse peritoneal cells (5×10^3 cells/well) as feeders. After 12 days in tissue culture medium (RPMI-1640 medium with 20% fetal bovine serum, 4 mM glutamine, and 50 μM 2-mercaptoethanol containing HAT and 10 μM ouabain), growth of hybrid cells was apparent microscopically, and control cultures of each parental line showed no surviving cells. The fusion frequency was calculated to be greater than 1 in 10^5, using the Poisson equation. When KR-4 was fused with nontransformed B cells, the fusion frequency was much lower (4×10^{-7}).

Fifty-four of 56 B6 X KR-4 hybrid cells were positive by ELISA for anti-TT antibody production. The four most positive hybrids were cloned by limiting dilution, and the cloning efficiency of these hybrids (64%) was considerably higher than that of the anti-TT lymphoblastoid line B6. The majority of the clones also continued to secrete anti-TT antibody in levels up to 6 μg/ml. As expected, the hybrid cells were near tetraploid, and expressed HLA antigens co-dominantly from both parental lines. A number of hybrids have now been stable in culture for over 2 years. Thus, it seems that fusion of antibody-producing lymphoblastoid cells with our fusion partner KR-4 serves to increase fusion frequencies, augment and stabilize antibody production, and increase cloning efficiency.

III. ADVANTAGES AND DISADVANTAGES OF THIS TECHNIQUE

The EBV hybridoma technique offers several advantages over other human-human hybridoma systems (listed in Table 1). A number of groups, including ours (35, 36,41,43,46,47), have found that stimulation of lymphocytes with EBV or other polyclonal activators, such as pokeweed mitogen, will increase fusion frequencies. The EBV has the added advantage in that it selectively immortalizes B cells. As

Table 1 Advantages of the EBV Hybridoma Technique

1. Selects for B cells prior to fusion
2. Can immortalize and expand a population of B cells; these cells can then be frozen for future use
3. Antigen-specific B cells can be preselected prior to fusion
4. High fusion frequencies (1 in 10^{-5})
5. High levels of immunoglobulin production (up to 100 μg/ml in some cases)
6. High levels of antibody production can be maintained (although in some cases, frequent recloning is necessary)

such, EBV infection is an excellent method for selecting B lymphocytes out of a mixed population of cells. For example, we have been able to establish EBV lines from tumor-infiltrating B cells by directly infecting tumor tissue with the virus. The hybridization frequency of KR-4 with lymphoblastoid cells is 1×10^{-5}. Non-transformed peripheral blood lymphocytes have a much lower fusion frequency with KR-4, only 4×10^{-7} (35). This is, in part, explained by the fact that only 1 in 10 peripheral blood mononuclear cells is a B cell. As well, KR-4 seems to fuse preferentially with EBV-transformed cells (47), which is not surprising, since it is itself an EBV-transformed cell line. KR-4 is now available through the ATCC and has been used successfully by other investigators (48).

The EBV hybridoma method is the most convenient of human hybridoma systems. The EBV-transformed cells can be expanded and frozen away, to be fused when it is convenient to do so. As well, it is possible to select and expand antigen-specific B cells prior to fusion. The levels of immunoglobulin produced using this system are among the highest reported for human MAbs, up to 100 μg/ml. Some of the hybrids have been stable for many months in culture, although others must be repeatedly subcloned to maintain stability (see section IV).

The major stimulus for development of human hybridoma systems has been the anticipation that human MAbs will be preferable to murine MAbs for the treatment of human diseases. It is natural that there be some concern expressed about the use of products of virus-infected human cell lines for human therapy. However, we do not believe that this will prove to be a problem. The EBV is a ubiquitous virus in North America, with 80-90% of all adults showing serological evidence of prior infection. Subjects who have had EBV infection, whether clinical or subclinical, will continue to harbor the EBV genome in some of their lymphocytes. As Crawford *et al.* (49) have pointed out, this means that 80-90% of transfused blood products will contain EBV. Only rarely does this prove to be a problem. Even if there is EBV present in the human MAbs produced by this method, it is possible to purify the immunoglobulins, and inactivate any DNA that might be remaining in the preparation, as has been outlined previously (49).

In fact, an EBV-infected hybridoma cell line has already been used in a clinical trial, with no untoward effects. Watson *et al.* (50) devised a simple chamber in which human hybridomas could be grown *in vivo*. This chamber was implanted subcutaneously into the abdominal wall of a patient with an advanced malignant glioma. Human hybridoma cells producing antibodies that react with malignant gliomas (40), and derived initially from this particular patient's lymphocytes, were grown in this chamber. The hybridoma cells expressed EBNA, but did not secrete the virus. The subcutaneous chamber remained in place for more than 3 months without causing any problems. Monoclonal antibody secreted by the hybridoma was detected in the circulation, but there was no change in the patient's EBV titer. The U.S. Food and Drug Administration has now approved a clinical trial of a human MAb that is the product of an EBV-positive lymphoblastoid cell line (51).

The problems encountered with the EBV hybridoma technique are common to all human hybridoma systems. Our KR-4 fusion partner secretes small amounts of IgG-k, and this interferes with specific antibody production. Despite efforts by many groups, there is still no widely available nonsecreting human fusion partner.

Another problem with all human hybridoma systems is the lack of adequate numbers of antigen-specific B cells. It is not always ethically possible to immunize human subjects against a specific antigen, especially when the antigen of interest is a tumor-associated antigen. For this reason, a number of groups (47,52, 53) are exploring the feasibility of *in vitro* immunization. Another group (54) has used precursor enrichment techniques to increase the numbers of antigen-specific cells for the production of human monoclonal antibodies.

In the mouse system, it is possible to greatly amplify the production of MAbs by growing the hybridomas as ascites tumors in syngeneic mice. Obviously, it is not possible to do this with humans. Attempts have been made to grow human hybridomas in immunodeficient (nude) mice, as discussed in section IV, but, in general, human myeloma and lymphoblastoid lines do not grow well in nude mice. In addition, nude mice are very expensive, so even if all technical problems were overcome, this system would likely not be suitable for large-scale production of human MAbs.

We have encountered considerable variability in the stability of antibody secretion of our human hybridomas (see section IV). Some of the hybridomas are stable for years, while others have to be repeatedly recloned to maintain spefic antibody production. This process can be tedious, time-consuming, and expensive.

IV. ATTEMPTS CURRENTLY UNDERWAY TO IMPROVE THIS TECHNOLOGY

KR-4 is an excellent fusion partner in terms of fusion frequencies and levels of antibody secretion. However, because of the significant problems of instability of antibody production and secretion of endogenous immunoglobulin, we sought to develop better fusion partners. We attempted to improve the features of our KR-4 fusion partner by hybridizing it with the human myeloma line RPMI-8226 (33). In this way, we hoped to create a new line with the high growth rate and fusion frequencies of KR-4, but with the capacity to support high levels of immunoglobulin production expected of a myeloma line. This approach is not new and, in fact, a widely used mouse myeloma fusion partner is itself a hybrid between two murine myeloma cell lines (55).

We have now selected for further study a hybrid myeloma KR-12 (56). This line secretes gamma and kappa chains of the KR-4 parent and lambda light chains of the RPMI-8226 parent. It has been selected for 6-thioguanine and ouabain resistance, so that it can be fused with human lymphoblastoid cell lines. It has the ultrastructural features of a plasma cell line, with a large amount of rough endoplasmic reticulum and prominent golgi apparatus. However, it has the desirable growth characteristics of a lymphoblastoid line, with a doubling time of 24-28 hours, and fusion frequencies comparable with those of the KR-4 parent (1 in 10^{-5} with lymphoblastoid lines, and 8 in 10^{-7} with unstimulated lymphocytes).

KR-12 has now been fused with the anti-TT-secreting lymphoblastoid line B6 (54). The resultant hybrids secrete up to 30 μg/ml of immunoglobulin, although only up to 10 μg/ml of this is specific anti-TT antibody. These hybrids have been stable after more than a year in continuous culture.

Most of the widely used mouse myeloma lines do not produce or secrete their own immunoglobulins and, as such, they are able to support the secretion of specific antibodies without contamination or dilution with irrelevant immunoglobulins. Although there have been reports of low secretors or even nonsecretory human fusion partners (43,46,57,58), these are not widely available. One of us (Kozbor, unpublished results) has selected for a non-Ig-producing variant of the hybrid myeloma KR-12, using two approaches. First, the Ig-positive cells were repeatedly killed with rabbit anti-human Ig and complement, and second, Ig-negative variants were selected using the fluorescence-activated cell sorter. After many such selections, some clones have been obtained that are negative for surface Ig expression, but lines that do not synthesize any detectable heavy or light chains have not yet been observed. Further studies are now in progress to determine the usefulness of these fusion partners.

One of the remaining limitations of the human MAb techniques developed thus far is the lack of sufficient numbers of antigen-specific B-cells. We have shown that naturally occurring tumor-specific antibodies in cancer patients occur at an extremely low frequency (19). The chances of success in obtaining specific human MAbs still depends largely on either the prior deliberate immunization of human subjects (which is not always possible or ethically feasible) or the presence of naturally occurring autoreactive B cells. This severely limits the number of antigens to which MAbs can be formed.

The chances of finding antibody-producing cells of desired specificity can be greatly improved by enriching antigen-specific lymphocytes prior to fusion. This can be done using *in vitro* immunization or by precursor enrichment techniques. A variety of methods for *in vitro* immunization of mouse spleen cells have been described (59-61), and the various factors to be considered have been reviewed (62). These techniques have now been effectively coupled with murine hybridoma technology (63-68). *In vitro* immunization has been used with some success in human hybridoma systems for production of human MAbs to tetanus toxoid antigen (47), sheep erythrocytes (53), and a variety of other antigens (52). However, this technique is not yet developed for routine applications. An alternative approach used by Winger *et al.* (54) has been to enrich for antigen-specific B cells using panning or rosetting techniques.

Another major obstacle to be overcome is that of bulk production of human MAbs. In the murine system, hybridomas can be easily grown as ascites in syngeneic mice, thus increasing the yields of MAbs 1000-fold. It is obviously not feasible to grow human hybridomas in syngeneic animals, so immunodeficient (nude) mice have been used to avoid xenograft rejection. In general, however, human myeloma and lymphoblastoid cells do not grow well in nude mice (69, 70). We have observed that human hybridomas can be induced to grow as ascites in nude mice by first growing them as solid subcutaneous tumors in irradiated nude mice, readapting the cells to tissue culture, and then injecting them as ascites into irradiated, pristane-primed nude mice (56,71,72). We found that after one passage as a subcutaneous tumor, hybrids formed with either KR-4 or KR-12 became more tumorigenic and would grow as ascites tumors in some of the mice. One of the KR-4 X B6 hybrids secreted 0.7 mg/ml of human Ig, with 0.3 mg of this being specific for TT. After a second passage *in vivo,* Ig production increased up to 1.5 mg/ml, with up to 0.7 mg/ml of this being specific IgM. The KR-12 X B6 hybrids secreted even higher levels, with up to 5.1 mg/ml being specific IgM. The higher levels of Ig production in ascites can only be partially explained by a 20-30-fold higher cell density in the ascites fluid as compared with tissue culture. An interesting observation was that the KR-4 hybrids adopted a myelomalike morphology when grown as ascites. This may have contributed to the increased immunoglobulin production. Despite our limited success, it is unlikely that ascites growth of human hybridomas will prove to be an efficient or economically practical means for large-scale production of human MAbs. Nude mice are expensive and difficult to maintain, and the volume of ascites that they produce is small (usually < 2 ml). Furthermore, less than half of the animals will form ascites.

There is work currently in progress to adapt large-scale tissue culture techniques for the bulk production of human MAbs. To be economically feasible, a serum-free culture system is essential. We have now adapted a number of hybridomas, secreting antibodies to TT or to lung tumor cells, to growth in serum-free medium containing albumin and transferrin (73). Efforts are currently underway to develop a completely protein-free system.

V. APPLICATION OF THIS METHOD TO PRODUCE SPECIFIC MONOCLONAL ANTIBODIES

A. Lung Cancer

In a variety of human neoplasms, including melanoma (74,75), breast cancer (76,77), and sarcoma (78,79), a naturally occurring host antibody response to the tumor has been demonstrated. Therefore, it should be possible to select and immortalize tumor-reactive antibody-producing B cells using human hybridoma techniques. It has already been demonstrated in the mouse system that it is possible to produce monoclonal antibodies to a naturally occurring murine tumor (80). Because of the potential therapeutic advantages of human MAbs, there has been a great deal of effort directed toward producing human MAbs reactive with human tumors.

We have chosen to study human lung cancer because of its tremendous importance as a public health hazard and because there is evidence from a number of sources of a host immune response (81,82). Since in most cases of lung cancer there is a history of exposure to carcinogens, it may be analogous to the highly immunogenic methylcholanthrene-induced tumors in mice (83).

We have now established over 30 EBV-transformed cell lines from lymph nodes, tumors, effusions, and peripheral blood of patients with all major histological types of lung cancer (19). Initially, we attempted to clone several of these EBV lines. We found that the cloning efficiency of the different cell lines was quite variable, but generally they were very difficult to clone, even with the use of mouse spleen feeder cells or conditioned medium from other EBV lines. Supernatants from 140 clones were tested for reactivity against glutaraldehyde-fixed tumor cells using an ELISA system. Only one of these 140 clones showed any positivity. We concluded that B lymphocytes secreting antibody specific for tumor antigens occur at a very low frequency and cannot be easily cloned out of a polyclonal EBV-transformed population. A more productive approach has been to use the EBV-hybridoma technique. We have now done more than 150 fusions, and screened supernatants from more than 10,000 hybrids for reactivity with fixed tumor cells. From this experience, we can make the following conclusions. When uncloned EBV lines are fused with KR-4, the proportion of positive hybrids is highly variable, ranging from 0-20%. The source of donor lymphocytes appears to be important. In general, lymphocytes obtained from tumor-draining lymph nodes yield the highest proportion of positive hybrids. The frequency of positive hybrids decreases with increasing passage number of the EBV line, although fusion frequency is unaffected. The vast majority of positive hybrids showed apparently nonspecific reactivity in that they also reacted with the autologous EBV lines. Nearly all of the hybridomas produced IgM, and levels of immunoglobulin production ranged from less than 1 to 100 μg/ml.

To overcome the problem of the very low frequency of tumor-specific B cells in patients with lung cancer, we have now changed our previous strategy in one respect. After establishment of an EBV line and prior to fusion, the cells were plated at 100 cells/well, and the supernatants were screened for reactivity against fixed lung tumor cells. Selected positive wells were then expanded, and these prescreened "mini-clones" were used for fusion.

We have produced several hybridomas (all from one patient) that show some specificity for lung cancer cells. The lymphocytes were obtained from a draining lymph node of a patient undergoing surgery for adenocarcinoma of the lung. After an EBV line was established, the cells were plated at 100 cells/well. Growth was apparent in all wells, and the supernatants were screened for reactivity against a lung tumor line. There were several positive wells, and the most positive one was expanded, frozen, and later fused with KR-4. On initial screening by ELISA, done 1 month after fusion, 33% of the growth-positive wells showed reactivity against lung tumor cells. Several hybridomas have now been repeatedly subcloned and screened against a wider panel of tumor cells (Fig. 1). An antibody titration curve is shown in Figure 2. After more than a couple of months in culture, the clones began to lose their specificity. The problem usually can be circumvented by frequent cloning. The pattern of tumor cell reactivity of many of our subclones is similar, suggesting that they may have originated from the same B cell.

B. Leprosy

Leprosy is an insidious infectious disease affecting 15-20 million people worldwide. It is caused by a poorly understood organism, *Mycobacterium leprae,* an obligatory intracellular parasite. Leprosy has been difficult to study since, until recently (84), there has been no animal model for the disease, and it is still not

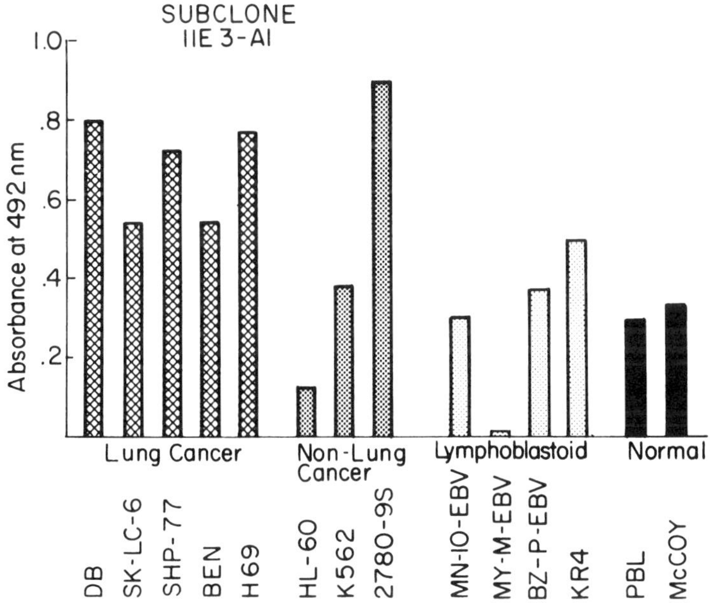

Figure 1 Supernatants from a subclone, designated 11E 3-A1, were screened against a panel of glutaraldehyde-fixed human cells, using an ELISA system. The cell lines used were as follows: DB (large cell lung cancer), SK-LC-6 (large cell lung cancer), SHP-77 (large cell variant of small cell lung cancer), BEN (squamous cell lung cancer), H69 (small cell lung cancer), HL-60 (promyelocytic leukemia), K562 (erythroleukemia), 2780-9S (ovarian carcinoma), MN-10-EBV (lymphoblastoid cell line used for construction of the hybridoma from which subclone 11E 3-A1 was derived), MY-M-EBV (lymphoblastoid cell line derived from bone marrow), BZ-P-EBV (lymphoblastoid cell line derived from peripheral blood), KR4 (lymphoblastoid fusion partner), PBL (peripheral blood leukocytes), and McCoy (fibroblast cell line).

possible to grow the organism in culture (85). Clinically, leprosy is a spectrum of diseases (86), from the tuberculoid form in which cell-mediated immunity is intact but circulating antibodies are low, to the more serious lepromatous leprosy in which cell-mediated immunity is depressed but B-cell function is unaffected (87-91).

The advent of hybridoma technology has facilitated the antigenic analysis of *M. leprae.* A number of murine MAbs has now been produced that react specifically with *M. leprae,* but not with other species of mycobacteria (92-94). Patients

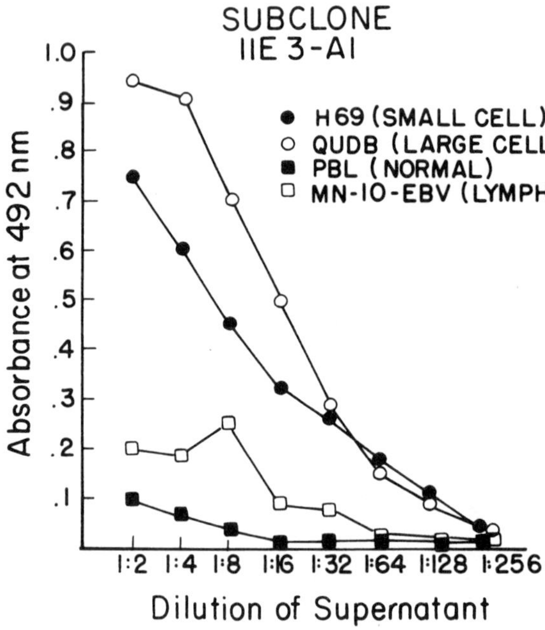

Figure 2 Serial dilutions of supernatants from subclone 11E 3-A1 were screened against glutaraldehyde-fixed human cell lines, using an ELISA system.

with lepromatous leprosy have high levels of serum antibodies that unfortunately do not seem to have a favorable influence on the course of the disease (95,96).

Using the EBV hybridoma technique, we attempted to produce human MAbs from patients with leprosy (97). Lymphocytes were obtained from four patients undergoing therapy for lepromatous leprosy. The EBV lines were established and fused with KR-4. Hybrid cells were screened against three different extracts of *M. leprae,* including a soluble sonicate antigen, a detergent extract of insoluble sonicated *M. leprae,* and a phenolic glycolipid antigen. A total of 1760 hybrids were screened, and the proportion of positive wells varied from 5 to 14% depending on the type of extract used. Positive hybrids were cloned and rescreened for specific antibody production. The frequency of positive clones was no higher after cloning and rescreening, suggesting that antibody production is initially unstable. However, after several more cloning steps, the stability increased, and antibody production has remained stable after several months in culture.

We also cloned and screened the EBV lines directly in an attempt to produce lines enriched for antigen-specific B cells, which might yield a higher frequency of positive hybrids when fused with KR-4. However, this approach proved unfruitful, since only 42 of 10,000 clones were positive, and these lost their reactivity within 6 weeks. Some of the positive hybridomas have now been screened against extracts of four other mycobacteria. Nine clones of 122 screened against this panel showed reactions specific for *M. leprae.*

Thus, we have shown that it is possible to apply this technique to produce human cell lines secreting antibodies reactive with *M. leprae.* Analysis of these antibodies should enable us to determine which mycobacterial antigens are recognized by the human immune system. Our ultimate goal is to develop reagents that may be of use in the treatment or prevention of this disease.

VI. SUMMARY

The EBV hybridoma system has many advantages over other methods for producing human MAbs. The process of EBV immortalization prior to fusion is a simple method for selecting only B cells. This enables one to immortalize and expand a population of B cells, which can be frozen for future use or fused immediately. It has also been shown that EBV-stimulated cells fuse more readily than do unstimulated lymphocytes. The process of fusion of the EBV lines with KR-4 serves to increase and stabilize antibody production. The fusion frequencies that can be achieved are greater than those obtained with other human hybridoma systems.

Using this technique, we have been able to produce human monoclonal antibodies to a variety of antigens, including tetanus toxoid, lung tumor antigens, and mycobacterial antigens. Lymphocytes have been derived from naturally immune patients, vaccinated normal donors, and *in vitro* immunization. These human hybridomas can be grown as ascites tumors in nude mice or in serum-free medium for bulk production. Attempts are currently underway to develop non-Ig-secreting, plasmacytomalike cell lines as human fusion partners. Since many of the technical problems encountered in human hybridoma technology can now be overcome, this technology should soon be applied to the diagnosis and therapy of a wide variety of human diseases.

REFERENCES

1. A. Rosen, P. Gergely, M. Jondal, G. Klein, and S. Britton. Polyclonal Ig production after Epstein-Barr virus infection of human lymphocytes *in vitro. Nature, 267*:52 (1977).
2. M. Steinitz, G. Klein, S. Koskimies, and O. Makela. EB virus-induced B lymphocyte cell lines producing specific antibody. *Nature, 269*:420 (1977).
3. V. R. Zurawski Jr., E. Haber, and P. M. Black. Production of antibody to tetanus toxoid by continuous human lymphoblastoid cell lines. *Science, 199*: 1439 (1978).

4. M. Steinitz, I. Seppala, K. Eichman, and G. Klein. Establishment of a human lymphoblastoid cell line with specific antibody production against group A streptococcal carbohydrate. *Immunobiology, 156*:41 (1979).
5. D. Kozbor, M. Steinitz, G. Klein, S. Koskimies, and O. Makela. Establishment of anti-TNP antibody producing human lymphoid lines by preselection for hapten binding followed by EBV-transformation. *Scand. J. Immunol., 10*: 187 (1979).
6. S. Koskimies. Human lymphoblastoid cell line producing specific antibody against Rh antigen D. *Scand. J. Immunol., 11*:73 (1980).
7. A. W. Boylston, B. Gardner, I. R. Anderson, and N. C. Hughes-Jones. Production of human IgM anti-D in tissue culture by EB virus transformed lymphocytes. *Scand. J. Immunol., 12*:355 (1980).
8. D. H. Crawford, M. J. Barlow, J. F. Harrison, L. Winger, and E. R. Huehns. Production of human monoclonal antibodies to rhesus D antigen. *Lancet i*: 386 (1983).
9. M. Steinitz, G. Izak, S. Cohen, M. Ehrenfeld, and J. Fletcher. Continuous production of monoclonal rheumatoid factor by EBV-transformed lymphocytes. *Nature, 287*:443 (1980).
10. S. Tsuchiya, S. Yokoyama, O. Yoshie, and Y. Ono. Production of diphtheria antitoxin antibody in Epstein-Barr virus induced lymphoblastoid cell lines. *J. Immunol., 124*:9970 (1980).
11. R. F. Irie, P. C. Jones, D. L. Morton, and N. Sidell. *In vitro* production of human antibody to a tumour associated fetal antigen. *Br. J. Cancer, 44*: 262 (1981).
12. S. Hirohashi, Y. Shimosato, and Y. Ino. Antibodies from EB-virus transformed lymphocytes of lymph nodes adjoining lung cancer. *Br. J. Cancer, 46*:802 (1982).
13. D. B. Watson, G. F. Burns, and I. R. Mackay. *In vitro* growth of B lymphocytes infiltrating human melanoma tissue by transformation with EBV: evidence for secretion of anti-melanoma antibodies by some transformed cells. *J. Immunol., 130*:2442 (1983).
14. I. Kamo, S. Furukawa, A. Tada, Y. Mano, Y. Iwasaki, and T. Furuse. Monoclonal antibody to acetylcholine receptor: cell line established from thymus of patient with myasthenia gravis. *Science, 215*:995 (1982).
15. D. Crawford, R. E. Callard, M. I. Muggeridge, D. M. Mitchell, E. D. Zanders, and P. C. L. Beverly. Production of human monoclonal antibody to X31 influenza virus nucleoprotein. *J. Gen. Virol., 64*:697 (1983).
16. M. Steinitz, S. Koskimies, G. Klein, and O. Makela. Establishment of specific antibody producing human lines by antigen preselection and Epstein-Barr (EBV) technique. *Clin. Lab. Immunol., 2*:1 (1979).
17. D. Kozbor and J. C. Roder. Requirements for the establishment of high-titered human monoclonal antibodies using the Epstein-Barr virus technique. *J. Immunol., 127*:1275 (1981).
18. T. Sasaki, T. Muryoi, Y. Sekiguchi, E. Tamate, K. Yoshinaga, and Y. Kitagawa. Monoclonal human anti-DNA antibodies from EB virus-transformed lympho-

cytes of systemic lupus erythematosus (SLE) patients. *J. Clin. Immunol. 5*: 246 (1985).

19. S. P. C. Cole, B. G. Campling, I. H. Louwman, D. Kozbor, and J. C. Roder. A strategy for the production of human monoclonal antibodies reactive with lung tumor cell lines. *Cancer Res., 44*:2750 (1984).
20. G. Kohler and C. Milstein. Continuous cultures of fused cells secreting antibody of predefined specificity. *Nature, 256*:495 (1975).
21. L. Olsson and L. Kaplan. Human-human hybridomas producing monoclonal antibodies of predefined specificity. *Proc. Natl. Acad. Sci. (USA), 77*: 5429 (1980).
22. C. M. Croce, A. Linnenbach, W. Hall, Z. Steplewski, and H. Koprowski. Production of human hybridomas secreting antibodies to measles virus. *Nature, 288*:488 (1980).
23. R. Levy and J. Dilley. Rescue of immunoglobulin secretion from human neoplastic lymphoid cells by somatic cell hybridization. *Proc. Natl. Acad. Sci. (USA), 75*:2411 (1978).
24. D. Kozbor, J. C. Roder, T. H. Chang, Z. Steplewski, and H. Koprowski. Human anti-tetanus monoclonal antibody secreted by EBV-transformed human B cells fused with murine myeloma. *Hybridoma, 1*:323 (1982).
25. R. Nowinski, C. Berglund, J. Lane, M. Lostrom, I. Bernstein, W. Young, S. Hakomori, L. Hill, and M. Cooney. Human monoclonal antibody against Forssman antigen. *Science, 210*:537 (1980).
26. J. Schlom, D. Wunderlich, and Y. A. Teramoto. Generation of human monoclonal antibodies reactive with human mammary carcinoma cells. *Proc. Natl. Acad. Sci. (USA), 77*:6841 (1980).
27. K. Sikora and R. Wright. Human monoclonal antibodies to lung cancer antigens. *Br. J. Cancer, 43*:696 (1981).
28. J. Satoh, B. S. Prabhakar, M. V. Haspel, F. Ginsberg-Fellner, and A. L. Notkins. Human monoclonal auto-antibodies that react with multiple endocrine organs. *N. Engl. J. Med., 309*:217 (1983).
29. R. J. Cote, D. M. Morrisey, A. W. Houghton, E. J. Beattie, H. F. Oettgen, and L. J. Old. Generation of human monoclonal antibodies reactive with cellular antigens. *Proc. Natl. Acad. Sci. (USA), 80*:2026 (1983).
30. P. G. Abrams, J. A. Knost, G. Clarke, S. Wilburn, R. K. Oldham, and K. A. Foon. Determination of the optimal human cell lines for development of human hybridomas. *J. Immunol., 131*:1202 (1983).
31. A. Imam, M. M. Drushella, C. A. Taylor, and Z. A. Tokes. Generation and immunological characterization of human monoclonal antibodies to mammary carcinoma cells. *Cancer Res., 45*:263 (1985).
32. M. V. Haspel, R. P. McCabe, N. Pomato, N. J. Janesch, J. V. Knowlton, L. C. Peters, H. C. Hoover, and M. G. Hanna Jr. Generation of tumor cell-reactive human monoclonal antibodies using peripheral blood lymphocytes from actively immunized colorectal carcinoma patients. *Cancer Res., 45*:3951 (1985).

33. Y. Matsuoka, G. E. Moore, Y. Yogi, and D. Pressman. Production of free light chains of immunoglobulin by a hemopoietic cell line derived from a patient with multiple myeloma. *Proc. Soc. Exp. Biol. Med., 125*:1246 (1967).
34. K. Nilsson, H. Bennich, S. G. O. Johansson, and J. Ponten. Established immunoglobulin producing myeloma (IgE) and lymphoblastoid (IgG) cell lines from an IgE myeloma patient. *J. Clin. Exp. Immunol.,* 7:477 (1970).
35. D. Kozbor, A. E. Lagarde, and J.C. Roder. Human hybridomas constructed with antigen-specific Epstein-Barr virus transformed cell lines. *Proc. Natl. Acad. Sci.* (*USA*), *79*:6651 (1982).
36. Y. Shoenfeld, S. C. Hsu-Lin, J. E. Gabriels, L. E. Silberstein, B. C. Furie, B. Furie, B. D. Stollar, and R. S. Schwartz. Production of autoantibodies by human-human hybridomas. *J. Clin. Invest., 70*:205 (1982).
37. D. S. Dwyer, R. J. Bradley, C. K. Urquhart, and J. F. Kearney. Naturally occurring anti-idiotypic antibodies in myasthenia gravis patients. *Nature, 301*:611 (1983).
38. G. S. Eisenbarth, A. Linnenbach, R. Jackson, R. Scearce, and C. M. Croce. Human hybridomas secreting anti-islet autoantibodies. *Nature, 300*:264 (1982).
39. P. A. W. Edwards, C. M. Smith, A. M. Neville, and M. J. O'Hare. A human-human hybridoma system based on a fast-growing mutant of the ARH-77 plasma cell leukemia-derived line. *Eur. J. Immunol., 12*:641 (1982).
40. K. Sikora, T. Alderson, J. Phillips, and J. V. Watson. Human hybridomas from malignant gliomas. *Lancet, i*:11 (1982).
41. H. M. Warenius, J. W. Taylor, B. E. Durack, and P. A. Cross. The production of human hybridomas from patients with malignant melanoma. The effect of pre-stimulation of lymphocytes with pokeweed mitogen. *Eur. J. Cancer Clin. Oncol., 19*:347 (1983).
42. K. Sikora, T. Alderson, J. Ellis, J. Phillips, and J. Watson. Human hybridomas from patients with malignant disease. *Br. J. Cancer, 47*:135 (1983).
43. J. W. Larrick, K. E. Truitt, A. A. Raubitschek, G. Senyk, and J. C. N. Wang. Characterization of human hybridomas secreting antibody to tetanus toxoid. *Proc. Natl. Acad. Sci.,* (*USA*), *80*:6376 (1983).
44. H. H. Handley and I. Royston. A human lymphoblastoid B cell line useful for generating immunoglobulin secreting human hybridomas. In M. S. Mitchell and H. F. Oettgen (eds.). *Hybridomas in Cancer Diagnosis and Treatment.* Raven Press, New York (1982).
45. D. Kozbor, D. Dexter, and J. C. Roder. A comparative analysis of the phenotypic characteristics of available fusion partners for the construction of human hybridomas. *Hybridoma, 2*:7 (1983).
46. L. Olsson, H. Kronstrom, A. Cambon-De Mouzon, C. Honsik, T. Brodin, and B. Jacobsen. Antibody producing human-human hybridomas. 1. Technical aspects. *J. Immunol. Meth., 6*:17 (1983).
47. D. Kozbor and J. C. Roder. *In vitro* stimulated lymphocytes as a source of human hybridomas. *Eur. J. Immunol., 14*:23 (1984).

48. D. O. Haskard and J. R. Archer. The production of human monoclonal autoantibodies from patients with rheumatoid arthritis by the EBV-hybridoma technique. *J. Immunol. Meth., 74*:361 (1984).
49. D. H. Crawford, E. R. Huehns, and M. A. Epstein. Therapeutic use of human monoclonal antibodies. *Lancet i*:1040 (1983).
50. J. V. Watson, T. Alderson, K. Sikora, and J. Phillips. Subcutaneous culture chamber for continuous infusion of monoclonal antibodies. *Lancet, i*:99 (1983).
51. M. Hanna. Personal communication. (1985).
52. J. Cavagnaro and M. Osband. Successful *in vitro* primary immunization of human peripheral blood mononuclear cells and subsequent fusion with human myeloma cells to produce human-human hybridomas secreting specific monoclonal antibody (abstr.). *Hybridoma, 2*:128 (1983).
53. L. E. Strike, B. H. Devens, and R. L. Lundak. Production of human-human hybridomas secreting antibody to sheep erythrocytes after *in vitro* immunization. *J. Immunol., 132*:1798 (1984).
54. L. Winger, D. Winger, P. Shastry, A. Russell, and M. Longenecker. Efficient generation in vitro, from human peripheral blood cells, of monoclonal Epstein-Barr virus transformants producing specific antibody to a variety of antigens without prior deliberate immunization. *Proc. Natl. Acad. Sci. (USA), 80*:4484 (1983).
55. M. Shulman, C. D. Wilde, and G. Kohler. A better cell line for making hybridomas secreting specific antibody. *Nature, 276*:269 (1978).
56. D. Kozbor, P. Tripputi, J. C. Roder, and C. M. Croce. A human hybrid myeloma for production of human monoclonal antibodies. *J. Immunol., 133*:3001 (1984).
57. R. E. Ritts, A. Ruiz-Arguelles, K. G. Weyl, A. L. Bradley, B. Weihmeir, D. Jacobsen, and B. L. Strehlo. Establishment and characterization of a human non-secretory plasmacytoid cell line and its hybridization with human B cells. *Int. J. Cancer, 31*:133 (1983).
58. L. E. Strike, S. A. Murray, W. H. Fletcher, and R. L. Lundak. Evaluation of immunoglobulin-secreting human-human hybridomas by scanning electron microscopy (abstr.). *Fed. Proc., 41*:594 (1982).
59. R. I. Mishell and R. W. Dutton. Immunization of dissociated spleen cell cultures from normal mice. *J. Exp. Med., 126*:423 (1967).
60. J. Marbrook. Primary immune response in cultures of spleen cells. *Lancet ii*:1279 (1967).
61. Z. Jonak and R. H. Kennett. *In vitro* immunization of mouse spleen cells. In R. H. Kennett, K. B. Bechtol, and T. J. McKearn (eds.). *Monoclonal Antibodies and Functional Cell Lines.* Plenum Press, New York (1984).
62. C. L. Reading. Theory and methods for immunization in culture and monoclonal antibody production. *J. Immunol. Meth., 53*:261 (1982).
63. H. Hengartner, A. L. Luzzati, and M. Schreier. Fusion of *in vitro* immunized lymphoid cells with X63Ag8. *Curr. Top. Microbiol. Immunol., 81*:92 (1978).
64. R. A. Luben and M. A. Mohler. *In vitro* immunization as an adjunct to the

production of hybridomas producing antibodies against the lymphokine osteoclast activating factor. *Mol. Immunol. 17*:635 (1979).
65. R. A. Luben, P. Brazeau, P. Bohlen, and R. Guillemin. Monoclonal antibodies to hypothalamic growth hormone-releasing factor with picomoles of antigen. *Science, 218*:887 (1982).
66. C. A. K. Borrebaeck. *In vitro* immunization for the production of antigen-specific lymphocyte hybridomas. *Scand. J. Immunol., 18:*9 (1983).
67. J. Van Ness, U. K. Laemmli, and D. E. Pettijohn. Immunization *in vitro* and production of monoclonal antibodies specific to insoluble and weakly immunogenic proteins. *Proc. Natl. Acad. Sci.* (*USA*), *81*:7897 (1984).
68. D. Buchman, D. Miller, and G. Koch. Monoclonal antibodies to digoxin: comparison of *in vitro* and *in vivo* immunization. *Hybridoma, 4*:173 (1985).
69. K. Nilsson, B. C. Giovanella, J. S. Stehlin, and G. Klein. Tumorigenicity of human hematopoietic cell lines in athymic nude mice. *Int. J. Cancer, 19*: 337 (1977).
70. B. Giovanella, K. Nilsson, L. Zech, O. Yim, G. Klein, and J. S. Stehlin. Growth of diploid, Epstein-Barr virus-containing human lymphoblastoid cell lines heterotransplanted into nude mice under immunologically privileged conditions. *Int. J. Cancer, 24*:103 (1979).
71. S. P. C. Cole, B. G. Campling, T. Atlaw, D. Kozbor, and J. C. Roder. Human monoclonal antibodies. *Mol. Cell. Biochem., 62*:109 (1984).
72. D. Kozbor, W. Abramow-Newerly, P. Tripputi, S. P. C. Cole, J. Weibel, J. C. Roder, and C. M. Croce. Specific immunoglobulin production and enhanced tumorigenicity following ascites growth of human hybridomas. *J. Immunol. Meth., 81*:31 (1985).
73. S. P. C. Cole, E. H. Vreeken, and J. C. Roder. Antibody production by human X human hybridomas in serum-free medium. *J. Immunol. Meth., 78*: 271 (1985).
74. A. C. Morgan Jr., and R. F. McIntyre. Monoclonal antibodies to human melanoma-associated antigens: an amplified enzyme-linked immunosorbent assay for the detection of antigen, antibody, and immune complexes. *Cancer Res., 43*: 3155 (1983).
75. E. Seibert, C. Sorg, R. Happle, and E. Macher. Membrane-associated antigens of human malignant melanoma. III. Specificity of human sera reacting with cultured melanoma cells. *Int. J. Cancer, 19*:172 (1977).
76. D. R. Howard and C. R. Taylor. A method of distinguishing benign from malignant breast lesions utilizing antibody present in normal human sera. *Cancer, 43*:2279 (1979).
77. K. M. A. Sheik, F. P. Quismorio, G. J. Friou, and Y. Lee. Ductular carcinoma of the breast. Serum antibodies to tumour-associated antigens. *Cancer, 44*: 2083 (1978).
78. W. F. Sindelar. Demonstration of specific serologic reactivity in human osteosarcoma. *Cancer, 51*:444 (1983).
79. F. R. Eilber and D. L. Morton. Sarcoma-specific antigens: detection by com-

plement fixation with serum from sarcoma patients. *J. Natl. Cancer Inst., 44*: 651 (1970).
80. C. R. Simrell and P. A. Klein. Antibody responses of tumor-bearing mice to their own tumours captured and perpetuated as hybridomas. *J. Immunol., 132*:2386 (1979).
81. B. S. Kelly, U. Stredulinsky, J. Vanden Hoek, and J. G. Levy. Antibodies in the sera of patients with bronchogenic carcinoma that react with antigen from a tumour cell line. I. An assay system. *Cancer Immunol. Immunother., 12*:5 (1981).
82. E. Paluch and H. L. Ioachim. Lung carcinoma-reactive antibodies isolated from tumor tissues and pleural effusions of lung cancer patients. *J. Natl. Cancer Inst., 61*:319 (1978).
83. R. W. Baldwin and M. R. Price. Neoantigen expression in chemical carcinogenesis. In F. F. Becker (ed.). *Cancer, A Comprehensive Treatise. Vol. 1.* Plenum Press, New York (1975).
84. W. F. Krichheimer and E. E. Storrs. Attempts to establish the armadillo (*Dasypus novemcinctus Linn.*) as a model for the study of leprosy. *Int. J. Lepr., 39*:693 (1971).
85. C. H. Binford, H. M. Meyers, and G. P. Walsh. Leprosy, state of the art. *J. Am. Med. Assoc., 247*:2283 (1982).
86. D. S. Ridley and W. H. Jopling. Classification of leprosy according to immunity. A five group system. *Int. J. Lepr., 34*:255 (1966).
87. J. A. J. Grabosz, H. Derblom, and T. Godal. IgE serum levels in leprosy. *Acta Pathol. Microbiol. Scand., 81*:806 (1973).
88. W. E. Bullock, M. F. Ho, and M. J. Chen. Studies of immune mechanisms in leprosy. *J. Lab. Clin. Med., 75*:863 (1970).
89. P. Jha, K. Balakrishnan, G. P. Talwar, and L. K. Bhutani. Status of humoral immune responses in leprosy. *Int. J. Lepr., 39*:14 (1971).
90. K. Saha, M. M. Mittal, and S. N. Ray. Consequences of small pox vaccination in leprosy patients. *Infect. Immun., 8*:301 (1973).
91. J. L. Turk and M. F. R. Waters. Immunological significance of changes in lymph nodes across the leprosy spectrum. *Clin. Exp. Immunol. 8*:363 (1971).
92. D. B. Young, S. R. Khanolkar, L. L. Barg, and T. H. Buchanan. Generation and characterization of monoclonal antibodies to the phenolic glycolipid antigen of *Mycobacterium leprae. Infect. Immun., 43*:183 (1984).
93. T. P. Gillis and T. M. Buchanan. Production and partial characterization of monoclonal antibodies to *Mycobacterium leprae. Infect. Immun., 37*:172 (1982).
94. J. Ivanyi, S. Sinha, R. Aston, D. Cussell, M. Keen, and U. Sengupta. Definition of species-specific and cross-reactive antigenic determinants of *Mycobacterium leprae* using monoclonal antibodies. *Clin. Exp. Immunol., 52*: 528 (1983).
95. S. Chaparas. The immunology of mycobacterial infections. *CRC Critical Reviews in Microbiology,* 139 (1982).

96. T. Godal. Immunological aspects of leprosy-present status. *Progr. Allergy, 25*:211 (1978).
97. T. Atlaw, D. Kozbor, and J. C. Roder. Human monoclonal antibodies against *Mycobacterium leprae*. *Infect. Immun., 49*:104 (1985).

2
Production of Human Monoclonal Antibodies by *In Vitro* Immunization

MAY-KIN HO
E. I. Du Pont de Nemours & Company, North Billerica, Massachusetts

Mouse monoclonal antibodies (MAbs) have been used widely for the identification of infectious agents and diagnosis of various disease states. However, the use of human MAbs has been limited because relatively few of these MAbs have been produced. Human antibodies offer several advantages when compared with xenoantibodies. First, human lymphocytes might recognize antigenic determinants not readily detected by xenogeneic lymphocytes. This phenomenon has been observed with antibodies against human histocompatibility antigens. Human antibodies tend to recognize polymorphic determinants, whereas xenoantibodies tend to react with framework determinants on these antigens. Second, human antibodies can participate in certain immune reactions *in vivo* more efficiently than can mouse or rat antibodies. Lastly, anti-mouse reactions have been observed when mouse MAbs were administered to humans (1-5). Human MAbs are probably less immunogenic *in vivo*.

Since the development of the first human MAb in 1977 (6), a number of human MAbs has been produced against bacteria, viruses, tumor cells, and other antigens (reviewed in reference 7). Almost all of these MAbs were produced by fusion or viral transformation of lymphocytes obtained from immune donors. This approach has proved successful in generating clinically relevant antibacterial or antiviral MAbs, especially if neutralizing antibodies are produced by the infected individuals. However, little can be done to manipulate the specificity, affinity, and isotype of the antibody-producing cells or the resulting MAbs. In the area of cancer, most attempts to obtain MAbs against tumor-associated antigens (TAA) by immortalization of cells from tumor-bearing patients were unsuccessful (8,9). It seems that the frequency of TAA-specific B lymphocytes is extremely low in these patients. Therefore, it is highly desirable to have a procedure whereby human B lymphocytes can be sensitized to produce the desired antibodies. In this chapter, the immunization of normal human splenic lymphocytes *in vitro* against several protein antigens and the fusion of the sensitized cells to produce human MAbs are described.

I. WHY *IN VITRO* IMMUNIZATION?

The desired antibody-forming cells were obtained by immunization *in vitro* for the following reasons: (a) The immunization process can be readily manipulated *in vitro* to allow the generation of MAbs with the desired specificity, affinity, and isotype. For example, the immunogen could be presented in different forms to elicit a preferential IgG response (see section III.A.2). (b) *In vitro* culture might yield antibodies against self-antigens that are poorly or nonimmunogenic *in vivo.* Previously, *in vitro* sensitization has been used to produce mouse MAbs against a variety of weak immunogens, such as osteoclast-activating factor (10) and calmodulin (11). (c) Immunization *in vitro* eliminates the hazards of exposing humans to potentially harmful substances, such as virulent bacteria, toxins, or tumor cells. (d) *In vitro* sensitization requires only a few days, whereas immunization *in vivo* usually takes more than a few weeks.

II. IMMUNIZATION OF HUMAN LYMPHOCYTES

A. Bombesin-Tetanus Toxoid as Model Antigen

1. MAb to Bombesin and Tetanus Toxoid

For immunization of human B lymphocytes *in vitro,* the tetradecapeptide bombesin was used as the model antigen because of its low immunogenicity, defined composition, and tumor association. Bombesinlike substances are found in human fetal lung and small cell lung carcinoma, but not in adult lung (reviewed in reference 12). [Lys^3]-bombesin (Bachem, Burlingame, CA) was conjugated to the protein carrier tetanus toxoid (TT) (purified from concentrates from Massachusetts State Public Health Laboratories) via 1-ethyl 3-(3-dimethyl aminopropyl) carbodiimide hydrochloride (ECDI) (Calbiochem, San Diego, CA) according to a modified method of Goodfriend *et al.* (13). Because most individuals have been exposed to TT through vaccination, the use of bombesin-tetanus toxoic (BTT) conjugates allowed the study of both primary (anti-bombesin) and secondary (anti-TT) responses simultaneously.

First, two previously reported sensitization procedures (14,15) employing peripheral blood lymphocytes (PBL) were adapted. Both protocols worked well for the more immunogenic antigens, such as sheep red blood cells and trinitrophenol conjugated to keyhole limpet hemocyanin (TNP-KLH). When PBL were cultured with BTT, there was an occasional anti-TT response, but most of the antibodies were IgM. However, no anti-bombesin response was detected. The failure to generate primary responses with PBL prompted the development of another method of immunization. This procedure involved separating human spleen cells on nylon wool columns to obtain a nylon-nonadherent (T-enriched) and a nylon-adherent (B-enriched) fraction. One million each of the two cell fractions were cocultured with 20% phytohemagglutinin (PHA)-activated lymphocyte culture supernatant (LCS), 10% human AB serum (Biobee, Boston, MA), 7.5 μg/ml *E. coli* lipopolysaccharide (LPS) (Difco, Detroit, MI), and various concentrations of BTT in 1 ml of RPMI-1640 in a 16-mm culture well. After 6 days, the cultured cells were fused with NS-1 cells at a lymphocyte:myeloma ratio of 2:1, using 45% polyethylene glycol (PEG) (MW 3350) as described previously (16). The fused cells were plated at 1×10^5 lymphocytes/well with 1.5×10^4 of 2000R-irridated allogeneic human PBL as feeder cells. The culture medium was RPMI-1640 supplemented with 20% fetal calf serum, 2 mM glutamine, 1 mM sodium pyruvate, 5% NCTC-109, 10 μg/ml gentamycin, 10^{-4} M hypoxanthine, 4×10^{-7} M aminopterin, and 1.6×10^{-5} M thymidine. After 2-3 weeks, the resulting hybrids were screened for binding to BTT by ELISA. To determine whether the BTT-positive hybrids were against bombesin or TT, their binding to bombesin conjugated to bovine thyroglobulin (BTG), an irrelevant carrier, as well as to free TT and free thyroglobulin (TG) were assayed. Table 1 shows the reactivity of three hybrids (8A2, 8D12, and 14G8). Monoclonal antibodies 8A2 and 8D12 were reactive with BTT and TT. The former was an IgG antibody and the latter was an IgM antibody. These results suggested that MAb 8A2 and 8D12 were specific for TT. Monoclonal antibody 14G8 was an IgM antibody that reacted with BTT and BTG, but not TT or TG. This MAb seemed to be an anti-bombesin, but the unlikely possibility exists that the eoptope recognized by MAb 14G8 is part of the coupling agent ECDI. To determine the true specificity of putative anti-bombesin hybrids, competitive inhibition studies were performed. The antibodies were preincubated with various inhibitors before being used in ELISA for binding to BTT. As seen in Figure 1A, the binding of the putative IgM-secreting anti-bombesin MAb BM-1 was inhibited by preincubation with BTT, unconjugated bombesin, and BTG conjugated via ECDI or glutaraldehyde. Free TT or TG (not shown) was not inhibitory. Therefore, BM-1 was a genuine anti-bombesin MAb. In contrast, an IgG anti-TT MAb was inhibited by BTT and TT, but not BTG and TG (Fig. 1B).

Table 1 Reactivity of Human MAbs Against Bombesin-Tetanus Toxoid

	OD_{488}				
MAb	BTT	BTG	TT	TG	Isotype
8A2	1.9	0	1.7	0	IgG
8D12	1.8	0.1	1.8	0.1	IgM
14G8	1.0	0.7	0.1	0	IgM

Ninety-six well microtiter plates were coated with 400 ng/well of bombesin-tetanus toxoid (BTT), bovine thyroglobulin (BTG), free tetanus toxoid (TT), or free thyroglobulin (TG) in carbonate buffer, pH 9.6, overnight at 4°C. Fifty μl of human MAb diluted 1:4 in PBS-1% BSA were added to each well and incubated for 3 hours at 37°C. The plates were washed with PBS, and 50 μl of horseradish peroxidase (HRP)-conjugated goat anti-human Ig was added to each well. After 1 hour at 37°C, the enzyme was detected by addition of 100 μl of o-phenylene diamine and 0.15% hydrogen peroxide. Optical densities at 488 nM were determined in an Artek automatic ELISA reader.

Figure 1 Inhibition of binding of anti-bombesin (A) or anti-tetanus toxoid (B) human MAbs. Concentrations of human MAb giving half-maximal binding to BTT were preincubated with various concentrations of inhibitors for 3 hours at 37°C before being used in an ELISA on BTT-coated plates as described in Table 1. The inhibitors used were: BTT conjugated by ECDI (●—●), BTG conjugated by ECDI (△—△), BTG conjugated by glutaraldehyde (▲—▲), unconjugated TT (□—□), unconjugated [Lys^3]-bombesin (■—■), and dilution beffer, PBS-1% BSA (○—○).

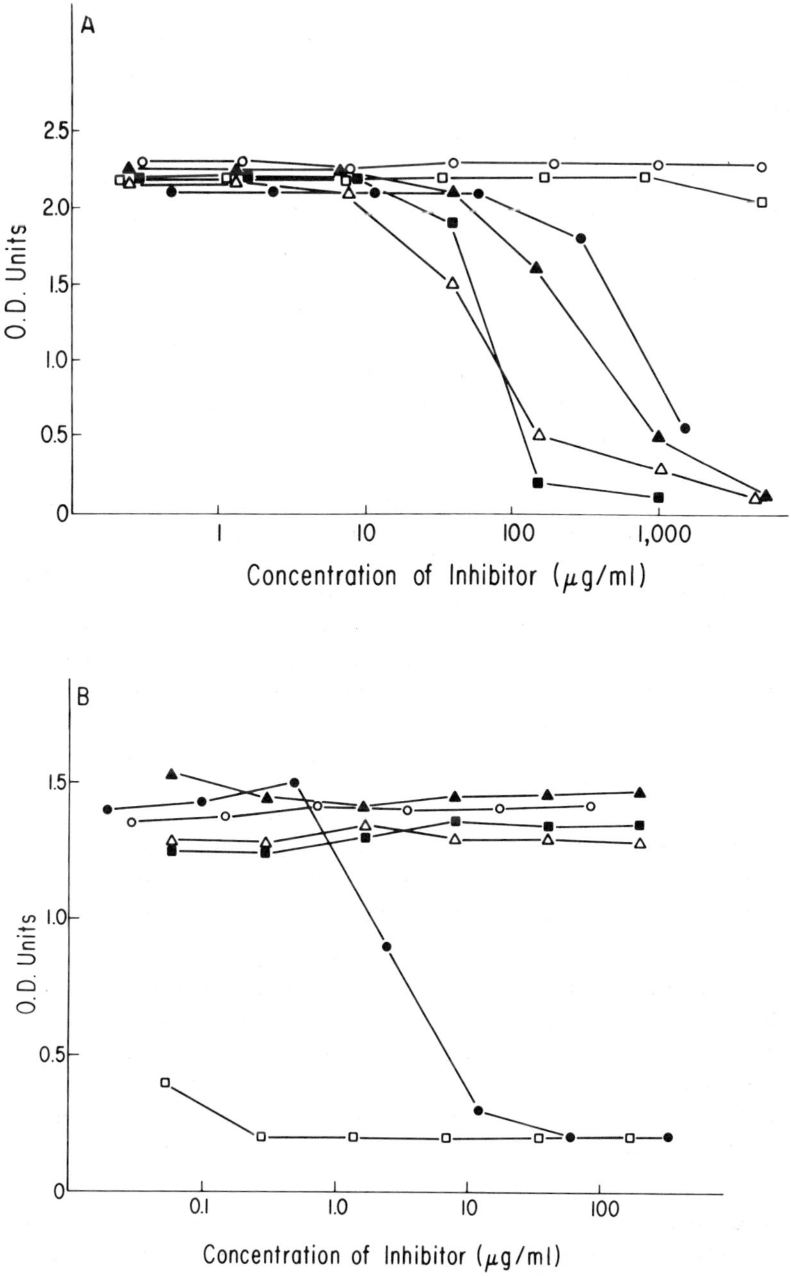
A
O.D. Units
2.5
2.0
1.5
1.0
0.5
0
1
10
100
1,000
Concentration of Inhibitor (μg/ml)
B
O.D. Units
1.5
1.0
0.5
0
0.1
1.0
10
100
Concentration of Inhibitor (μg/ml)

2. Factors Affecting Optimal Immunization Against TT

The factors related to optimal immunization against BTT were examined. As the magnitude of anti-bombesin response was low (<2.2% of wells; see summary in section III.A.3), only data on anti-TT responses where significantly large numbers of specific hybrids could be obtained were included.

Source and Manipulation of Cells. Lymphocytes from peripheral blood, tonsil, spleen, lymph node, and bone marrow potentially can be used in immunizations *in vitro*. However, peripheral blood lymphocytes were found to be a consistently poor responder in this system. This may be due to the low percentage and/or the relatively mature state of the B lymphocytes in peripheral blood. In contrast, splenic lymphocytes proved to be an abundant and responsive population for immunization against bombesin and TT. Tonsillar cells responded well to TT, but poorly to bombesin. Because of the relatively low number of lymphocytes recovered from lymph node and bone marrow, experience with these lymphocytes is limited.

For optimal immunization, manipulation of the lymphocyte subpopulations is required. Nylon wool separation and reconstitution of the nonadherent and adherent fractions were essential for anti-TT responses. The frequency of hybrid growth was not affected when unseparated splenocytes were used. However, a dramatic decrease in the percentages of TT-specific hybrids was observed (Fig. 2). Phenotypic analysis showed that the nylon-spearated and reconstituted splenocytes contained a higher ratio of $T4^+$ cells to B lymphocytes than in the untreated spleen cells. However, the percentage of $T8^+$ cells in the reconstituted population was similar to that of the unseparated cells. This suggests that removal of $T8^+$ suppressor cells probably was not critical to optimal anti-TT production. Indeed, lysis of $T8^+$ cells with complement did not increase the anti-TT responses of spleen cells (unpublished data). This finding is in contrast to the studies by Hoffman (14) and Cavagnaro and Osband (15), who found that removal of T suppressor cells from peripheral blood lymphocytes could enhance antibody responses *in vitro*.

Serum Requirements. Previous studies on anti-sheep red blood cell responses (14,15,17-20) showed that human serum was essential for optimal antibody production *in vitro*. Therefore, the anti-TT responses of cultures containing human AB serum were compared with those containing fetal calf serum (FCS). Even though the cell recovery after immunization and the percentage of hybrid growth were not significantly different between the two types of cultures, cultures with human AB serum generally gave 2-10 times higher anti-TT responses than did those with FCS.

Growth Factors and Lipopolysaccharide. The LCS used in the immunization procedure in this study was prepared by culturing peripheral blood lymphocytes from individual donors at 1×10^6/ml in RPMI-1640 supplemented with 5% FCS

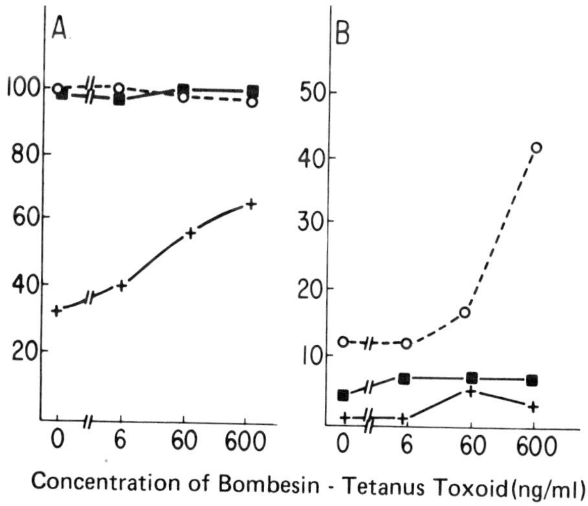

Figure 2 Effects of nylon wool separation and LCS on anti-TT responses *in vitro*. Human splenocytes were sensitized with indicated concentrations of BTT in the presence of 20% LCS, human AB serum, and LPS for 6 days (Group 1, ○- - -○). The sensitized cells were fused to NS-1, and the percentages of culture wells showing hybrid growth (A) and TT-specific hybrids (B) were determined. Two other groups of cells were sensitized, as for Group 1, except that untreated spleen cells were used instead of nylon-separated cells in Group 2 (■——■), and LCS was omitted in Group 3 (+——+).

and 0.1% PHA-P (Difco Inc.) for 48 hours. Supernatants with interleukin-2 (IL-2) activity were pooled and stored at 4°C. In addition to IL-2, these preparations also contain B-cell growth factor (BCGF) activity determined by a *Staphylococcus aureus* costimulator assay. To test whether LCS was essential for *in vitro* immunization, the anti-TT responses in the presence and absence of LCS were studied. Omission of LCS from the immunization process led to a decrease in overall hybrid frequencies as well as in the percentages of specific hybrids (Fig. 2). The recovery of cells after immunization was also lowered in the absence LCS (not shown). In addition to IL-2 and BCGF, the LCS preparations may well contain other factors essential for proliferation and differentiation of TT-specific B cells. To further define the mediators involved, studies utilizing purified and/or recombinant growth factors will be performed. In contrast to LCS, the requirement for lipopolysaccharide (LPS) was not as critical for optimal immunization. For some donors, LPS could enhance the anti-TT responses by one to two times, whereas for others, no enhancement was observed.

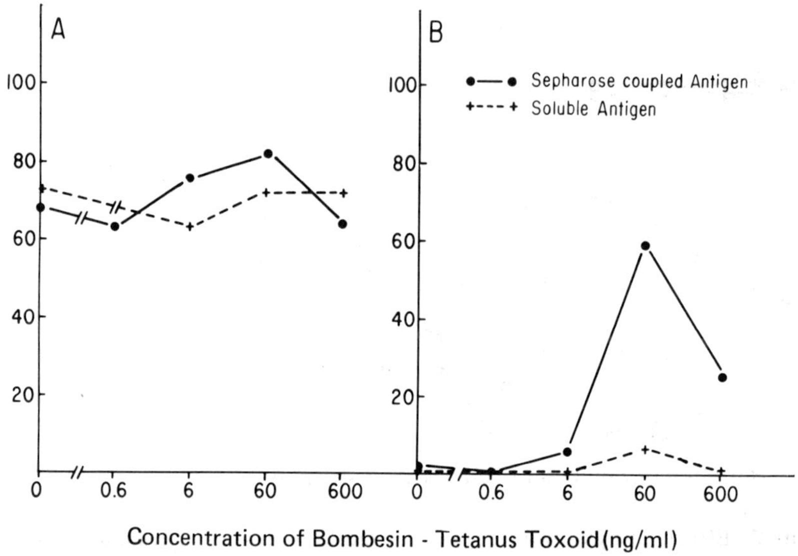

Figure 3 Comparison of soluble antigen with Sepharose-conjugated antigen. Human spleen cells were sensitized with indicated concentrations of soluble BTT (+--+) or bombesin and TT conjugated to Sepharose 4B (●—●) before fusion with NS-1. The percentages of wells showing hybrid growth (A) and anti-TT (B) were determined.

Concentration and Form of Antigen. There is considerable donor to donor variation in optimal antigen concentration. The optimal dose ranged from 5 ng/ml to 5 μg/ml of soluble TT. Therefore, it is advisable to titrate a wide range of antigen concentrations for each donor. Antigen on solid supports, such as Sepharose beads, tends to be more immunogenic and elicit higher IgG responses than do soluble antigens. Figure 3 shows the effect of Sepharose-conjugated TT on the splenocytes from a low responder of TT. The cells from this donor yielded 7% TT-specific wells when stimulated with 60 ng/ml BTT. The specific response was dramatically increased to 59% when 60 ng/ml of Sepharose-coupled antigen was used. In both cases, greater than 90% of the specific MAbs were IgG. This indicated that the number of TT-specific B cells secreting IgG was greatly expanded during *in vitro* culture when insoluble antigen was used. In one or two experiments, IgM anti-TT response was also increased, but this was not consistently observed. Similar enhancement of anti-TT response by insoluble antigen was also found with tonsillar lymphocytes. The responses observed with both splenocytes and tonsillar cells were antigen-specific. Only 1-3% of anti-TT-posi-

Table 2 Summary of Experiments on *In Vitro* Sensitization of Human Splenocytes Against Bombesin-Tetanus Toxoid

	IgM Anti-bombesin	Anti-tetanus toxoid		
		Total	IgM	IgG
A. Soluble antigen				
No. donors	5	6	4	4
No. experiments	7	8[a]	5[a]	5[a]
% specific wells[b]	1.0 ± 0.7	13.7 ± 10.8	6.5 ± 5.2	2.7 ± 3.7
B. Sepharose-coupled antigen				
No. donors	2	2	2	2
No. experiments	2	2	2	2
% specific wells[b]	0.9 ± 0	61.1 ± 34.0	37.5 ± 37.5	28.3 ± 1.2

[a]Eight experiments were performed, but isotype analysis was conducted for only five experiments.
[b]Percentages of wells that contained hybrids secreting antibodies specific for either bombesin or tetanus toxoid. Results are expressed as mean ± standard deviation.

tive wells were detected when antigen was omitted from the cultures or when mock conjugated Sepharose beads were used as immunogen.

Kinetics. The optimal time of immunization before fusion is partly dependent upon the fusion parent used. Cells harvested after 6 days of culture fused at a higher frequency (70-100%) with NS-1 than those harvested after 4 days (50-70%). Moreover, significant numbers of specific hybrids were observed only from fusions of the former. For other fusion parents, such as WI-L2 729HF2, the optimal time of harvesting cells was shifted to 4-5 days. Cells cultured for 6 days generally did not fuse well with this parent.

3. Summary of *In Vitro* Immunizations

The above approach was used to sensitize lymphocytes from seven spleens and two tonsils. A summary of the studies on splenocytes is presented in Table 2. Generally, three to four concentrations of antigen were used for each donor, and cultures with no antigen were included in all experiments as controls. Greater than 70% of the experiments yielded MAbs to bombesin, but all the MAbs were IgM. The response against bombesin was antigen-specific because no anti-bombesin was detected when the immunogen BTT was omitted from the cultures. The mean percentage of bombesin-specific wells was 1.0%. The relatively small percentage may represent a low number of precursors with bombesin specificity.

This is not unexpected in view of the small molecular size (MW 1592) and, hence, the limited number of epitopes on bombesin.

As for anti-TT, the magnitude of response was much higher. An average of 13.7% and 61.1% of the wells showed anti-TT in immunizations involving soluble and Sepharose-conjugated antigen, respectively. Both IgM and IgG MAbs were detected. The use of Sepharose-coupled antigen yielded significantly higher responses than did use of soluble antigens.

B. MAb to Tumor Cell Antigens

It was also attempted to generate human monoclonal antibodies to antigens on tumor cells by immunizing human splenocytes with tumor cell lysates. The sensitized cells were fused with NS-1 as described above. Hybrids were screened by a cellular ELISA. Briefly, tumor or normal cell lines were plated at 5×10^4 cells/well in tissue culture wells. After incubating at 37°C overnight, the cells were fixed with methanol. Hybrid culture supernatant fluids were added (50 μl/well) and incubated for 3 hours at 37°C. The presence of human MAbs binding to the cells was determined by the addition of horseradish peroxidase (HRP)-conjugated goat anti-human immunoglobulin. Hybrids were initially selected for preferential binding to tumor cell lines, but not normal fibroblasts. Using detergent-solubilized lysates of two human breast tumor lines, MCF-7 and MDA MB231, as immunogen, several human MAbs that showed preferential binding to tumor lines were generated. One of these MAbs, 1G8, is an IgM antibody. It is reactive with MCF-7, MDA MB231, and A549, a human lung adenocarcinoma line, but not with two normal fibroblast lines, Flow 5000 and HSF. To define the 1G8 antigen, A549 and Flow 5000 cells were biosynthetically labeled with ^{35}S-methionine and solubilized with detergent. The cells lysates were incubated with 1G8 and goat anti-human IgM conjugated to Sepharose. The immunoprecipitates were then analyzed by sodium dodecylsulfate (SDS) polyacrylamide gel electrophoresis. The 1G8 antigen is composed of two polypeptides of 58Kd and 46Kd (Fig. 4). The migration of the 1G8 polypeptides is similar to that of another tumor antigen, 89E5, previously identified by a mouse MAb developed in our laboratory (Carney *et al.*, unpublished data). The 89E5 MAb was derived by immunization of mice with A549 tumor cells. Immunoperoxidase studies showed that 89E5 MAb is reactive with a wide range of epithelial tumors (Carney *et al.*, unpublished data). These preliminary studies suggest that human MAbs to tumor cell antigens can be generated by *in vitro* immunization. Cross-clearing with the two antibodies before immunoprecipitation will determine whether the human MAb 1G8 and the mouse MAb 89E5 are recognizing the same antigen.

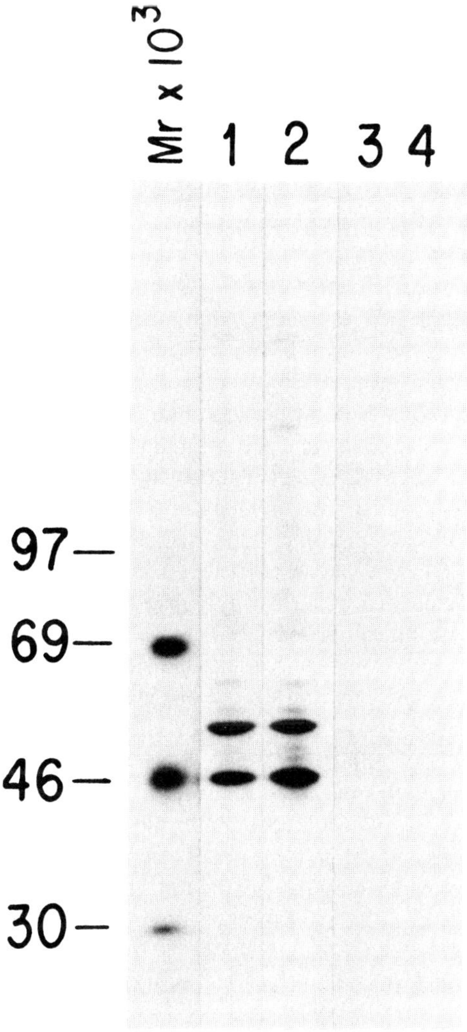

Figure 4 SDS-PAGE of 1G8 human MAbs and 89E5 mouse MAbs. Cells of human lung adenocarcinoma line, A549, were biosynthetically labeled with ^{35}S-methionine and detergent-solubilized. Immunoprecipitations were performed using 1G8 human IgM plus Sepharose-conjugated goat anti-human IgM (lane 1) or 89E5 mouse IgG1 monoclonal antibody directly conjugated to Sepharose (lane 2). Controls were immunoprecipitated with normal human IgM plus Sepharose-conjugated goat anti-human IgM (lane 3) or Sepharose coupled with MOPC21 mouse myeloma protein (lane 4). The precipitates were eluted with reducing sample buffer and analyzed on 5-15% SDS-PAGE.

III. IMMORTALIZATION OF SENSITIZED LYMPHOCYTES

A number of fusion partners, including NS-1, SP2/0, P3Ag8.653, WI-L2 729HF2, LICR LON HMy-2, UC729, and GM-4672, were also evaluated (7). NS-1 consistently fused at an equal or higher frequency than the other partners. The hybrids derived from NS-1 also grew more robustly. Because our initial aim was to determine the conditions for *in vitro* immunization, it was more important to "capture" as many antibody-producing cells as possible rather than to have long-term stable hybrids. Therefore NS-1 was used in the studies reported above. Generally, 70-100% of the wells showed visible hybrid growth within 3 weeks after fusion. As observed by other investigators, human-mouse hybrids tend to be unstable. Approximately one-third of our human X NS-1 hybrids lose their ability to secrete human Ig after 6 weeks in culture. However, approximately 40-50% of the hybrids that retain Ig secretion after 6 weeks can be stabilized by vigorous subcloning. Therefore, the stability problem can be partially overcome. High cloning efficiency of human X NS-1 hybrids is dependent on the presence of feeder layers. It was found that 5-10 X 10^4 mouse thymocytes, 2000R-irradiated allogeneic human peripheral blood lymphocytes, or irradiated human MRC-5 fibroblasts (obtained from ATCC) were similarly efficient in supporting clonal growth. Another disadvantage associated with NS-1 hybrids is the secretion of mouse K chain in association with human Ig heavy (H) chains. If this occurs with both heavy chains of a human IgG molecule resulting in an H_2K_2 structure, then the antibody specificity is lost. The percentage of specific Ig secreted by each hybrid differs because the ratio of H_2L_2 (active molecules with both human H and light (L) chains) to H_2K_2 and HLK molecules varies. For most *in vitro* studies, a mixture of HL and HK molecules can be used. For *in vivo* studies, it is preferable to eliminate the molecules containing mouse K chains so as to decrease the anti-mouse reactions and increase the specific activity of the antibody preparation. This can be accomplished by passing the MAb through an anti-mouse K affinity column. All of the four human fusion partners tested (namely, WI-L2 729HF2, LICR LON HMy2, UC729, and GM-4672) will secrete parental Ig chains after fusion, even though the amounts vary. Because all the Ig chains involved are of human origin, it is difficult to separate the inactive or semi-active Ig molecules from the specific Ig. Theoretically, an affinity purification step involving anti-allotypic or anti-idiotypic reagent can be used, but it is impractical. Therefore, it is highly desirable to have a nonsecreting and efficient fusion partner. Recently, several nonsecreting heteromyeloma parents (products of mouse fusion partners and human lymphocytes), such as SHM D33 (21,22) and SBC-H20 (23), have been developed. They seem to fuse well and yield stable hybrids. Fusions between *in vitro* sensitized cells and these parents are currently being evaluated at our laboratory. In our experience, SP2/0 and P3Ag8.653 fusion partners are not as efficient as NS-1 in fusion. The resulting hybrids also tend to be unsatble. However, other investigators (24) have had good success in using subclones of P3Ag8.653 as fusion partners.

IV. PURIFICATION OF HUMAN MAbs

To obtain large amounts of human MAbs, attempts were made to grow the human X NS-1 hybrids in ascites. Generally, 2-3 $\times$ 10^6 hybrid cells are injected intraperitoneally into nude mice, which have been primed with pristane 2 weeks before injection. A limited study showed that only 30% of the hybrids could be grown in this form. Another approach is to grow the hybrids in suspension culture in spinner flasks. To reduce contamination with extraneous fetal calf protein, the hybrids are first adapted to growth in low serum conditions within a 3-4-week period. Typically, hybrids are weaned sequentially in RPMI-1640-10% FCS, RPMI-1640-5% FCS, followed by serum-free media such as Nutricyte (International Enzymes, Fallbrook, CA) and HB102 (DuPont-NEN, Boston, MA) supplemented with 5%, 3%, and 1% FCS. A low level of FCS is retained in the culture media because (a) some hybrids grow much more slowly in totally serum-free conditions, and (b) the small amounts of serum proteins that are present can act as carriers to enhance the recovery of immunoglobulins (Ig) during purification. Using this approach, it is possible to recover 10-30 mg of human Ig from each liter of culture supernatant fluids.

For purification of human Ig from culture supernatant fluids, the Ig is concentrated 30 to 50 times by ultrafiltration through Pellicon membranes (Millipore, Bedfore, MA). This step can be completed in 1 hour, with 95% recovery of Ig. The immunoglobulins (Ig) were then purified by conventional gel filtration and ion exchange chromatography or fast-protein liquid chromatography (FPLC). We have not tried high pressure liquid chromatography (HPLC), which others have used successfully for purification of human MAbs (M. Glassy, personal communication).

V. PERSPECTIVES

A procedure for immunization of human B lymphocytes *in vitro* has been described. This procedure allowed the production of the first human MAb to a peptide antigen, bombesin. In addition to generating a primary antibody response, the immunization procedure can also induce secondary responses (e.g., to TT). Previous studies on human antibody response against TT and diphtheria toxoid (25,26) showed that antibody-producing cells are found in the peripheral blood only for a short and well-defined time period after *in vivo* boosting. There are only a few weeks during which the antigen-specific antibody-producing cells can be "captured." Using the procedure described here, this time restraint is eliminated. It was possible to elicit anti-TT responses from all the donors tested, independent of their vaccination histories. Therefore, this procedure might be used to recall and expand lymphocytes against other antigens that the donors have been exposed to previously. All the immunogens used thus far are protein antigens. It would be interesting to study sensitization against other types of antigens, such as carbohydrates and lipids, especially in view of the prevalence of TAA which are glycolipids (27).

As mentioned, human lymphocytes can recognize polymorphic determinants that are weakly or poorly immunogenic in animals. It might be possible to produce human MAbs against those tumor antigens that bear only minor differences to normal cellular antigens. Similarly, strain-specific bacterial or viral antigens may be more immunogenic for human lymphocytes than for lymphocytes of other species. Another interesting question is whether one can generate human MAbs against antigens that are not immunogenic *in vivo*. *In vitro* immunization could be used to produce neutralizing antibodies against bacterial antigens, such as group B meningococcal polysaccharides, which have been shown to be nonimmunogenic in humans (28). Previously, mouse MAbs to weak immunogens have been obtained by *in vitro* sensitization (10,11).

The immunization process reported here can serve as an *in vitro* model for dissecting the elements involved in antigen-specific activation and differentiation of human B lymphocytes. Examinations of the lymphocyte subpopulation and growth factors required for immunization *in vitro* will be undertaken. Information in this area is critical to the understanding of immune regulation, as well as to the optimization of the immunization procedure. In accordance with primary responses, only IgM anti-bombesin MAbs have been generated thus far. Identification and addition of appropriate differentiation factors to the cultures might lead to IgG antibodies.

ACKNOWLEDGMENTS

I am deeply indebted to N. Rand, Dr. J. H. Murray, M. Sullivan, and K. Kato for their contributions to the studies presented here. I am also grateful to Dr. H. Rabin for critical review of the manuscript, and M. Godfroy for skilled secretarial assistance.

REFERENCES

1. R. A. Miller, D. G. Maloney, R. Warnke, and R. Levy. Treatment of B cell lymphoma with monoclonal anti-idiotype antibody. *N. Engl. J. Med., 306*: 517 (1982).

2. R. A. Miller, A. R. Oseroff, P. T. Stratte, and R. Levy. Monoclonal antibody therapeutic trials in seven patients with T-cell lymphoma. *Blood, 62*: 988 (1983).
3. H. F. Sears, D. Herlyn, Z. Steplewski, and H. Koprowski. Effects of monoclonal antibody immunotherapy on patients with gastrointestinal adenocarcinoma. *J. Biol. Resp. Modifiers, 3*:138 (1984).
4. P. A. Farrands, M. V. Pimm, M. J. Embleton, A. C. Perkins, J. D. Hardy, R. W. Baldwin, and J. D. Hardcastle. Radioimmunodetection of human colorectal cancers by an anti-tumor monoclonal antibody. *Lancet, ii*:397 (1982).
5. R. K. Oldham, K. A. Foon, A. C. Morgan, C. S. Woodhouse, R. W. Schroff, P. G. Abrams, M. Fer, C. S. Schoenberger, M. Farrell, E. Kimball, and S. A. Sherwin. Monoclonal antibody therapy on malignant melanoma: *in vivo* localization in cutaneous metastasis after intravenous administration. *J. Clin. Oncol., 2*:1235 (1984).
6. M. Steinitz, G. Klein, S. Koskomies, and O. Makel. EB virus-induced B lymphocyte cell line producing specific antibody. *Nature, 269*:420 (1977).
7. J. W. Larrick and D. W. Buck. Practical aspects of human monoclonal antibody production. *Bio Techniques, 2*:6 (1984).
8. R. J. Cote, D. M. Morrissey, A. N. Houghton, E. J. Beattie, Jr., H. F. Oettgen, and L. J. Old. Generation of human monoclonal antibodies reactive with cellular antigens. *Proc. Natl. Acad. Sci.* (*USA*), *80*:2026 (1983).
9. A. N. Houghton, H. Brooks, R. J. Cote, M. C. Taormina, H. F. Oettgen, and L. J. Old. Detection of cell surface and intracellular antigens by human monoclonal antibodies. Hybrid cell lines derived from lymphocytes of patients with malignant melanoma. *J. Exp. Med., 158*:53 (1983).
10. R. A. Luben and M. A. Mohler. *In vitro* immunization as an adjunct to the production of hybridomas producing antibodies against the lymphokine osteoclast activity factor. *Mol. Immunol., 17*:635 (1980).
11. R. L. Pardue, R. C. Brady, G. W. Perry, and J. R. Dedman. Production of monoclonal antibodies against calmodulin by *in vitro* immunization of spleen cells. *J. Cell. Biol., 96*:1149 (1983).
12. F. Cuttitta, D. N. Carney, J. Mulshine, T. W. Moody, J. Fedorko, A. Fischler, and J. D. Minna. Bombesin-like peptides can function as autocrine growth factors in human small cell lung cancer. *Nature, 316*:823 (1985).
13. T. L. Goodfriend, L. Levine, and G. D. Fasman. Antibodies to bradykinin and angiotensin: a use of carbodiimides in immunology. *Science, 144*: 1344 (1964).
14. M. K. Hoffmann. Antigen-specific induction and regulation of antibody synthesis in cultures of human peripheral blood mononuclear cells. *Proc. Natl. Acad. Sci.* (*USA*), *77*:1139 (1980).
15. J. Cavagnaro and M. E. Osband. Successful *in vitro* primary immunization of human peripheral blood mononuclear cells and its role in the development of human-derived monoclonal antibodies. *Bio Techniques, 1*:30 (1983).

16. G. Galfre, C. Milstein, and B. Wright. Rat X rat hybrid myeloma and a monoclonal anti-Fd portion of mouse IgG. *Nature, 277*:131 (1979).
17. J. Misiti and T. A. Waldmann. *In vitro* generation of antigen-specific hemolytic plaque-forming cells from human peripheral blood mononuclear cells. *J. Exp. Med., 154*:1069 (1981).
18. A. S. Fauci and K. R. Pratt. Activation of human B lymphocytes. I. Direct plaque-forming cell assay for the measurement of polyclonal activation and antigenic stimulation of human B lymphocytes. *J. Exp. Med., 144*:674 (1976).
19. A. L. Luzzati, C. Ramoni, and G. B. Ferrara. Antigen-specific antibody response induced in cultures of human blood lymphocytes in presence of polyethylene glycol. *Eur. J. Immunol., 11*:943 (1981).
20. L. E. Strike, B. H. Devens, and R. L. Lundak. Production of human-human hybridomas secreting antibody to sheep erythrocytes after *in vitro* immunization. *J. Immunol., 132*:1798 (1984).
21. N. N. H. Teng, K. S. Lam, F. C. Riera, and H. S. Kaplan. Construction and testing of mouse-human heteromyelomas for human monoclonal antibody production. *Proc. Natl. Acad. Sci. (USA), 80*:7308 (1983).
22. N. N. H. Teng, H. S. Kaplan, J. M. Hebert, C. Moore, H. Douglas, A. Wunderlick, and A. I. Braude. Protection against gram-negative bacteria and endotoxemia with human monoclonal IgM antibodies. *Proc. Natl. Acad. Sci. (USA), 82*:1790 (1985).
23. S. K. H. Foung, S. Perkins, A. Raubitschek, J. Larrick, G. Lizak, D. Fishwald, E. G. Engleman, and F. C. Grumet. Rescue of human monoclonal antibody production from an EBV-transformed B cell line by fusion to a human mouse hybridoma. *J. Immunol. Meth., 70*:83 (1984).
24. E. Oh, K. Burnet, J. Kayden, and K. Waldron. Characterization and antigen identification of a human monoclonal antibody to colon carcinoma. *Fed. Proc., 44*:792 (1985).
25. R. H. Stevens. Regulation of human B lymphocyte function in secondary humoral immune responses. *Immunol. Today, 3*:144 (1982).
26. D. J. Volkman, S. P. Allyn, and A. S. Fauci. Antigen-induced *in vitro* antibody production in humans: tetanus toxoid-specific antibody synthesis. *J. Immunol., 129*:107 (1982).
27. S. I. Hakomori. Aberrant glycosylation in cancer cell membranes as focused on glycolipids: overview and perspectives. *Cancer Res., 45*:2405 (1985).
28. F. A. Wyle, M. S. Artenstein, B. L. Brandt, E. C. Tramont, D. L. Kasper, P. L. Altieri, S. L. Berman, and L. P. Lowenthal. Immunologic response of man to group B meningococcal polysaccharide vaccine. *J. Infect. Dis. 126*: 514 (1972).

3

In Vitro Sensitization for the Production of Human Monoclonal Antibodies

MARCIA BIEBER
Cancer Biology Research Laboratory, Stanford, California

NELSON N. H. TENG
Stanford University School of Medicine, Stanford, California

The development of hybridoma technology by Kohler and Milstein (1) opened a new era, not only in immunology, but in all fields of biological science. Hybridoma cell lines formed by the fusion of mutant mouse myeloma cells with spleen cells from an immunized mouse assure the permanent availability of monoclonal antibody of defined specificity. The clinical use of these xenoantibodies in human patients, however, will be limited by the fact that they themselves will be immunogenic upon repeated administration. For therapeutic applications in man, the availability of human monoclonal antibodies would be advantageous.

In developing mouse monoclonal antibodies, mice can be optimally immunized and the spleen removed, yielding lymphoid cells highly enriched in actively proliferating, antigen-primed B cells. Since this is not possible in humans, methods have been developed to immunize and use peripheral blood as the source of antigen-sensitized B cells (2,3). However, antigens used in these methods must be nonhazardous. Another method for obtaining B cells for fusion is the use of lymph nodes removed from patients at the time of surgery (4-6). The difficulty in this approach is recovering and expanding the B cells actively responding to the desired antigens. For these and other reasons, it is desirable to develop a system for *in vitro* antigen sensitization of human lymphocytes. Several groups (7-10) have developed methods for *in vitro* sensitization. We have utilized various methods for sensitization and amplification of the B-cell immune response to obtain *in vitro*-sensitized human monoclonal antibodies.

I. MATERIALS AND METHODS

A. Cell Preparation

Normal spleens were obtained from trauma patients or patients with spherocytosis. Uninvolved spleens from patients undergoing exploratory laparotomy for B-cell lymphoma were also used. The tissue was minced in RPMI-1640 medium, and the mononuclear cells (MNCs) were isolated by centrifugation on Ficol Hypaque. The MNCs were frozen using 4-5 $\times$ 10^7/ml in 20% fetal calf serum (FCS) and 20% DMSO, and stored in liquid nitrogen. Peripheral blood MNCs were obtained from Ficol Hypaque centrifugation of heparinized blood from normal donors. These cells were used fresh. T cell-enriched suspensions and non-T cells were obtained by rosetting MNCs with neuraminidase-treated sheep erythrocytes (SRBC). The T-cell fraction contained 90-95% E rosettes. For some experiments, the T cells were irradiated in a cesium irradiator. T cells were panned on cimetidine-coated plates (Seragen Inco, Boston, MA) to remove H_2 receptor-positive cells.

B. Mitogens and Antigens

The following mitogens were utilized. *Staphylococcus aureus* Cowan I (SAC) (Calbiochem, San Diego, CA), PHA (Burroughs Wellcome Co., Research Triangle Park, NC), PWM (Difco, Detroit, MI), lipopolysaccharides, phenolic extraction, and *E. coli* 0111:B4 and *Salmonella typhosa* (Sigma Chemical Co., St. Louis, MO). Muramyl dipeptide (MDP-N-acetylmuramyl-L alanyl D-isoglutamine) (Calbiochem), wheat germ agglutinin, 8-mercaptoguanosine and cimetidine (Sigma Chemical Co.), keyhold limpet hemocyanin (KLH), DNP-human albumin (Calbiochem), and sperm whale myoglobin (Sigma Chemical Co.) were used as antigens.

C. Growth Factors

Forty-hour supernatant was harvested from peripheral blood lymphocytes (PBLs) or spleen cells, stimulated with PHA, 2 μg/ml, or PWM, 1:100 dilution, and cultured at 1.5 $\times$ 10^6/ml in RPMI-1640 with 5% FCS (Irvine Scientific, Santa Ana, CA) and 5 $\times$ 10^{-5} M mercaptoethanol. Supernatants from three-way mixed lymphocyte cultures were also used (11).

D. Assays

DNP-human albumin, albumin, KLH, and sperm whale myoglobin were coupled to SRBC using pyridyldithiopropronic acid, N-hydroxysuccinimide ester (SPDP) (Sigma Chemical Co.) (12). Direct and indirect hemolytic plaque assays were done using the technique of Cunningham and Szenberg (13). ELISA was performed on Linbro plates. Antigen was coated on the plates. Antibody binding to the antigen was determined with peroxidase-labeled goat anti-human IgG or IgM (Tago, Inc., Burlingame, CA). As a substrate, ABTS (2,2-azinodi-3-ethyl-benzthiazoline) sulfonic acid (Sigma Chemical Co.) was used, and optical density was read on a Titertek Multiscan.

E. Fusion

Fusions using the SHM D33 or SHM D36 lines were performed according to a previously published protocol (14).

II. RESULTS

Sensitization of PBLs *in vitro* has been unsuccessful. Good results were obtained with lymphocytes from normal spleens (trauma) or uninvolved spleens from patients with lymphoma at staging laparotomy. Sensitization *in vitro* was determined using the Cunningham plaque assay, with antigen coupled to SRBC. ELISA was also used to assay culture supernants. The initial work to establish the optimal culture conditions utilized DNP-human albumin as antigen. DNP coupled to SRBC was also effective as an antigen, having the same range of response of DNP-human albumin. Antigen priming of human B cells required the presence of antigen-presenting cells and helper T cells and the inactivation of suppressor T cells. Mononuclear cells from the spleen contain a high percentage of Ia-positive B cells and accessory cells as compared with PBLs. These Ia-positive cells act as antigen-presenting and accessory cells and may explain why spleen cells can be sensitized *in vitro* (15-17). Suppressor T cells had to be removed or inactivated (6,7). T and B cells, including monocyte-type cells, were separated by E rosetting, and the T cell population was irradiated with 1100 rads in a cesium irradiator (18). The T lymphocytes were also panned on cimetidine-coated plates to remove the H_2-positive T suppressor cells (19). Both methods worked well to inactivate or remove suppressor cells. Adding cimetidine (10^{-5} M) to the mononuclear cells or panning unseparated mononuclear cells was inadequate. Most experiments utilized the irradiated T cells. Several variations of cell concentration, proportion of T to non-T cells, volume, and flat wells versus round tubes were compared. Best results were obtained using 1 to 2×10^6 non-T cells and 1.5 to 3×10^6 treated cells. Normal human serum (NHS) was found to be essential in the early stages of sensitization (6). Normal human sera was pooled from 10-20 normal donors and frozen at -70°C. It was heat-inactivated before use. Commercial human sera gave poor results.

A variety of additives were added at early (time 0) and later (day 4) stages of culture in an effort to improve sensitization. None of the following additives alone or combined, enhanced sensitization of B cells in this system: 8-mercaptoguanosine (20), wheat germ agglutin (21), lithium carbonate (22), monocyte-conditioned medium (23), T-cell growth factors, and either 40-hour supernatants from PHA-stimulated lymphocytes (24,25) or MLC supernatants (11).

When T-cell growth factors, SAC, PHA, or PWM were added at time 0, sensitization was inhibited. However, lipopolysaccharide (LPS), 1-5 μg/ml, or muramyl dipeptide (MDP), 1-5 μg/ml, were needed at time 0, probably to enhance stimulation of antigen-presenting cells and interleukin-1 (IL-1) release. The combination of LPS and MDP was synergistic and improved sensitization two-to three-fold. In addition, 2-mercaptoethanol, 5×10^{-5} M, was added to the medium. Antigen can either be soluble or linked to SRBC. Soluble antigen at a concentration of 1-10 μg/ml gave equal or better sensitization to that obtained with SRBC antigen. Higher or lower antigen concentrations did not produce sensitization. Antibody response to the antigen was not detected when antigen was not present in the culture.

After incubation for 2 to 3 days, the medium was removed and replaced with fresh medium containing 15% fetal calf serum, with PHA, 1 μg/ml, and SAC, 0.01% (28). The change of medium washed out the antigen (29,30,8) but removal of antigen was not needed to obtain sensitization. However, removal of the NHS allowed the supernatants to be tested for human antibody on ELISA. Although addition of mitogens early in culture inhibited sensitization (6,31), by day 3 or 4 it was necessary to provide growth and differentiation factors. The combination of SAC, 0.01%, and PHA, 1 μg/ml, (32) was the most efficient. The SAC induced B-cell amplification and the PHA stimulated helper T cells to secrete T- and B-cell lymphokines. Addition of T- and B-cell growth factors (from 40-hour supernatants) plus the SAC/PHA competition did not enhance and often inhibited sensitization. Growth factor supernatant alone did allow sensitization, possibly from mitogen carryover, but the SAC/PHA combination gave better results (Table 1). Dexamethasone, 10^{-7} M added at day 4, increased sensitization (number of plaque-forming cells) two- to four-fold in some patients (33). The effect of dexamethasone at day 4 may be due to inhibition of prostaglandin-mediated suppression (34). Dexamethasone added at time 0 did not enhance sensitization and sometimes inhibited the response. Surprisingly, in the few comparison fusions done, the increased number of plaques by dexamethasone-treated cells did not yield an increase in antigen-specific hybridomas.

After addition of mitogens at day 3 or 4, the cells were fed several times with Iscove's 15% FCS and assayed on days 7-11. Assay was by direct and indirect plaquing of antigen-coupled SRBC. The number of anti-SRBC plaques was subtracted from the antigen-SRBC plaques. In some donors, the number of anti-SRBC antibody-forming cells was high. Antibodies to SRBC may be due to recall of cross-reactive antibodies (35). The SRBC membranes left on the T lymphocytes after rosetting and some contamination of the lymphocytes with SRBC provide the antigen for recall.

Table 1 *In Vitro* Sensitization with DNP-Human Albumin–Additives for Enhancing Sensitization Added at Time 0/Day 4

	Number of DNP SRBC PFC/10^6 lymphocytes[a]		
Time 0	Patient 1[b]	Patient 2	Patient 3
Control conditions[c] (w̄ PHA/SAC day 4)	80	0	120
plus			
LPS μg/ml time 0	220	290	630
MDP 5 μg/ml time 0	280	220	570
LPS and MDP time 0	460	510	720
Dexamethasone 10^{-7} M (w̄ LPS)	100	0	
40 hr "lymphokine" supernatant[d]	0	0	0
Day 4	**Patient 1[e]**	**Patient 4**	**Patient 5**
Control conditions‡ (w̄ LPS/MDP time 0)	50		50
PHA	200		190
PWM	150		0
PHA/SAC	350	800	540
PWM/SAC	180	300	310
40 hr "lymphokine" supernatant	200	330	
48 hr MLC supernatant	200	0	
PHA/SAC w̄ dexamethasone 10^{-7} M	90	790	1100
PHA/SAC w̄ 40 hr "lymphokine" supernatant	–	750	400

[a]PFC assayed day 8 (or day 9, patients 3 and 4) DNP-SRBC plaques minus SRBC plaques.
[b]Representative results shown.
[c]1.5 × 10^6 non-T cells/ml and 2•10^6 T cells/ml (irradiated 1100R) in 1 ml Iscove medium, 5% NHS. DNP-human albumin 2-5 μg/ml time 0.
[d]PBL 1.5 × 10^6/ml Iscove, 5% FCS, PHA 2 μg/ml for 40 hr.
[e]Separate experiment.

ELISA was also used to assay the supernatant for antigen-specific antibody. The peak of plaque-forming cells on days 8-9 coincided with the best fusion-frequency response. At the end of 8 days, the culture viability was about 50-60%, with approximately 2.5 × 10^6 live cells/well. Fewer cells or lower viability indicated an unsuccessful experiment. The live cells were 60-70% surface Ig-positive and about 1 per 100 was positive for cytoplasmic immunoglobulin. By plaque assay, 200-1000 anti-DNP-secreting cells per 10^6 live cells have been obtained in culture.

The cells were fused at a 1:2 to 1:5 ratio with the SHMD33 line. Fusion seemed to be selective for the sensitized, dividing B cells as up to 8% of hybrids secreting immunoglobulin were positive for DNP.

Using this system, *in vitro* sensitization was accomplished with DNP-human albumin (20 or 35 haptens/molecule), keyhole limpet hemocyanin, and sperm whale myoglobin, which represents haptenated protein and nonhuman proteins. The response to strong foreign antigens *in vitro* may not be de novo sensitization, but may be a form of cross-reactive recall. It has also been shown that different processes are involved in the T-cell response to soluble antigen versus cells (36, 37). Different presentation and culture conditions may be needed to obtain *in vitro* sensitization to tumor membrane or viral antigens.

ACKNOWLEDGMENT

This work was supported in part by Grant CA 36422 from the National Cancer Institute.

REFERENCES

1. G. Kohler and C. Milstein. Continuous cultures of fused cells secreting antibody of predefined specificity. *Nature, 256*:495 (1975).
2. H. C. Lane, D. J. Volkman, G. Whalen, and A. S. Fauci. *In vitro* antigen-induced, antigen-specific antibody production in man. Specific and polyclonal components, kinetics, and cellular requirements. *J. Exp. Med., 154*:1043 (1981).
3. J. W. Larrick, K. E. Truitt, A. A. Raubitschek, G. Senyk, and J. C. N. Wang, Characterization of human hybridomas secreting antibody to tetanus toxoid. *Proc. Natl. Acad. Sci.* (*USA*), *80*:6376 (1983).
4. M. C. Glassy, H. H. Handley, H. Hagiwara, and I. Royston. UC729-6, a human lymphoblastoid B-cell line useful for generating antibody-secreting human-human hybridomas. *Proc. Natl. Acad. Sci.* (*USA*), *80*:6327 (1983).
5. B. J. Cote, D. M. Morrissey, A. N. Houghton, E. J. Beattie, H. F. Oettgen, and L. J. Old. Generation of human monoclonal antibodies reactive with cellular antigens. *Proc. Natl. Acad. Sci.* (*USA*), *80*:2026 (1983).
6. C. M. Crose, A. Linnenback, W. Hall, Z. Steplewski, and H. Koprowski. Production of human hybridomas secreting antibodies to measles virus. *Nature, 288*:488 (1980).
7. C. Morimoto, E. I. Reinherz, and S. F. Schlossman. Regulation of *in vitro* primary anti-DNP antibody production by functional subsets of T lymphocytes in man. *J. Immunol., 127*:69 (1981).
8. C. Morimoto, J. Distaso, Y. Borel, S. F. Schlossman, and E. I. Reinherz. Communicative interactions between subpopulations of human T lymphocytes required for generation of suppressor-effector function in a primary antibody response. *J. Immunol. 128*:1645 (1982).

9. J. Misiti and T. A. Waldmann. *In vitro* generation of antigen-specific hemolytic plaque-forming cells from human peripheral blood mononuclear cells. *J. Exp. Med., 154*:1069 (1981).
10. M. K. Hoffman. Antigen-specific induction and regulation of antibody synthesis in cultures in human peripheral blood mononuclear cells. *Proc. Natl. Acad. Sci. (USA), 77*:1139 (1980).
11. M. Peters and A. S. Fauci. Selective activation of antigen-specific human B cells by non-specific factors in the absence of antigen. *J. Immunol. 130*: 678 (1983).
12. L. D. Leserman, J. Barbet, and F. Kourilsky. Targeting to cells of fluorescent liposomes covalently coupled with monoclonal antibody or protein A. *Nature, 228*:602 (1980).
13. A. J. Cunningham and A. Szenberg. Improvements in the plaque technique for detecting single antibody forming cells. *J. Immunol., 14*:599 (1968).
14. N. N. H. Teng, K. S. Lam, F. Calvo Rivera, and H. S. Kaplan. Construction and testing of novel mouse-human heteromyelomas for human monoclonal antibody production. *Proc. Natl. Acad. Sci. (USA), 88*:7308 (1983).
15. T. L. Gerrard and A. S. Fauci. Activation and immunoregulation of antigen-specific human B lymphocyte responses. Multifaceted role of the monocyte. *J. Immunol., 128*:2367 (1982).
16. D. L. Thiele and P. E. Lipsky. The accessory function of phagocytic cells in human T cell and B cell responses. *J. Immunol., 129*:1033 (1982).
17. D. I. Beller and K. Ho. Evaluation of the control of macrophage Ia expression *in vitro*. *J. Immunol. 129*:971 (1982).
18. B. L. Kotzin, C. J. Benike, and E. G. Engleman. Induction of immunoglobulin-secreting cells in the allogeneic mixed leukocyte reaction: regulation by helper and suppressor lymphocyte subsets in man. *J. Immunol., 127*:931 (1981).
19. J. Cavagnaro and M. Osband. Successful *in vitro* primary immunization of human peripheral blood mononuclear cells and its role in the development of human-derived monoclonal antibodies. *Bio Techniques, 1*:30 (1983).
20. M. G. Goodman and W. O. Weigle. Induction of immunoglobulin secretion by a simple nucleoside derivative. *J. Immunol., 128*:2399 (1982).
21. W. C. Greene, C. K. Goldman, S. T. Marshall, T. A. Fleisher, and T. A. Waldman. Stimulation of immunoglobulin biosynthesis in human B cells by wheat germ agglutinin. *J. Immunol., 129*:799 (1981).
22. A. P. Weetman, A. M. McGregor, J. H. Lazarus, B. Rees Smith, and R. Hall. Enhancement of immunoglobulin synthesis by human lymphocytes with lithium. *Clin. Immunol., 22*:400 (1982).
23. M. Finelt and M. K. Hoffman. A human monocyte function test: Release of B-cell differentiation factor (BDF). *Clin. Immunol. Immunopathol., 12*: 281 (1979).
24. S. Gillis, M. Fern, W. Ou, and K. A. Smith. T cell growth factor: parameters of production and a quantitative microassay for activity. *J. Immunol., 120*: 2027 (1978).

25. M. Howard, J. Farrar, M. Hiflicker, B. Johnson, K. Takatsu, T. Hamakoa, and W. E. Paul. Identification of a T cell-derived B cell growth factor distinct from interleukin 2. *J. Exp. Med., 155*:914 (1982).
26. C. Leclerc, D. Juy, and L. Chedid. Inhibitory and stimulatory effects of a synthetic glycopeptide (MDP) on the *in vitro* PFC response factors affecting the response. *Cell Immunol. 42*:336 (1979).
27. A. Togawa, J. J. Oppenheim, and S. B. Mizel. Characterization of lymphocyte activating factor (LAF) produced by human mononuclear cells. *J. Immunol. 122*:2112 (1979).
28. O. Saiki and P. Ralph. Induction of human immunoglobin secretion. I. Synergistic effect of B-cell mitogen Cowan I plus T cell mitogens. *J. Immunol. 127*:1044 (1981).
29. R. H. Stevens and A. Saxon. Antigen-induced suppression of human *in vitro* pokeweed mitogen-stimulated antibody production. *Cell Immunol., 55*:85 (1980).
30. W. Borkowsky and F. T. Valentine. The proliferative response of human lymphocytes to antigen is suppressed preferentially by lymphocytes precultured with the same antigen. *J. Immunol., 122*:1867 (1979).
31. G. Golding, D. R. Burger, and M. B. Rittenberg. Lectin-induced regulation of human thymus-independent anti-TNP responses *in vitro. J. Immunol., 129*:942 (1982).
32. R. J. M. Falkoff, L. P. Zhu, and A. S. Fauci. Separate signals for B cell proliferation and differentiation in response to staphylococcus aureus: evidence for a two-signal model of B cell activation. *J. Immunol. 129*:97 (1982).
33. A. Fauci, R. Pratt, and G. Whalen. Activation of human B lymphocytes IV. Regulatory effects of corticosteroids on the triggering signal in the plaque-forming cell response of human peripheral blood B lymphocytes to polyclonal activation. *J. Immunol., 119*:598 (1977).
34. R. J. Flower and G. J. Blackwell. Anti-inflammatory steroids induce biosynthesis of a phospholipase A_2 inhibitor which prevents prostaglandin generation. *Nature, 278*:456 (1979).
35. P. Marrack, S. D. Graham, Jr., E. Kushnir, H. J. Leibson, N. Roehm, and J. W. Kappler. Nonspecific factors in B cell responses. *Immunol. Rev., 63*:33 (1982).
36. H. Z. Streicher, I. J. Berkower, M. Busch, F. R. N. Gund, and J. A. Berzofsky. The role of antigen conformation in determining requirements for antigen processing for T cell activation. In E. Sercarz, H. Cantor, and I. Chess (eds.). *UCLA Symposium on Molecular and Cellular Biology*. Alan R. Liss, Inc., New York (1984).
37. A. Finnergan, B. W. Needleman, and R. J. Hodes. Antigen processing requirements for T cell activation: differential requirements for presentation of soluble conventional antigen vs cell surface MHC determinants. *J. Immunol., 134*:2960 (1985).

4

Human Monoclonal Antibodies and the LICR-LON-HMy2 System

MICHAEL J. O'HARE and PAUL A. W. EDWARDS*
Ludwig Institute for Cancer Research (London Branch), Sutton, Surrey, England

It is now 10 years since Kohler and Milstein (1) described the production of murine monoclonal antibodies of predefined specificity, and a few years since the search for a comparable system for making human monoclonal antibodies began. However, the systems that have been developed still leave something to be desired in various respects, not least in their labor-intensive nature.

Fusing human lymphocytes with hypoxanthine/aminopterin/thymidine (HAT)-sensitive human B-cell lines is probably still the most widely used method of making human monoclonal antibodies. Several appropriate parental lines have been developed during the past 5 years, the majority being of lymphoblastoid type and, unlike murine systems, Epstein-Barr nuclear antigen (EBNA)-positive, rather than true myeloma (plasmacytoma) cell lines. Some cell lines of this type have appeared under a variety of different designations as they have passed through different hands, or have been separately derived from the same original stocks. This has lead, unfortunately, to a superficial impression that there are a large number of different human cell lines for monoclonal antibody production, whereas in fact the number is still quite limited.

The LICR-LON-HMy2 cell line was introduced by us in 1982. It has been widely distributed and used successfully to make human monoclonal antibodies

---

**Present affiliation*: University of Cambridge, Cambridge, England in a number of independent laboratories. We have recently described in some detail the practical aspects of making human monoclonals with this line (2), as well as comparative aspects of its performance and characteristics with respect to other systems. In this brief chapter we will, therefore, confine ourselves to:

1. a summary of the properties of this line,
2. an update of the state of the art with respect to newer cell lines and techniques that were not covered in our previous publications,
3. a preliminary description of the use of electrofusion techniques to improve hybrid yield, and
4. an update of our assessment of the future directions in human monoclonal research.

Our assessment of the performance of HMy2 is based, in part, on comparative studies that we carried out with other parental lines, as well as the results of a brief questionnaire that we distributed to certain laboratories to which we have sent HMy2.

We would, however, first like to reiterate certain caveats concerning the general properties of human, as distinct from rodent, monoclonal antibodies. These are, essentially, that there is no firm evidence that human antibodies can be generated with unique specificities that are not available from the rodent systems; that rodent antibodies are by no means totally unsuited for therapeutic administration, provided that appropriate regimes are adopted to minimize anti-mouse (or rat) immune responses in the patient; and that it is still the case that even the best human monoclonal-generating systems are less efficient, in terms of overall hybrid yield than comparable rodent systems.

I. LICR-LON-HMy2

A. Origin

This cell line (3,4) is a HAT-sensitive (HPRT-) variant prepared by us from stocks of the ARH-77 cell line. The latter line was derived by Burk *et al.* (5) from a patient with a plasma cell leukemia. This is a form of multiple myeloma in which the majority of tumor cells are found in the circulation, rather than as solid deposits; nonetheless, the tumor cells are more or less fully differentiated plasma cells with high concentrations of intracytoplasmic immunoglobulin (5). In this case, the myeloma paraprotein was IgG (lambda). Characterization of early cultures of ARH-77 confirmed secretion of this paraprotein (5). However, as distributed to us (and other laboratories) at higher passage numbers, the ARH-77 line turned out to be a lymphoblastoid, not a myeloma line. This was apparent from the fact that it was EBNA-positive; furthermore, it secreted IgG (kappa) and, thus, did not match the original patient's myeloma. It was from these late passage ARH-77 stocks (derived presumably from the overgrowth of the original cultures by an EB-transformed lymphocyte) that we selected our HAT-sensitive variant HMy2, originally in the belief that we were working with a myeloma cell line (hence, HMy2). The true situation became apparent prior to our initial publication (3), when our variant was fully characterized and compared, in turn, with the ARH-77 stocks that we had received and the original publication (5).

B. Nomenclature

We have detailed the exact history of HMy2 because it is still sometimes incorrectly referred to as a myeloma line in other publications. There also apparently remains some doubt as to when and where the transition from putative myeloma to lymphoblastoid line occurred (see, for example, reference 6). Unlike other cell lines for human monoclonal antibody production, HMy2 has not, fortunately, undergone significant changes in nomenclature in other laboratories, although it has been called LICR-2 (7,8), and a substrain was designated CAM-1 (9). We have derived an ouabain-resistant substrain called HMy2OR, which will grow at concentrations of up to 10^{-5} M ouabain (i.e., two orders of magnitude greater than wild-type cells). Its fusion characteristics are identical to the original stocks, and it is suitable for the immortalization of EB-transformed lymphocytes, as advocated by Kozbor *et al.* (10).

C. Characteristics

As distributed by us to other laboratories, the HMy2 line is of proved human origin by isoenzyme and karyotypic analyses (with a pseudodiploid mode [4] and certain marker chromosomes). A full karyotype has been illustrated elsewhere (2). Stocks usually contain a small pseudotetraploid component. In one subline we have, however, observed a transition to the pseudotetraploid mode (3), a phenomenon which does not seem to impair the capacity of the line to form lymphocyte hybrids, but which could lead to confusion when chromosome content or DNA profiles are used to identify hybrids.

Pseudodiploid stocks yield hybrids with near-tetraploid or subtetraploid modes (3). Because long-term passaged stocks of some proved hybrids are significantly subtetraploid, this indicates a degree of initial chromosomal instability which has relevance to the stability of new antibody production. Although this feature of human monoclonal production has not received extensive attention with other systems, it is not unique to HMy2 (see for example references 10,11). In the case of HMy2, we believe that such instability is an early phenomenon because passaged stocks of selected hybrids have shown no continuous progressive loss of chromosomes. It does, however, militate against very early screening of fusion products for new antibody secretion.

As mentioned, the HMy2 parent line secretes IgG (kappa), but at relatively low levels (0.5 $\mu g/10^6$ cells/24 hr). New antibody-producing hybrids will, therefore, inevitably secrete "hybrid" antibody molecules produced by more or less random association of parent and lymphocyte-derived chains. This will reduce the effective titer of the lymphocyte antibody, because at worst only 1/16th of the molecules will possess both antibody-binding sites of the type specified by the lymphocyte. As far as we are aware, at the time of writing, all parent human lines for human monoclonal production suffer from this disadvantage. Some lines are clearly low-level secretors rather than chain-loss variants, but this does not preclude enhanced production of parental chains in hybrids, with corresponding loss of new antibody activity. For example, hybrids formed with the RH-L4 lymphoma line, which in its unfused state synthesizes but does not secrete IgG, secrete parental light and heavy chains (12). Antibody secretion by HMy2 hybrids ranged from 0.5 to 8 $\mu g/ml$ (3) in our experience, although others (8) have reported higher values.

Interestingly, a comparative study (8) of secretion levels in hybrids derived from lymphoblastoid (including HMy2) versus a true myeloma parent (SKO-007) has shown no significant difference in either range or means, thus dispelling the common assumption that lymphoblastoid lines are inherently less capable of yielding high-secreting hybrids.

One of the principal advantages of HMy2 as a fusion parent is its extraordinary robustness. It can be passaged at very low densities ($> 10^3/ml$) and allowed to grow to very high densities ($< 2\text{-}5\ 10^5/ml$) without problems. Although some other lines such as WI-L2 derivatives (see below) are reasonably robust, this is not, in our experience, true for such lines such as GM-1500 derivatives (e.g., GM-4672), which require frequent feeding and maintenance at high densities to preserve viability. While HMy2 and to a lesser extent WI-L2-type cells grow well as isolated cells until they reach high densities, GM-1500-type cells are more typically lymphoblastoid, growing as tightly-packed clumps with few viable isolated cells (Fig. 1). This characteristic seems to be shared by many of its hybrids and has, in some hands, impeded attempts at recloning them by limiting dilution methods (13). In general, HMy2 hybrids do not suffer from this problem.

We, and others, have observed virtually no HAT-resistant revertants when using HMy2 (< 1 in 10^9 per generation). In contrast, the myleoma-derived SKO-007 has been reported (14) to give a low but not insignificant yield of revertants (1 in 10^5). However, like a number of human lines, death of HAT-sensitive HMy2 cells is not particularly rapid when compared with that of rodent myeloma cells, and aminopterin levels must be maintained for several weeks to ensure that no re-

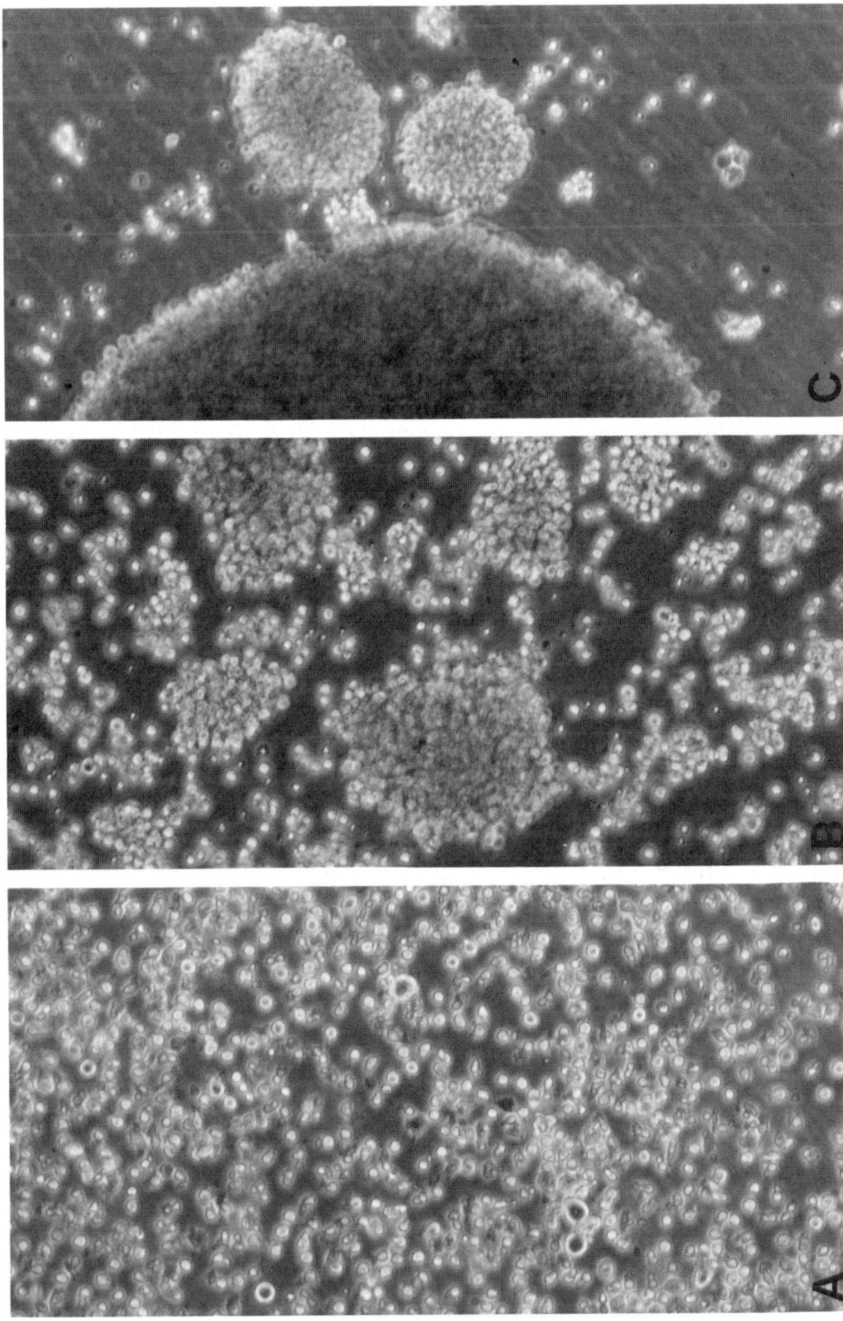

Figure 1 Phase-contrast photomicrographs (magnification ×120) of HMy2OR (A), UC729-6 (B), and GM-4762 (C).

growth of parent cells occurs to contaminate hybrids. Despite its EBNA-positive phenotype, we have no substantive evidence that it gives rise to transformed lymphocytes by releasing live virus. Neither the parental line nor its hybrids produce live virus, as demonstrated by viral capsid antigen (VCA) screening (T. Alderson and K. Sikora, personal communication). Analysis of the percentage of lambda (lymphocyte-derived) and kappa (parental) light chains in HMy2 hybrids supports the contention that the majority are true hybrids (3,15). This may not necessarily be the case for other lymphoblastoid lines. Although this may seem an academic point, the general stability of EB-transformed lines leaves something to be desired (see below).

HMy2 will grow when inoculated subcutaneously in nude mice (2). Adaptation of hybrids to subcutaneous growth, followed by intraperitoneal injection, therefore, seems likely to give ascites forms. This procedure has been used to enhance human antibody yields with hybrids generated from the WI-L2-derived LTR228 line (16), and has also been successfully applied to GM-1500-derived hybridomas (6). HMy2 also grows well in the serum-free medium HL-1 (Ventrex, Portland, ME), after a period of adaptation.

HMy2 has proved consistently hybridizable in our experience over a period of several years of continuous subcultivation, and also in a number of independent laboratories (see reference 2), using conventional polyethylene glycol methods (2). Routine testing for mycoplasma contamination, as described by Edwards and O'Hare (2), is important because infected cultures will not form hybrids. HMy2 performed relatively well in comparative study of different parent lines (17). It is, however, our more recent experience (18) that one of the WI-L2-derived HAT-sensitive lymphoblastoid cell lines, UC-729-6 (19), consistently yields a significantly greater number of individual hybrids compared with HMy2, using the same human lymphocytes with the same polyethylene glycol fusion protocol. The fusion characteristics of all WI-L2-derived HAT-sensitive lines seem comparable (17) irrespective of their origin and designation. Such lines include UC-729-6 (19), 729-HF2 (20), and LTR228 (21). UC-729-6 is generally available. It is ironic that the HPRT-negative WI-L2 stocks were generated simply to study regulation of purine synthesis (18) several years before the search for human hybridoma systems began.

On balance, therefore, these lines seem to provide the best available option at present, at least as far as absolute hybrid yield is concerned. We would, however, reserve judgment on the long-term stability of such hybrids and the actual percentage that secrete new antibody (see for example, reference 17). We have also noted in fusions with UC-729-6 and HMy2, using the same lymph node lymphocytes, that comparative hybrid yields are not invariably directly proportional. Although there are many purely technical reasons that could account for such discrepancies, there remains a possibility that the different lines fuse preferentially with different lymphocyte populations, which might influence, for example, the relative numbers of hybrids secreting different antibody classes. In any case, the best results with these lines still fall short, in our experience, of the overall hybrid yield from mouse or rat fusions where frequencies can reach 1 in 10^4 lymphocytes fused. Results with so-called human "myeloma analogues" reportedly yielding one hybrid in 10^3 cells fused (22) remain to be independently confirmed.

II. NEW CELL LINES

Despite a proliferation of designations, as just noted, there have been few genuinely novel parental cell lines introduced during the last 2 years. Exceptions have been the use of human-mouse heteromyelomas, as devised by Bron *et al.* (23), and the hybridization of the GM-1500-derived HAT-sensitive KR-4 cell line with the wild-type RPMI-8226 myeloma and reselection of a new HAT-sensitive variant, designated KR-12 (24). This cell line reportedly gives fusion frequencies equivalent to the KR-4 parent (1 in 10^6 unstimulated peripheral blood lymphocytes), but secretes over 10 times the Ig of the lymphoblastoid parent, as do its hybrids (up to 30 μg/ml). The increased number of chromosomes apparently does not impede long-term stability of antibody secretion (24). Overall, however, these levels are not significantly greater than those obtained with the original lymphoblastoid KR-4 parent (24). The ultimate practical value of this, and other analogous exercises with mouse-human hybrids reselected for HAT sensitivity (25) may, therefore, legitimately be doubted. Furthermore, the mixed antibody problem remains with both strategies.

III. NEW TECHNIQUES AND RECENT DEVELOPMENTS

These problems lead to the question of whether human-human fusions can be improved by use of alternative fusion techniques, or whether different methods of making human monoclonals are to be preferred. In some respects, it seems to us that this question is no closer to a definitive answer than it was 2 or 3 years ago. However, there has been one major advance that may outdate current methods, and this is the engineering of "human" antibodies by recombinant DNA techniques. Another novel technology for which important claims have been made is electrofusion, and we will describe some preliminary observations that we have made using this method.

There have also been certain observations in the field of EBV transformation that have reinforced the suspicion that many so-called transformants are not, in fact, truly immortal lines.

A. EB Transformation

The principal advantage of direct EB transformation of human lymphocytes is the absence of irrelevant antibody associated with hybridization with Ig-secreting B cell lines. Furthermore, there is no evidence that such generally pseudodiploid lymphoblastoid cell lines are subject to the karyotypic drift that plagues heterospecific and, to a lesser extent, human-human hybridomas. However, while there is no doubt that EBV can truly immortalize some lymphocytes, there remain some problems associated with the long-term propagation of such cultures. It has generally been thought that the virus will transform the majority of B cells exposed to it (26). Certainly in the short-term, most cells respond proliferatively and vigorously, with early cloning essential if specific antibody-producing cells are not to be overgrown by others.

However, even under optimal culture conditions, many such cultures either cease to produce antibody or cannot be established as permanent cell lines. For example, in a recent study (27), only one continuous culture of an anti-tetanus toxoid-producing EBV-transformed line was established from a total of over 2×10^7 lymphocytes initially cultured, albeit without preselection of reactive lymphocytes. Such cell lines do, in some instances, continue to produce low levels of infectious virus (28). However, it has been cogently argued that there is no evidence from conventional antibody therapy or blood transfusions that EBV contamination of blood preparations constitute any risk (29), and that human monoclonal antibodies from EBV-transformed lymphocytes can be effectively purified free from viral DNA (28,29).

The major problem with this technique is the tendency of many productive cultures to peter out. This is particularly clear in the experiments in which EB transformants are plated at limiting dilutions from the outset to obviate "swamping" by nonspecific antibody-producing clones (30). Even under these conditions, recloning efficiencies of 1% or less can be encountered. In a recent interesting study Melamed *et al.* (31) noted a progressive loss of growth capacity in a cloned lymphoblastoid line producing anti-Rhesus D, together with evidence of terminal differentiation to a plasma cell-like state. Normal lymphocytes in culture have a very limited proliferative capacity when compared with fibroblasts, which can divide 30-40 times (equivalent to at least 10^8 cells per clone) before reaching the so-called "Hayflick limit," when they senesce. It may be that many so-called EB transformants are actually cells whose lifespan *in vitro* has been extended to this limit, but not beyond. The technique of back-hybridization of such lines with HAT-sensitive lymphoblastoid hybridoma parents has been devised by Kozbor *et al.* (10) to circumvent this problem.

Inadvertant contamination of EB-transformed lines with mycoplasma derived from the virus-containing supernatant may also contribute to the failure to reclone such lines.

B. EB Transformation with Back Hybridization

The ouabain-resistant KR-4 lymphoblastoid cell line (10) was derived from GM-1500 A12. The dominant resistant phenotype confers on these cells and hybrids constructed from them the capacity to grow in concentrations of ouabain (10^{-5} M) that kill wild-type cells such as transformed lymphocytes. Our HMy2OR variant was derived to serve the same purpose. It seems likely that this strategy will see increasing use in the future because not only are EBV lines stabilized, but specific antibody yields may also be increased (10) and the specificity of the new antibody can be identified in the transformed lymphoblastoid clones prior to their crisis or senescence phase (although the mixed antibody problem again recurs).

C. Electrofusion Methods

Methods for the fusion of bacterial, protozoal, plant, and animal cells by the application of ultrashort pulses of electricity have been developed over the past 5 years, notably by Zimmermann (32). However, it is only in the last 2 years that this technique has been applied to the production of hybridomas (33-35). Its supposed potential in this area has resulted in the construction of at least two commercial versions of the Zimmermann electrofusion apparatus. We are in the process of evaluating one of these systems (from GCA Corporation, USA) for making human hybridomas.

Two stages are usually involved in electrofusion. The cells are suspended in a weakly conductive isotonic medium (300 mM sucrose, mannitol, or inositol, with 0.5 mM $CaCl_2$ and $MgCl_2$) and first subjected to a high-frequency alternating current. Over a period of 10-20 seconds, this results in the alignment of cells due to dielectrophoresis, forming so-called "pearl chains" composed of a mixture of parent cell lines and lymphocytes (Fig. 2A). Once alignment is complete, a series (2-3 pulses) of ultrashort squarewave DC shocks causes a transient membrane permeability. The pores so created enable amalgamation of neignboring cell membranes to form a series of heterokaryons (Fig. 2B). These are transferred to growth medium for synkaryons subsequently formed to grow out as hybridomas. The problem is to establish the optimal combination of electrical parameters for any given cell mixture, as the effects of the applied voltage are dependent on parameters such as cell diameter (32).

In the case of HMy2, pearl-chaining with human lymphocytes is accomplished by applying an AC voltage of 200 V/cm at a frequency of 1.0 MHz. Preliminary experiments have shown that the optimum DC voltage is 2.5 kV/cm applied in three consecutive pulses of 20 μs duration, separated by 1 second. These results are closely comparable with those reported for murine fusions (34,35). Above this DC voltage ($>$ 3.0 kV/cm), the cells are rendered permanently and lethally

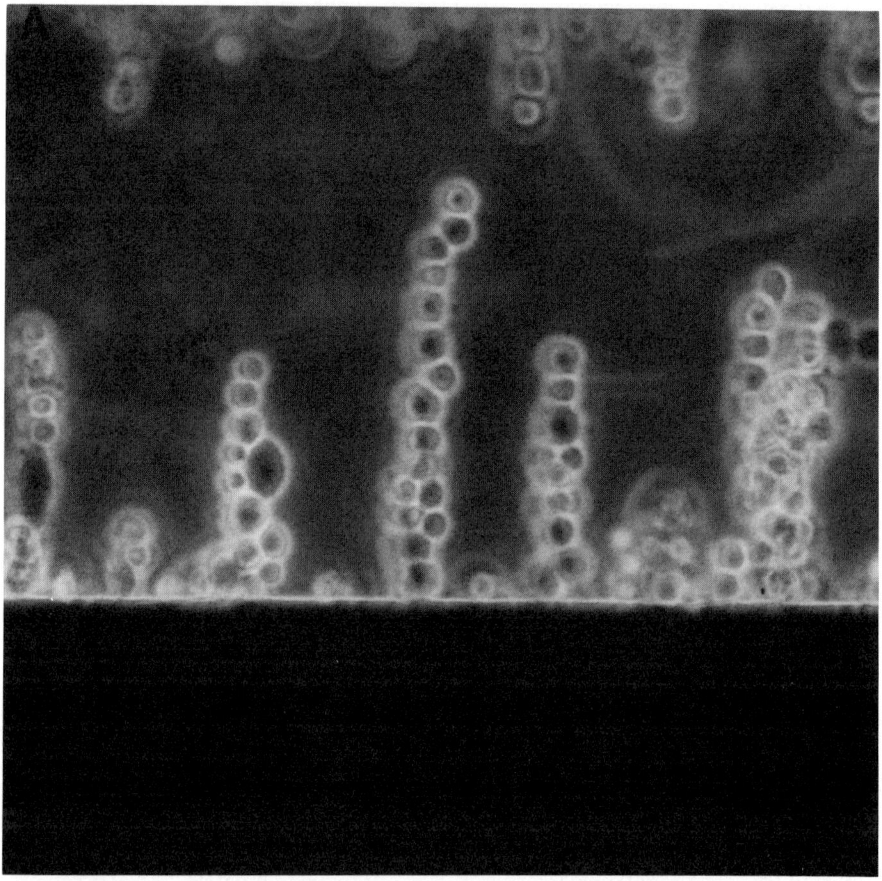

Figure 2 (A) Pearl-chaining of HMy2 with lymphocytes with AC alignment field (1 MHz, 200 V/cm) (magnification ×400).

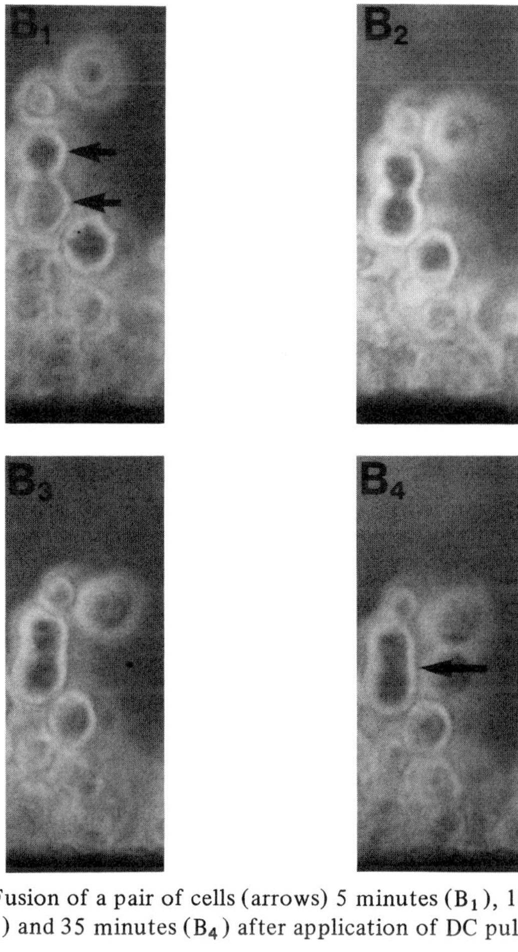

Figure 2 (B) Fusion of a pair of cells (arrows) 5 minutes (B_1), 15 minutes (B_2), 25 minutes (B_3) and 35 minutes (B_4) after application of DC pulses (magnification X600).

permeable, and below it (< 2.0 kV/cm) no heterokaryons are formed. Up to 2×10^6 HMy2 cells plus 10^7 lymphocytes can be treated simultaneously in a specially constructed chamber with helically wound platinum electrodes 200 μ apart and 75 cm in length, capable of accommodating 200 μl of fluid, and available from either GCA Corporation or Krüss GmbH (West Germany).

To date, however, it is our experience that hybrid yields are not significantly increased by electrofusion methods; if anything, they are lower than with polyethylene glycol (PEG). This may reflect our relative inexperience or the inappropriate handling of cells after fusion. Others have recently reported (36) success with production of human hybridomas from WI-L2-derived parent cell lines using electrofusion. Based on our microscopic observations of the actual fusions (Fig. 2B), we (and others) remain skeptical of the capacity of this system to greatly enhance hybrid yields. However, with murine cells it was reported (35) to give approximately one hybrid from 3×10^4 lymphocytes, yields comparable with the best results obtained with PEG. Its principal advantage actually seems to lie in its capacity to fuse very small numbers of cells (e.g., lymphocytes sorted by FACS on the basis of reactivity with an antigen). It has also recently been used with the murine hybridoma system for fusion of hapten-directed lymphocyte-myeloma pairs (37), the dielectrophoretic step being omitted. It may, therefore, be of value in conjunction with improved methods of *in vitro* human lymphocyte immunization and selection. It is this latter aspect of human fusion protocols that probably has provided the main barrier to the recovery of antibodies of predefined or useful specificities, as compared with murine systems.

D. Mouse-Human Fusions

Some laboratories continue to make heterospecific hybrids, using well characterized lines, such as NS1, NSO, and P3x63-Ag8.653, as the fusion partner for human lymphocytes. Two advantages accrue from this strategy; first that the use of true nonsecretor mouse lines obviates the "mixed antibody" problem, and second that rodent cell lines are intrinsically ouabain-resistant, rendering them directly suited for back-fusions with, for example, EB-transformed lymphoblastoid lines. Loss of human chromosomes from such hybrids remains a problem. Individual mouse-human hybrids show considerable karyotypic heterogeneity (38), and frequent recloning is reportedly necessary to minimize karyotypic drift and maintain human antibody secretion. However, Gigliotti *et al.* (39) reported that a heterospecific hybrid producing anti-tetanus toxin antibody has remained stable for at least 18 months after fusion, although only about 10% of the original positive hybrids were stable to long-term growth and cloning.

It has recently been shown that heterohybridomas will produce human Ig when grown as ascites in nude mice (40).

E. Recombinant Techniques

Possibly the most significant development has been the application of recombinant DNA techniques to the problem of creating antibodies with predefined specificities available from rodent systems, but without the immunogenic characteristics of the entire rodent molecules, which lead to human allergic and immune responses when used therapeutically (41). Morrison *et al.* (42) have engineered chimeric immunoglobulin chains, consisting of the binding sites (V) of the mouse myeloma protein, combined with the constant regions (C) of human immunoglobulin. Chimeric light- and heavy-chain genes were first constructed, inserted into pSV2-gpt and pSV2-Neo plasmid vectors, and then sequentially transfected into mouse myeloma cells. The new genes were expressed in selected cells (transfectomas) at a level comparable with a poor hybridoma; no quantitative data on levels of new chimeric antibody secretion were given, although active tetrameric chimeric immunoglobulin molecules made up of two heavy and two light chimeric chains were secreted in ascites fluid. The advantage of lymphoid cells as recipients of these gene constructs is that it assures any posttranslational modifications of antibody molecules that are necessary for assembly and secretion. Combination of these constructs with available hormone-responsive promotor sequences and the replacement of the human intronic-controlling elements in some constructs with their mouse equivalents could lead to a more productive system in the future.

These techniques are relatively straightforward and, apparently, efficient. Takeda *et al.* (43) have also constructed chimeric mouse-human heavy chain genes. However, by inserting these genes in a retrovirus-based vector, they have been able to generate the DNA sequence corresponding to processed mRNA with introns removed as translated, which could, in principle, be expressed in any host cell including bacteria. Yeast cells are another possible host. Some expression of immunoglobulin sequences has recently been achieved in yeast cells, yielding functional antibody, but at very low levels (44).

IV. CONCLUSIONS

HMy2 represents a stage in the development of hybridoma systems for human monoclonal antibody production. It has proved easy to handle and has yielded useful information on the reactivity of antibodies derived from cancer patients (3,7,8), but suffers from the problem of relatively low hybrid yields. At the end of the day, however, the specificity of human monoclonal antibodies derived from cancer patients remains disappointing, with reactivity directed largely at banal intracytoplasmic constituents such as intermediate filaments (7,8,15). Reactivity with tumor-related or membrane-associated antigens is only rarely encountered, irrespective of whether hybridoma (3,7,8,16) or EB transformation techniques (45) are used. Methods of *in vitro* immunostimulation, perhaps combined with *in vivo* immunotherapeutic regimes based on cell lines derived from individual patients' tumors, may eventually provide some of the desired cancer-related specificities. At the present time, therefore, attempts at therapeutic administration of human monoclonals in malignant disease via, for example, implanted chambers (46), must be deemed premature.

ACKNOWLEDGMENTS

We are grateful to all our colleagues who responded to the questionnaire concerning HMy2, and to Mr. C. Yiu for assistance with the electrofusion experiments reported here.

REFERENCES

1. G. Kohler and C. Milstein. Continuous culture of fused cells secreting antibody of predefined specificity. *Nature, 256*:495 (1975).
2. P. A. W. Edwards and M. J. O'Hare. The production of human monoclonal antibodies. In P. Beverley (ed.). *Methods in Haematology*. Vol. 13, Monoclonal Antibodies. Churchill Livingstone, New York (1985).
3. P. A. W. Edwards, C. M. Smith, A. M. Neville, and M. J. O'Hare. A human-human hybridoma system based on a fast-growing mutant of the ARH-77 plasma cell leukaemia-derived line. *Eur. J. Immunol., 12*:641 (1982).
4. M. J. O'Hare, C. M. Smith, and P. A. W. Edwards. A new human hybridoma system (LICR-LON-HMy2) and its use in the production of human monoclonal antibodies. In H. Peeters (ed.). *Protides of Biological Fluids.* Pergamon Press, Oxford (1983).
5. K. H. Burk, B. Drewinko, J. M. Trujillo, and M. J. Ahearn. Establishment of a human plasma cell line *in vitro. Cancer Res., 38*:2508 (1978).
6. S. P. C. Cole, B. G. Campling, T. Atlaw, D. Kozbor, and J. C. Roder. Human monoclonal antibodies. *Mol. Cell Biochem., 62*:109 (1984).
7. A. N. Houghton, H. Brooks, R. J. Cote, M. C. Taormina, H. F. Oettgen, and L. J. Old. Detection of cell surface and intracellular antigens by human monoclonal antibodies. Hybrid cell lines derived from lymphocytes of patients with malignant melanoma. *J. Exp. Med., 158*:53 (1983).
8. R. J. Cote, D. M. Morrissey, A. N. Houghton, E. J. Beattie, H. F. Oettgen, and L. J. Old. Generation of human monoclonal antibodies reactive with cellular antigens. *Proc. Natl. Acad. Sci.* (*USA*), *80*:2026 (1983).
9. K. Sikora, T. Alderson, J. Ellis, J. Phillips, and J. Watson. Human hybridomas from patients with malignant disease. *Br. J. Cancer, 47*:135 (1983).
10. D. Kozbor, A. E. Lagarde, and J. C. Roder. Human hybridomas constructed

with antigen specific Epstein-Barr virus transformed cell lines. *Proc. Natl. Acad. Sci.* (*USA*), *79*:6651 (1982).
11. J. F. Kearny. Hybridomas and monoclonal antibodies. In W. E. Paul (ed.). *Fundamental Immunology*. Raven Press, New York (1984).
12. L. Olsson, R. B. Andreasen, A. Ost, B. Christensen, and P. Biberfield. Antibody producing human-human hybridomas. II. Derivation and characterisation of an antibody specific for human leukemia cells. *J. Exp. Med., 159*: 537 (1984).
13. D. E. Normansell and J. R. Lane. *In vitro* production of monoclonal human rheumatoid factors. *Ann. Clin. Lab. Med., 14*:64 (1984).
14. L. Olsson and H. Kaplan. Human-human monoclonal antibody-producing hybridomas: technical aspects. In J. J. Langone and H. van Vunakis (eds.). *Methods in Enzymology, Vol. 92.* Academic Press, New York (1983).
15. R. J. Cote, D. M. Morrissey, H. F. Oettgen, and L. J. Old. Analysis of human monoclonal antibodies derived from lymphocytes of patients with cancer. *Fed. Proc., 43*:2465 (1984).
16. K. E. Truitt, J. W. Larrick, A. A. Raubitschek, D. W. Buck, and S. W. Jacobson. Production of human monoclonal antibody in mouse ascites. *Hybridoma, 3*:195 (1984).
17. P. G. Abrams, J. A. Knost, G. Clarke, S. Wilburn, R. K. Oldham, and K. A. Foon. Determination of optimal human cell lines for development of human hybridomas. *J. Immunol., 131*:1202 (1983).
18. J. E. Lever, G. Nuki, and J. E. Seegmiller. Expression of purine overproduction in a series of 8-azaguanine resistant diploid human lymphoblast lines. *Proc. Natl. Acad. Sci.* (*USA*) *711*:2679 (1974).
19. M. C. Glassy, H. H. Handley, H. Haigwara, and I. Royston. UC 729-6, a human lymphoblastoid B-cell line useful for generating antibody-secreting human-human hybridomas. *Proc. Natl. Acad. Sci.* (*USA*), *80*:6327 (1983).
20. J. G. Heitzmann and M. Cohn. The WI-L2-729-HF2 human hybridoma system: stable hybrids at high frequency. *Mol. Biol. Med., 1*:235 (1983).
21. J. W. Larrick, K. E. Truitt, A. A. Raubitschek, G. Senyk, and J. C. N. Wang. Characterization of human hybridomas secreting antibody to tetanus toxoid. *Proc. Natl. Acad. Sci.* (*USA*), *80*:6376 (1983).
22. M. R. Posner, S. F. Schlossman, and H. Lazarus. Novel approach to construction of human 'myeloma analogues' for production of human monoclonal antibodies. *Hybridoma, 2*:369 (1983).
23. D. Bron, M. D. Fienberg, N. H. Teng, and H. S. Kaplan. Production of human monoclonal IgG antibodies against Rhesus (D) antigen. *Proc. Natl. Acad. Sci.* (*USA*), *81*:3214 (1984).
24. D. Kozbor, P. Tripputi, J. C. Roder, and C. M. Croce. A human hybrid myeloma for production of human monoclonal antibodies. *J. Immunol., 133*: 3001 (1985).
25. S. K. H. Foung, S. Perkins, A. A. Raubitschek, G. Lizak, D. Fishwild, E. G. Engleman, and F. C. Grumet. Rescue of human monoclonal antibody pro-

duction from an EBV-transformed B cell line by fusion to a human-mouse hybridoma. *J. Immunol. Meth., 70*:83 (1984).

26. E. Henderson, G. Miller, J. Robinson, and L. Heston. Efficiency of transformation of lymphocytes by Epstein-Barr virus. *Virology, 76*:152 (1977).
27. R. F. Tiebout, E. A. M. Stricker, R. Hagenaars, and W. P. Zeijlemaker. Human lymphoblastoid cell line producing protective monoclonal IgG, x anti-tetanus toxins. *Eur. J. Immunol., 14*:399 (1984).
28. D. H. Crawford, D. C. J. McDougall, M. Mulholland, G. D. Zanders, P. Tipett, and E. R. Huens. Further characterisation of a human monoclonal antibody to the Rhesus D antigen produced *in vitro*. *Behring Inst. Mitt., 74*:55 (1984).
29. D. H. Crawford, E. R. Heuns, and M. A. Epstein. Therapeutic use of human monoclonal antibodies. *Lancet, i*:1040 (1983).
30. L. Winger, C. Winger, P. Shastry, A. Russel, and M. Longenecker. Efficient generation *in vitro* from human peripheral blood cells of monoclonal Epstein-Barr virus transformants producing specific antibody to a variety of antigens with prior deliberate immunization. *Proc. Natl. Acad. Sci. (USA), 801*:4484 (1983).
31. M. D. Melamed, J. Gordon, S. L. Ley, D. Edgar, and N. C. Hughes-Jones. Senescence of human lymphoblastoid clone producing anti-Rhesus (D). *Eur. J. Immunol., 15*:742 (1985).
32. U. Zimmermann. Electric field-mediated fusion and related electrical phenomena. *Biochim. Biophys. Acta, 694*:227 (1982).
33. R. Bischoff, R. M. Eisert, J. Schedel, J. Vienken, and U. Zimmermann. Human hybridoma cells produced by electro-fusion. *FEBS Lett., 147*:64 (1982).
34. J. Vienken, U. Zimmermann, M. Fouchard, and D. Zagury. Electrofusion of myeloma cells on the single cell level. Fusion under sterile conditions without proteolytic enzyme treatment. *FEBS Lett., 163*:54 (1983).
35. J. Vienken and U. Zimmermann. An improved electrofusion technique for production of mouse hybridoma cells. *FEBS Lett., 182*:278 (1985).
36. G. E. Hubner, J. Trawinski, A. Zembrod, U. Opitz, B. G. D. Bodeker, G. Hewlett, and H. D. Schlumberger. Electro-fusion and growth promotion of human B cell hybridomas. *Biochem. Soc. Trans.*, (in press).
37. M. M. S. Lo, T. Y. Tsong, M. K. Conrad, S. M. Strittmatter, L. D. Hester, and H. S. Snyder. Monoclonal antibody production by receptor-mediated electrically induced cell fusion. *Nature, 310*:792 (1984).
38. H. C. Lane and A. S. Fauci. Establishment of human-human and human-mouse B cell hybrids and their use in the study of B cell activation. In B. F. Hayes and G. S. Eisenbarth (eds.). *Monoclonal Antibodies. Probes for the Study of Autoimmunity and Immunodeficiency*. Academic Press, New York (1983).
39. F. Gigliotti, L. Smith, and R. A. Insel. Reproducible production of protective human monoclonal antibodies by fusion of peripheral blood lymphocytes with a mouse myeloma cell line. *J. Infect. Dis., 149*:43 (1984).

40. P. G. Abrams, J. J. Ochs, S. L. Giardina, A. C. Morgan, S. B. Wilburn, A. R. Wilt, R. K. Oldham, and K. A. Foon. Production of large quantities of human immunoglobulin in the ascites of athymic mice: implications for the development of anti-human idiotype antibodies. *J. Immunol., 132*:1611 (1984).
41. H. F. Sears, B. Atkinson, J. Mattis, C. Ernst, D. Herlyn, Z. Steplewski, P. Hayry, and H. Koprowski. Phase-I clinical trial of monoclonal antibody in treatment of gastrointestinal tumors. *Lancet, i*:762 (1982).
42. S. L. Morrison, M. J. Johnson, L. A. Herzenberg, and V. T. Oi. Chimeric human antibody molecules: mouse antigen-binding domains with human constant region domains. *Proc. Natl. Acad. Sci.* (*USA*), *81*:6851 (1984).
43. S-I. Takeda, T. Naito, K. Hama, T. Noma, and T. Honjo. Construction of chimaeric processed immunoglobulin genes containing mouse variable and human constant region sequences. *Nature, 314*:452 (1985).
44. C. R. Wood, M. A. Boss, J. H. Kenten, J. E. Calvert, N. A. Roberts, and J. S. Emtage. The synthesis and *in vivo* assembly of functional antibodies in yeast. *Nature, 314*:446 (1985).
45. S. P. Cole, B. G. Campling, I. H. Louwman, D. Kozbor, and J. C. Roder. A strategy for the production of human monoclonal antibodies reactive with lung tumor cell lines. *Cancer Res., 44*:2750 (1984).
46. J. Watson, T. Alderson, K. Sikora, and J. Phillips. Subcutaneous culture chamber for continuous administration of monoclonal antibodies. *Lancet, i*:99 (1983).

5

Generation and Characterization of Human Monoclonal Anti-*Pseudomonas aeruginosa* Antibodies

JAMES W. LARRICK, SARAH HART,* DAVID S. LIPPMAN,* and MICHAEL GLEMBOURTT
Cetus Immune Corporation, Palo Alto, California

YAO-PI HSU and RICHARD B. MOSS
Stanford University Medical School, Palo Alto, California

Pseudomonas aeruginosa is a significant cause of severe nosocomial infections in patients receiving immunosuppressive therapy and in those with neoplastic diseases, cyctic fibrosis, and burns or other serious injuries (1). Despite therapy with appropriate antibiotics, the mortality rate from *P. aeruginosa* bacteremia is high in these debilitated patients (2). Treatment is often complicated by the patient's underlying disease, the availability of limited numbers of clinically effective antibacterial antibodies, and the absence of effective vaccines.

The pathogenesis of infections due to *P. aeruginosa* is poorly understood. Many different types of infections are recognized, from acute localized eye infections and chronic lung infections, to generalized systemic infections and septicemia. *P. aeruginosa* produces a myriad of structures and products, including lipopolysaccharides (LPS), pili, outer membrane proteins, alkaline protease, elastase, hemolysin, leukocidin, slime, exopolysaccharide, phospholipase C, exoenzyme S, and exotoxin A, that may contribute to its pathogenesis. The role that several of the virulence factors may play in the pathogenesis of *P. aeruginosa* infections has been demonstrated by the use of mutant strains deficient in only a single factor (3-7). Most of the investigations have centered on toxic extracellular products. The effect of loss or alteration of a somatic antigen on *P. aeruginosa* virulence has

**Present affiliation*: Biotherapy Systems, Inc., Mountain View, California been studied only in regard to motility; a nonmotile mutant was far less virulent for burned mice than was its parent strain (3). Several lines of evidence suggest that lipopolysaccharide contributes substantially to *P. aeruginosa* virulence. These include: (a) the toxic nature of *P. aeruginosa* LPS (7,8), (b) the fact that LPS may confer serum resistance (7) and, (c) the fact that antibody to LPS has been shown to be highly protective in experimental models (9-12). Although mutants that alter LPS structure have been reported for *P. aeruginosa* (13,14), the effect that such mutations have on virulence is unknown.

Numerous studies (9,10,15) have indicated that immunoglobulin G (IgG) antibody to lipopolysaccharide is protective in experimentally infected animals. A heptavalent vaccine containing LPS of the seven immunotypes of *P. aeruginosa* (16) is effective in inducing antibodies in humans (17). Attempts to immunize patients at high risk of *P. aeruginosa* infection with this vaccine, however, have been only moderately successful due, in part, to the potent endotoxin activity of LPS. Local and systemic adverse reactions to endotoxin, including fever, malaise, and pain at the site of injection, can limit vaccine dosage (8,18).

Pseudomonas aeruginosa infection is commonly associated with progressive pulmonary disease in patients with cystic fibrosis (19). Recent work from our laboratories (20), has indicated that patients with cystic fibrosis who were colonized with *P. aeruginosa* have substantial titers of antibody to various pathogenic factors of Pseudomonas. To investigate the possible role of defective antibodies in opsonophagocytosis in patients with cystic fibrosis and to prepare human monoclonal antibodies for passive immunotherapy of patients with severe *P. aeruginosa* infections, we used these patients as a source of immune B cells for the generation of human monoclonal antibodies that recognize *P. aeruginosa* lipopolysaccharides.

I. METHODS

A. Cell Lines

Human lymphoblastoid cell line LTR 228 and mouse and human plasmacytoma cell lines have been previously described (21-24). All cell lines were maintained in Iscove's DME medium supplemented with 10% fetal calf serum, 2 mM glutamine, and 5×10^{-5} M 2-mercaptoethanol. The cell lines were checked routinely for the presence of mycoplasma.

B. Fusion Protocol

Cells were combined and fused as described previously (25). Briefly, cells were fused with 40% polyethylene glycol 4,000 (BDH) and 10% dimethylsulfoxide in Hanks' balanced salt solution without calcium and with magnesium (2 mM). By using this technique, we consistently observed low incidence of cell death and formation of 3-8% heterokaryons. Cells were cultured 24 hours after fusion, prior to addition of hypoxanthine (100 μM)/azaserine (5 μg/ml) in Iscove's DME medium with 15% fetal calf serum. Fusions were plated at a density of 10^5 cells per microtiter well for hybrid selection. Cultures were subsequently fed every 3 days with selective medium. Hybrid colonies normally appeared after 10-21 days.

C. Epstein-Barr Virus Transformation

Epstein-Barr virus (EBV) transformations were performed essentially as described previously, (26) except that cells were usually cultured at a density of 10^4 per well in 96-well plates.

D. Cloning and Reverse-Plaque Techniques

Limiting-dilution (0.3 cells per well) cloning was performed in 96-well U-bottom plates (Costar) in Iscove's DME medium with 20% fetal calf serum.

For soft agar cloning, 1000 cells in 1 ml of 0.33% Sea-Plaque agarose (FMC, Rockland, ME) made in Iscove's DME medium with 20% fetal calf serum, were placed over a bed of 4 ml of SeaKem agarose (FMC) (0.4%) in 60 mm culture dishes (Falcon).

To select for high-producer hybrids, a reverse-plaque technique was used. Protein A-coated sheep erythrocytes (SRBCs) (1.0%) were added to the upper layer of soft agar according to the method of Gronowicz *et al.* (27).

E. Immunoblotting

Details of the procedure are essentially as described previously (28).

F. LPS-Specific ELISA

Immunlon I (Dynatech) flat-bottom microtiter plates were coated overnight with 50 μl of LPS (50 μg) in pH 9.6, $NaHCO_3$ buffer (50 mM). Plates were washed with PBS (containing calcium and magnesium) and 0.05% Tween 20 (Sigma Chemical Co., Detroit, MI). Subsequently, 100 μl of 1% BSA plus 0.05% Tween in PBS, followed by 100 μl of the antibody-containing supernatants, were added to each well. Supernatants were incubated for 30 minutes at 4°C. After another wash, peroxidase-conjugated goat anti-human immunoglobulin developing reagent (Tago Inc., Burlingame, CA) was added. After 30 minutes at 4°C and another wash, ABTS substrate plus H_2O_2 (0.03%) were added. Plates were read at OD_{405} after 30 minutes at 37°C.

G. Bacterial-Binding ELISA

Immunlon I flat-bottom microtiter plates were coated with 50 μl of 1.0% glutaraldehyde (Sigma Chemical Co.) in deionized water and incubated 4 hours at room temperature. Wells were aspirated with an eight-channel manifold. Sixty μl of 0.25% bacterial suspension was added to each well and incubated overnight. Plates were assayed as described for the LPS assay. *P. aeruginosa* bacterial strains from each Fischer-Devlin type were obtained from the American Type Culture Collection, Rockville, MD (Strain I.D. Nos. 27312-27318).

H. Opsonophagocytosis Assays

Opsonophagocytosis assays were performed essentially as described previously (29).

I. DNA Profiles

DNA profiles were performed based on a modified protocol of Gazitt *et al.* (30) and Cram *et al.* (31). Chicken erythrocyte nuclei (CEN) stored in 50% ethanol were used as internal standards for EPIC-V analysis and prepared according to Diamond and Braylon (32). Chicken erythrocyte nuclei were spun out of suspension at 100 *g* for 5 minutes at 4°C, and the 50% ethanol supernatant was aspirated. Chicken erythrocyte nuclei were then processed as described below. Cell lines (4×10^5) were aliquoted into 15 ml conical centrifuge tubes (Corning) and resuspended in 1 ml isotonic phosphate buffered saline, pH 7.4. The samples were centrifuged at 100 *g* for 5 minutes at 4°C. The supernatant was aspirated and 1 ml of ice-cold sodium citrate (1 mg/ml), pH 7.5, 11 mM $MgCl_2$, and 15 μg/ml RNase I-AS (Sigma Chemical Co.), (pretreated for 10 minutes at 95°C) were added to the cell pellet with gentle resuspension. The sample suspension was incubated for 10 minutes on ice for effective cell lysis. Subsequently, 10 μl propidium iodide (PI) (5 mg/ml) (Sigma Chemical Co.) in distilled water was added to the cell suspension and maintained at room temperature for 30 minutes. Samples were placed on ice and filtered through 37 μ nylon mesh (Small Parts, Inc.) before analysis on the EPIC-V.

An EPIC-V cell sorter equipped with a 76 μ nozzle (Coulter Electronics) was used for DNA content and forward-angle light scatter measurements. A 488 nm argon ion laser line at 1 watt light-regulated power was used for excitation, and the total fluorescent emission above 610 nm was measured. Forward-angle light scatter was obtained as a measure of cell size with a natural density, 2.0 O.D. filter (Melles Griot) placed in front of the scatter detector. Two-parameter (64 × 64 channel) DNA versus scatter histograms and 256-channel DNA histograms were generated with approximately 10,000 cells being analyzed per cell line.

Software- and hardware-based gated analysis, on DNA content and scatter, was done to reduce debris and cell aggregate events.

J. Surface Antigen Analysis

Cells were stained with fluorescent antibodies by the method of Loken and Stall (33). Fluorescein isothiocyanate-conjugated goat Fab$'_2$ anti-γ, anti-μ reagents were purchased from Tago Inc., Burlingame, CA.

K. DNA Techniques

DNA was extracted from isolated nuclei (34) for all cell lines. Nuclei were suspended in 1x TNE (50 mM *tris*-HCl, pH 7.5, 40 mM NaCl, and 10 mM EDTA) and extracted according to the method of Copeland *et al.* (35). DNAs were digested to completion with the appropriate restriction enzyme (New England Biolabs), electrophoresed in 0.7% agarose gels, and transferred to nitrocellulose (36). Filters were hybridized to a nick-translated EBV probe (provided by J. Pagano) in the presence of 10% dextransulphate as described by Wahl *et al.* (37). After hybridization filters were washed twice at 22°C in 2x SSC (0.015 M sodium citrate, 0.15 M NaCl), 0.1% SDS and twice at 68°C in 0.1x SSC, 0.1% SDS.

II. RESULTS

A number of workers have used Epstein-Barr virus for the immortalization of human B cells (38-49). The most successful approaches have been to either preselect the population of B cells to be transformed or to postselect the antigen-specific transformed populations by panning or rosetting techniques (45,47). Recently, we and others (23,43,50) have used EBV transformation combined with cell fusion to generate human monoclonal antibodies. Several observations have prompted this approach: (a) instability of immunoglobulin secretion by the EBV-transformed lines, (b) increased immunoglobulin secretion by hybridomas when compared with EBV lymphoblastoid cell lines, and (c) higher frequencies of rescue of the antigen-specific populations.

Table 1 demonstrates the use of EBV transformation and subsequent cell fusion for the generation of human monoclonal anti-*Pseudomonas aeruginosa* antibodies. We chose cystic fibrosis patients with serum anti-*Pseudomonas aeruginosa* titers (IgM, IgG, and IgA) greater than 1:2000 (20). When peripheral B cells from the patients were fused directly *ex vivo* or after pokeweed mitogen stimulation to a human fusion partner developed in our laboratory (21) or to a mouse-human fusion partner, no stable lines survived. However, using EBV transformation and cell fusion, several clones with anti-*Pseudomonas aeruginosa*

Table 1 Generation of Human Anti-*Pseudomonas aeruginosa* LPS Antibodies

Day 1

A. Draw 50 ml blood from preselected volunteers with high LPS antibody titers

B. Rosette cells with AET-treated SRBC (56)

C. EBV transformation with B958 supernatant

D. Plate at 1×10^4/well in 96-well plates

Day 20

Select positive wells by LPS-specific ELISA and expand or subculture highest titer wells

Day 27

Retest subcultures and fuse to mouse/human cell line F3B6

Days 40-47

Select positive wells by specific LPS ELISA and clone in soft agar or by limiting dilution

Day 61

Replica plaque-positive hybrids and expand positives

Day 75

Begin serum-free adaptation of hybridomas

binding were generated. Table 2 presents the whole bacteria ELISA results of two antibodies (L114 and CF6). In both cases, blood was drawn from cystic fibrosis patients, rosetted using AET-treated SRBCs transformed with Epstein-Barr virus and plated into 96-well microtiter plates. Wells were initially screened on the multivalent Parke-Davis vaccine, followed by bacterial ELISA's utilizing Pseudomonas strains from Fisher-Devlin types 1 through 7. Loss of antibody secretion is a common occurrence with EBV infection, reflecting the instability of antibody production in the young EBV transformants and their overgrowth by rapidly dividing nonproducers. After EBV transformants were screened and subcultured, they were fused to the 6-TG-resistant mouse/human cell line F3B6 (23). This cell line, containing predominantly mouse chromosomes, is ouabain-resistant. Ouabain (5×10^{-7} mM) was used in the selection medium to kill unfused EBV transformants. Unfused F3B6 cells were killed by the addition of hypoxanthine (100 μM) and azaserine (5 μg/ml) to the medium (51). Growing hybrids appeared within 10 to 21 days. Both of the antibodies that were selected for further characterization were of the IgM class. Many, but not all, of the antibodies generated by the EBV fusion technique have been of the IgM class. Ep-

Table 2 *Pseudomonas aeruginosa* Bacterial ELISA Using Human Monoclonal Antibodies CF6 and L114

	Pseudomonas aeruginosa bacteria (Fisher-Devlin type)						
	1	2	3	4	5	6	7
ATCC No.	27312	27313	27314	27315	27316	27317	27318
CF6	0[a]	0	0	+	0	0	0
L114	0	0	+	0	0	0	+

[a]Magnitude of numbers indicates the degree of monoclonal binding. 0 is negative, + is off scale, with the plate reader set at 2.0 absorbance full scale.

stein-Barr virus most frequently infects and transforms IgM-bearing B cells, but B cells secreting other classes of immunoglobulin can also be made into long-term lines using this technique (52).

With frequent cloning and plaque selection, we have been able to expand the anti-pseudomonas human hybridomas without loss of antibody secretion. Because a number of workers have reported that chromosomal loss frequently destroyed the antibody-secreting capacity of heterohybridomas, we measured DNA histograms on these cell lines after 10 months in culture. Figure 1 shows the parent cell lines compared with each hybrid clone. Both cell lines have segregated many chromosomes; they have much less than a tetraploid amount of DNA. Despite the decreased chromosome numbers, the two chromosomes required for antibody manufacture have still been retained (number 14 for mu heavy chain; number 2 for kappa light chain) since both hybrids continue to secrete anti-pseudomonas LPS antibody. Some workers (53,54) have suggested that chromosome 14 (carrying the heavy-chain genes) and chromosome 22 (carrying the λ light-chain genes) may be preferentially retained, whereas chromosome 2 (carrying the κ-chain genes) may be preferentially lost. We have routinely recloned our cell lines every few months to maintain high-secreting heterohybrids. An antigen-specific plaque technique and a nonspecific Ig reverse-plaque technique have both been useful for this purpose.

A potential drawback of EBV-transformed human antibody-producing cell lines is continued presence of the EBV genome. Using an EBV BAM II1-V probe (kindly provided by the laboratory of Dr. J. Pagano), we have performed Southern blots of CF6 and L114 cell lines. Figure 2 shows that the cell lines do not contain EBV genomes at a sensitivity of less than one copy per cell. Staining for EBNA was also negative (unpublished data).

The monoclonals were tested for binding to electrophoresed lipopolysac-

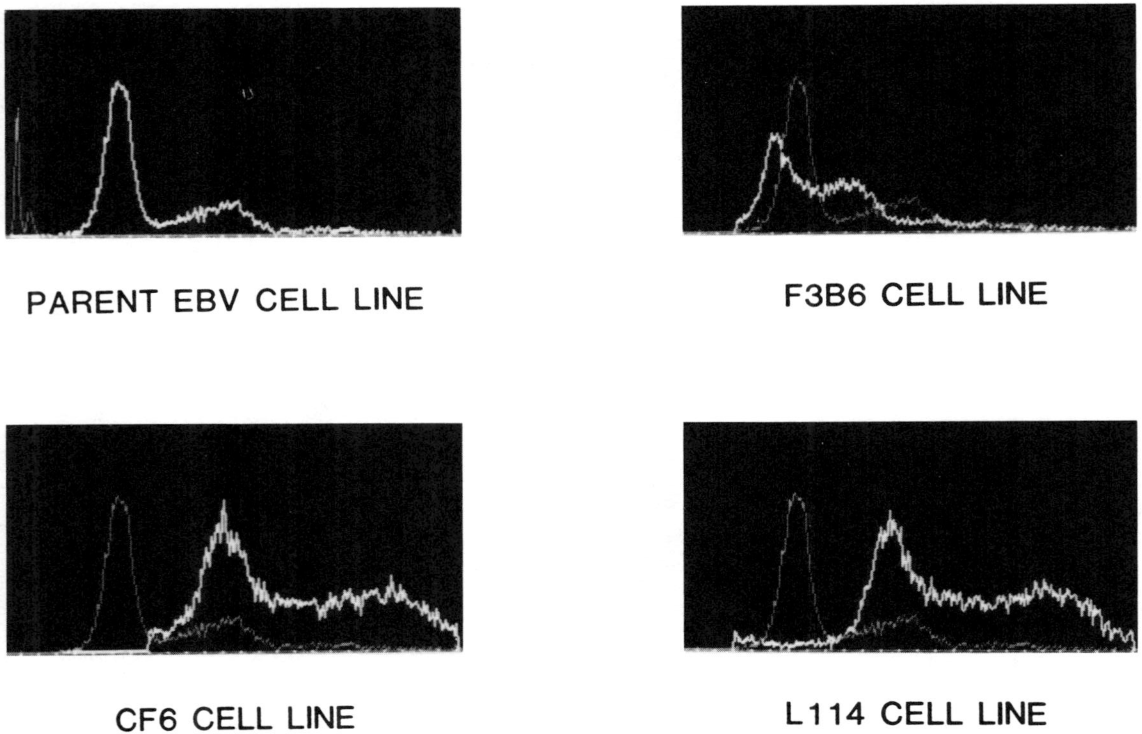

Figure 1 DNA histograms of human hybridomas CF6 and L113. Note the loss of DNA from hybrid lines compared with parent EBV cell line and fusion partner F3B6. The histograms (darker) of F3B6, CF6, and L114 are compared with a parent EBV cell line (lighter).

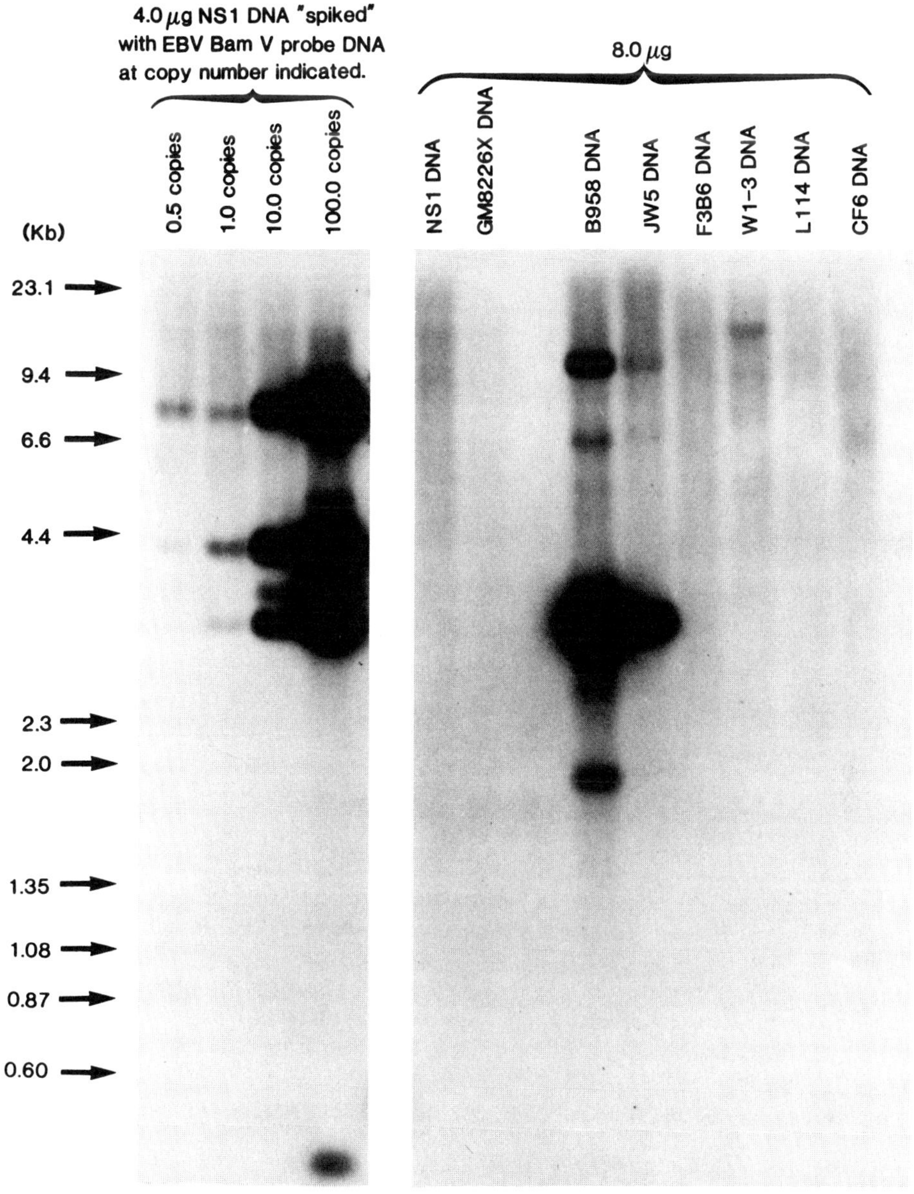

Figure 2 Southern blot of DNA from human hybridomas CF6 and L114. Blot was probed with the BAM H1-V region of EBV. *NS1* is a mouse plasmacytoma cell line. *GM8226X* is a human plasmacytoma cell line. *B958* is the marmoset cell line that produces EBV. *JW5* is an EBV-infected lymphoblastoid cell line. *F3B6* is the parent mouse/human cell lines. *WI-3*, *L114*, and *CF6* are human hybridomas.

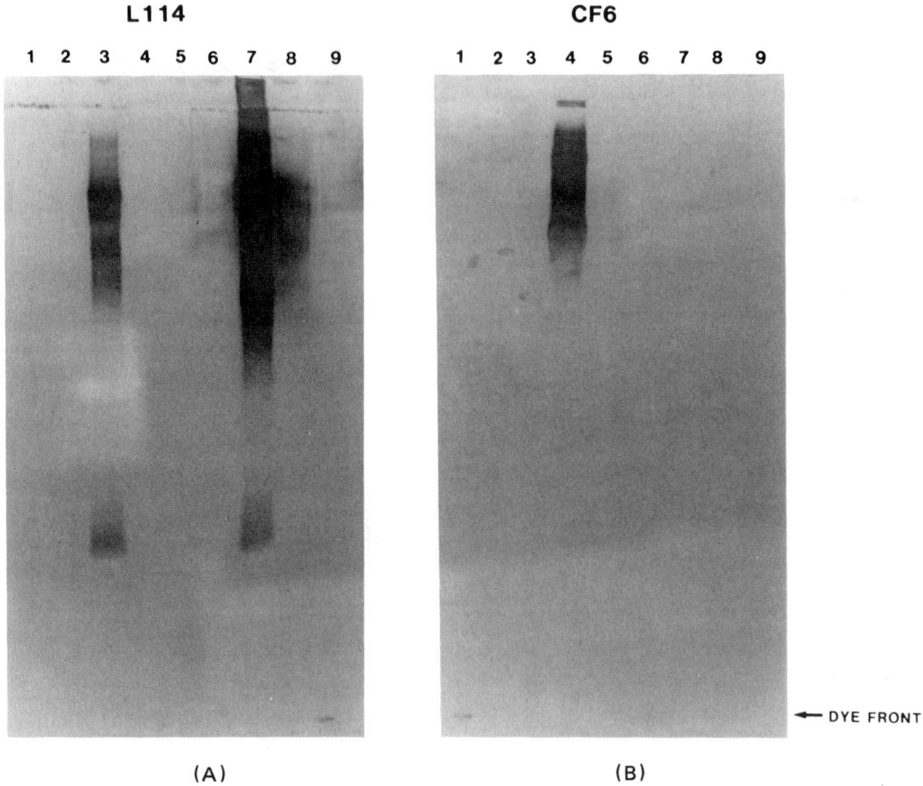

Figure 3 LPS immunoblots using purified human monoclonal antibody L114 (A) and CF6 (B). Lane 1: *Pseudomonas aeruginosa* (PA) LPS, Fisher-Devlin type 1. Lane 2: PA LPS type 2. Lane 3: PA LPS type 3. Lane 4: PA LPS type 4. Lane 5: PA LPS type 5. Lane 6: PA LPS type 6. Lane 7: PA LPS type 7. Lane 8: *E. coli* LPS type D31M4. Lane 9: *E. coli* LPS type 0127:B8.

charide. Immunoblots (Fig. 3) demonstrate specific binding of the monoclonals to the LPS corresponding to the bacterial binding (i.e., CF6 binds only type 4 LPS, and L114 recognizes a shared determinant between types 3 and 7).

We have also done limited testing of the function of these monoclonals in opsonophagocytic assays. These assays (Table 3) demonstrated diminished function compared with either normal serum or murine type-specific mono-

Table 3 Opsonic Function of Polyclonal and Monoclonal Antibodies for Autologous and Heterologous *Pseudomonas aeruginosa* Serotypes of Mucoid or Nonmucoid Morphology

	Pseudomonas aeruginosa strain						
	CFPM (1M)[a]	27312 (1NM)	CF HA (2M)	27314 (3NM)	CFDS (4M)	27315 (4NM)	CFAH (7M)
	Nonopsonic phagocytosis						
Antibody							
0	31[b]	21	35	36	17	26	41
	Opsonic phagocytosis						
NHS	24[c]	202	108	216	270	185	61
PS-IVIG	142	87	210	99	211	260	56
Murine IgM ∝ 1	83	134	15	ND	ND	-13	ND
Murine IgG_{2A} ∝ 1	95	99	2	ND	ND	-7	ND
Murine IgG_{2B} ∝ 1	-5	168	8	ND	ND	-1	ND
L114 ∝ 3, 7	ND	ND	ND	-9	-26	-14	-26
CF6 ∝ 4	ND	ND	ND	35	-32	-3	-28
C′	17	45	80	100	161	218	-3

[a]1-7 = Fisher serotype; M = mucoid phenotype; NM = nonmucoid phenotype.
[b]% uptake at 30 minutes of 10^7 cfu/ml ^{3}H-leucine-labeled PA by 10^6/ml normal human PBL.
[c]% change above nonopsonic PBL uptake baseline.

NHS = Normal human serum (5%); PS-IVIG = polyclonal Pseudomonas hyperimmune globulin (Cutter) (5%); C′ = human complement (0.1%); ND = not done.

clonals. Some workers have shown that serum from patients with cystic fibrosis also has reduced *in vitro* opsonophagocytic function. Whether this finding is a general result of the method used to generate these monoclonals or related to the defective opsonization of CF immunoglobulins is under investigation.

III. DISCUSSION

Recent work from our laboratory showed that patients with cystic fibrosis have very high titers of antibody to LPS of *Pseudomonas aeruginosa* (20). We have now used peripheral blood B cells from these individuals to generate two IgM type-specific anti-*Pseudomonas aeruginosa* human monoclonal antibodies. These monoclonals bind to Fisher-Devlin type 4 and to type 3 and 7 bacteria and immunoblot only these lipopolysaccharides. The cell lines stably produce over 10 μg/ml of specific monoclonal antibody. Although the cell lines were derived from EBV-transformed B cells, they no longer contain the EBV genome (Fig. 2).

Several studies (9,10) have shown that IgG antibody to LPS is protective in experimentally infected animals; however, data on IgM is lacking. Recently work from our laboratory (Larrick *et al.*, unpublished data) and from others (55) suggests that murine monoclonal antibodies are highly protective in burn models, and this protective capacity correlates with their capacity to opsonize bacteria. Both IgG and IgM monoclonals were opsonic in these assays (Larrick *et al.*, unpublished data).

Our preliminary studies indicate CF6 and L114 IgM human monoclonal antibodies had reduced *in vitro* opsonic capacity. To determine if this is a general feature of the EBV fusion technique or a result of our choice of donors for immune B cells, we have begun to generate monoclonals from normal individuals with histories of Pseudomonas infections. Because type-specific murine monoclonals have shown promising results both *in vitro* and *in vivo* in burn and infection models, it is likely that protective human monoclonals can be generated, and that these will have clinical utility. Whether the opsonization defect characteristic of cystic fibrosis can be ascribed to an abnormal structure of these CF-derived human monoclonals awaits further study.

ACKNOWLEDGMENTS

The technical assistance of Bradley Dyer, Karen Watson, George Senyk, Janet Wang, and Howard Weintraub is gratefully acknowledged. Joan Murphy and Dianne Jacobs provided expert secretarial assistance. Helpful discussions were provided by Drs. Barbara Iglewski, Matthew Pollack, and Andrew Raubitschek. Jack Bourla provided support at opportune times.

The laboratory of Dr. J. Pagano, University of North Carolina Cancer Center, Chapel Hill, NC, generously supplied the EBV probe.

REFERENCES

1. R. E. Wood. Pseudomonas, the compromised host. *Hosp. Pract., 11*:91 (1976).
2. M. R. Flick and L. E. Cluff. *Pseudomonas bacteremia*: review of 108 cases. *Am. J. Med., 60*:501 (1976).
3. T. C. Montie, D. Doyl-Huntzing, R. C. Craven, and I. A. Holder. Loss of virulence associated with absence of flagellum in an isogenic mutant of

Pseudomonas aeruginosa in the burned-mouse model. *Infect. Immun. 38*: 1296 (1982).
4. D. E. Ohman, R. P. Burns, and B. J. Iglewski. Corneal infections in mice with toxin A and elastase mutants of *Pseudomonas aeruginosa. J. Infect. Dis., 142*:547 (1980).
5. D. E. Ohman, S. J. Cryz, and B. J. Iglewski. Isolation of characterization of a *Pseudomonas aeruginosa* mutant PAO that produces altered elastase. *J. Bacteriol., 142*:836 (1980).
6. D. E. Ohman, J. C. Sadoff, and B. J. Iglewski. Toxin A-deficient mutants *Pseudomonas aeruginosa* PAI03: isolation and characterization. *Infect. Immun. 28*:899 (1980).
7. L. S. Young. Human immunity to *Pseudomonas aeruginosa.* II. Relationship between heat-stable opsonins and type-specific lipopolysaccharides. *J. Infect. Dis., 126*:277 (1972).
8. J. E. Pennington, H. Y. Reynolds, R. E. Wood, R. A. Robinson, and A. S. Levine. Use of a *Pseudomonas aeruginosa* vaccine in patients with acute leukemia and cystic fibrosis. *Am. J. Med., 58*:629 (1975).
9. S. J. Cryz, Jr., E. Furer, and R. Germanier. Protection against *Pseudomonas aeruginosa* infection in a murine burn wound sepsis model by passive transfer of antitoxin A, antielastase, and antilipopolysaccharide. *Infect. Immun. 39*:1072 (1983).
10. S. J. Cryz, Jr., E. Furer, and R. Germanier. Passive protection against *Pseudomonas aeruginosa* infection in an experimental leukopenic mouse model. *Infect. Immun. 40*:659 (1983).
11. S. J. Cryz, E. Furer, and R. Germanier. Protection against fatal *Pseudomonas aeruginosa* burn wound sepsis by immunization with lipopolysaccharide and high-molecular-weight polysaccharide. *Infect. Immun. 43*:795 (1984).
12. G. B. Pier, H. F. Sidberry, and J. C. Sadoff. Protective immunity reduced in mice by immunization with high-molecular weight polysaccharide from *Pseudomonas aeruginosa. Infect. Immun. 22*:919 (1978).
13. P. S. N. Rowe and P. M. Meadow. Structure of the core oligosaccharide from the lipopolysaccharide of *Pseudomonas aeruginosa* PAC1R and its defective mutants. *Eur. J. Biochem., 132*:329 (1983).
14. A. M. B. Kropinski, L. Chan, and F. J. Milazzo. Susceptibility of lipopolysaccharide-defective mutants of *Pseudomonas aeruginosa* PAO to dyes, detergents, and antibiotics. *Antimicrob. Agents Chemother., 13*:494 (1978).
15. M. W. Fisher. A polyvalent human Y-globulin immune to *Pseudomonas aeruginosa*: passive protection of mice against lethal infection. *J. Infect. Dis., 136*:S181 (1977).
16. M. W. Fisher, H. B. Devlin, and F. J. Gnabasik. New immunotype scheme for *Pseudomonas aeruginosa* based on protective antigens. *J. Bacteriol., 98*: 835 (1969).
17. R. Kohler and A. White. Detection of IgG antibodies to type-specific

Pseudomonas aeruginosa lipopolysaccharides by solid-phase radioimmunoassay. *J. Infect. Dis., 136*:112 (1977).
18. L. S. Young, R. D. Meyer, and D. Armstrong. *Pseudomonas aeruginosa* vaccine in cancer patients. *Ann. Intern. Med., 79*:518 (1973).
19. R. G. Doggett and G. M. Harrison. *Pseudomonas aeruginosa*: immune status in patients with cystic fibrosis. *Infect. Immun., 6*:628 (1972).
20. R. B. Moss, Y-P. Hsu, N. J. Lewiston, J. G. Curd, H. Milgrom, S. Hart, B. Dyer, and J. W. Larrick. Association of systemic immune complexes, complement activation, and antibodies to *Pseudomonas aeruginosa* lipopolysaccharide and exotoxin A with mortality in cystic fibrosis[1-3]. *Am. Rev. Respir. Dis., 133*:648 (1986).
21. J. W. Larrick, K. E. Truitt, A. A. Raubitschek, G. S. Senyk, and J. C. M. Wang. Characterization of human hybridomas secreting antibody to tetanus toxoid. *Proc. Natl. Acad. Sci. (USA), 80*:6376 (1983).
22. D. W. Buck, J. W. Larrick, A. A. Raubitschek, K. Truitt, G. Senyk, J. Wang, and B. J. Dyer. Production of human monoclonal antibodies. In R. J. Kennett, K. Bectol, and T. J. McKearn (eds.). *Monoclonal Antibodies and Functional Cell Lines.* Plenum Press, New York (1984).
23. J. W. Larrick, A. A. Raubitschek, B. Dyer, G. Senyk, S. Hart, D. Lippman, M. Jahnsen, J. Wang, and H. Weintraub. *In vitro* expansion of human B cells for production of human monoclonal antibodies. In E. Engleman, S. Foung, J. W. Larrick, and A. A. Raubitschek (eds.). *Human Hybridomas and Monoclonal Antibodies.* Plenum Press, New York (1985).
24. M. Shulman, C. D. Wilde, and G. Kohler. A better cell line for making hybridomas secreting specific antibodies. *Nature, 276*:269 (1978).
25. K. E. Truitt, J. W. Larrick, and A. A. Raubitschek. Fusion of nonadherent human cell lines. In R. J. Kennett, K. B. Bechtol, and T. J. McKean (eds.). *Monoclonal Antibodies and Functional Cell Lines.* Plenum Press, New York (1984).
26. S. K. H. Foung, S. Perkins, A. A. Raubitschek, J. Larrick, G. Lizak, D. Fishwild, E. G. Engleman, and F. C. Grumet. Rescue of human monoclonal antibody production from an EBV-transformed B cell line by fusion to a mouse/human hybridoma. *J. Immunol. Meth., 70*:83 (1984).
27. E. Gronowicz, A. Coutinho, and F. Melchers. A plaque assay for all cells secreting Ig of a given type or class. *Eur. J. Immunol., 6*:588 (1976).
28. J. Wang and J. Larrick. Immunoblotting. In E. G. Engleman, S. K. H. Foung, J. W. Larrick, and A. A. Raubitschek (eds.). *Human Hybridomas and Monoclonal Antibodies.* Plenum Press, New York (1985).
29. P. K. Peterson, J. Verhoef, D. Schneling, and P. G. Quie. Kinetics of phagocytosis and bacterial killing by human polymorphonuclear leukocytes and monocytes. *J. Infect. Dis., 136*:502 (1977).
30. Y. Gazitt, A. D. Deitch, P. A. Marks, and R. A. Rifkind. Cell volume changes in relation to the cell cycle of differentiating erythroleukemic cells. *Exp. Cell Res., 117*:413 (1978).
31. L. S. Cram, E. R. Gomez, C. O. Thoen, J. C. Forslund, and J. H. Jett. Flow

microfluorometric quantitation of the blastogenic response of lymphocytes. *J. Histochem. Cytochem.*, *24*:383 (1980).
32. L. W. Diamond and R. C. Braylan. Flow analysis of DNA content and cell size in non-Hodgkin's lymphoma. *Cancer Res.*, *40*:703 (1980).
33. M. R. Loken and A. M. Stall. Flow cytometry as an analytical and preparative roll in immunology. *J. Immunol. Meth.*, *50*:R85 (1982).
34. M. Ono, M. D. Cole, A. T. White, and R. C. C. Huang. Sequence organization of cloned intracisternal A-particle genes. *Cell*, *21*:465 (1980).
35. N. G. Copeland, A. D. Zelenetz, and G. M. Cooper. Transformation by subgenomic fragments of Rous sarcoma virus DNA. *Cell*, *19*:863 (1980).
36. E. M. Southern. Detection of specific sequences among DNA fragments separated by gel electrophoresis. *J. Mol. Biol.* *98*:503 (1975).
37. G. Wahl, M. Stern, and G. Stark. Efficient transfer of large DNA fragments from agarose gels to diazobenzyloxymethyl-paper and rapid hybridization by using dextran-sulfate. *Proc. Natl. Acad. Sci.* (*USA*), *76*:3683 (1979).
38. D. Crawford, R. E. Callard, M. I. Muggerridge, D. M. Mitchell, E. D. Zanders, and P. C. L. Beverley. Production of human monoclonal antibody to X31 influenza virus nucleoprotein. *J. Gen. Virol.*, *64*:697 (1983).
39. R. F. Irie, L. L. Sze, and R. E. Saxton. Human antibody to OFA-1, a tumor antigen, produced *in vitro* by Epstein-Barr virus-transformed human B-lymphoid cell lines. *Proc. Natl. Acad. Sci.* (*USA*), *79*:5666 (1982).
40. D. Kozbor and J. Roder. Requirements for the establishment of high-titered human monoclonal antibodies against tetanus toxoid using the Epstein-Barr virus technique. *J. Immunol.*, *127*:1275 (1981).
41. D. Kozbor and J. Roder. *In vitro* stimulated lymphocytes as a source of human hybridomas. *Eur. J. Immunol.*, *14*:23 (1983).
42. D. Kozbor and J. Roder. The production of monoclonal antibodies from human lymphocytes. *Immunol. Today*, *4*:72 (1983).
43. D. Kozbor, A. E. Lagarde, and J. C. Roder. Human hybridomas constructed with antigen-specific EBV transformed lines. *Proc. Natl. Acad. Sci.* (*USA*), *79*:6651 (1982).
44. D. Kozbor, J. C. Roder, T. J. Chang, Z. Steplewski, and H. Koprowski. Human anti-tetanus toxoid monoclonal antibody secreted by EBV-transformed human B cells fused with murine myeloma. *Hybridoma*, *1*:323 (1982).
45. D. Kozbor, M. Steinitz, G. Klein, S. Koskimies, and O. Makela. Establishment of anti-TNP antibody-producing human lymphoid lines by preselection for hapten binding followed by EBV transformation. *Scand. J. Immunol.*, *10*:187 (1979).
46. M. Steinitz, G. Klein, S. Koskimies, and O. Makela. EB virus-induced B lymphocyte cell lines producing specific antibody. *Nature*, *269*:420 (1977).
47. M. Steinitz, G. Klein, S. Koskimies, and O. Makela. Establishment of specific antibody producing human lines by antigen preselection and Epstein-Barr virus (EBV) transformation. *J. Clin. Lab. Immunol.*, *2*:1 (1979).
48. S. Tsuchiya, S. Yokoyama, O. Yoshie, and Y. Ono. Production of diptheria antitoxin antibody in Epstein-Barr virus induced lymphoblastoid cell lines. *J. Immunol.*, *124*:1970 (1980).

49. L. Winger, C. Winger, P. Shastry, A. Russell, and M. Longnecker. Efficient generation *in vitro,* from human peripheral blood cells, of monoclonal Epstein-Barr virus transformants producing specific antibody to a variety of antigens without prior deliberate immunization. *Proc. Natl. Acad. Sci. (USA), 80*:4484 (1983).
50. N. N. H. Teng, K. S. Lam, F. C. Riera, and H. S. Kaplan. Construction and testing of mouse/human heteromyelomas for human monoclonal antibody production. *Proc. Natl. Acad. Sci. (USA), 80*:7308 (1983).
51. G. Buttin, G. LeGuern, L. Phalente, E. C. C. Lin, L. Medrano, and P. A. Cazenave. Production of hybrid lines secreting monoclonal anti-idiotypic antibodies by cell fusion on membrane filters. In F. Melchers, M. Potter, and N. L. Warner (eds.). *Lymphocyte Hybridomas.* Springer-Verlag, Berlin, New York (1978).
52. N. A. Brown and G. Miller. Immunoglobulin expression by human B lymphocytes clonally transformed by Epstein-Barr virus. *J. Immunol., 128*:24 (1982).
53. C. M. Croce, M. Shander, J. Martinis, L. Circurel, G. G. D'Ancanar, T. W. Dolley, and H. Koprowski. Chromosome locations of the genes for human immunoglobulin heavy chains. *Eur. J. Immunol., 10*:486 (1979).
54. J. Erickson, J. Martinis, and C. M. Croce. Assignment of the genes for human immunoglobulin chains to chromosome 22. *Nature, 294*:123 (1981).
55. J. C. Sadoff, D. C. Wright, S. Futrowsky, H. Sidberry, H. Collins, B. Kaufman. Characterization of mouse monoclonal antibodies directed against *Pseudomonas aeruginosa* lipopolysaccharides. In D. P. Spert and R. E. W. Hancock (eds.). *Pseudomonas aeruginosa: New Therapeutic Approaches from Basic Research.* Karger, New York.
56. M. Madsen and H. E. Johnson. A methodological study of E-rosette formation using AET-treated sheep red blood cells. *J. Immunol. Methods, 27*: 61 (1979).

6

Construction of a Stable, Protective Human Monoclonal Antibody to the C Fragment of Tetanus Toxin

BRUCE D. FREIMARK
Scripps Clinic and Research Foundation, La Jolla, California

HOWARD OZER
University of North Carolina at Chapel Hill, and Lineberger Cancer Research Center, Chapel Hill, North Carolina

In 1975, Kohler and Milstein (1) demonstrated that monoclonal antibodies to predetermined antigens could be derived from murine lymphocytes immortalized in tissue culture by fusion to continuously proliferating tumor cell lines. This method has allowed the production of unlimited quantities of homogeneous antibodies against numerous antigens that have been of great value in both basic and applied clinical research. However, the generation of human monoclonal antibodies has been more difficult to achieve. Since Olsson and Kaplan's first report of production of human hybridomas secreting monoclonal antibodies of predetermined specificity, several pitfalls of this technology have been improved. This chapter addresses several key factors that have allowed successful fusion of human peripheral blood lymphocytes with tumor cell lines to establish anti-tetanus toxoid immunoglobulin-secreting human hybridomas.

I. HUMAN FUSION PARTNERS

The most significant problem in the construction of human immunoglobulin-secreting hybridomas has been selection of an efficient tumor cell fusion partner. Clearly, not all tumor cell lines are capable of generating stable hybrid formation.

Table 1 Characterization of HGPRT-Negative Human Tumor Cell Lines

Cell line	Origin of cell line	Antibody secretion	Membrane[a] markers	Successful[b] fusions
CCRF-CEM-8AZ	T cell ALL	–	TdT, Leu4	None
CCRF-HSB-2-8AZ	T cell ALL	–	Leu4	None
HPB-ALL-8AZ	T cell ALL	–	TdT,E^+,Leu4	None
Molt-4-8AZ	T cell ALL	–	E^+	None
KM-3-8AZ	Non-B, non-T ALL	–	TdT	None
K-562-8AZ	Non-B, non-T CML	–	EA	None
RPMI 1788-8AZ	Normal B cell	+	(κ,δ,μ),Ia^+,EBV	None
B35M-8AZ	Burkitt's lymphoma	–	(μ),Ia^+,cALL,EBV	None
Namalva-8AZ	Burkitt's lymphoma	–	(λ,μ),Ia^+,cALL,EBV	None
DG-75-8AZ	Burkitt's lymphoma	–	(κ,δ,μ),Ia^+,cALL	None
DND-39-8AZ	Burkitt's lymphoma	+	(λ,μ),Ia^+,cALL	None
BALL-1-8AZ	B cell ALL	–	(λ,δ,μ),Ia^+,EA	None
BALM-1-8AZ	B cell ALL	+	(κ,δ,μ),Ia^+,EAC	None
ARH-77-8AZ	Plasma cell leukemia	+	(λ,κ),Ia^+	None
UC-726-6-8AZ	Hereditary spherocytosis	+	(κ,δ,μ),Ia^+,EBV	Yes

[a]Membrane markers include: TdT = terminal deoxytidyl transferase; E = forms rosettes with sheep red blood cells; EA = forms rosettes with bovine red blood cells coated with antibody; heavy and light chain isotypes; EBV = Epstein Barr virus; cALL = common acute lymphocytic leukemia antigen; Leu4 = pan T-cell reactive monoclonal antibody (Becton Dickinson); Ia^+ = positive for HLA-D locus coded cell surface antigen.

[b]Represents at least two attempts to generate hybrids with peripheral blood lymphocytes.

The painstaking task of evaluating and selecting potential fusion partners has been encountered in several laboratories including our own. Table 1 summarizes our numerous attempts to construct hybrids from a variety of drug-marked human cell lines. Unfortunately, despite the overall failure of most cell lines to form hybridomas, there is no outstanding characteristic that distinguishes one successful fusion partner (UC-729-6) and all others tested. However, there is a striking observation in that many subclones of the WIL-2 cell line, which includes UC-729-6, yield hybrid growth with high efficiency (2-5). The only other human cell line from which several fusion partners have been derived with as much reported success is the lymphoblastoid cell line GM-1500 (6-9). Although WIL-2 and GM-1500 both express lymphoblastoid characteristics, there is no evidence to suggest that lymphoblastoid origin or phenotype confers improved cell fusion or more stable hybrid formation.

II. SELECTION MEDIA AND CLONAL EXPANSION

The hypoxanthine/aminopterin/thymidine (HAT) selection system described by Littlefield (10) is presently the most common method employed to isolate hybrids. However, due to the rather low formation of lymphocyte hybrids, particularly human-human hybrids, other selection systems have been evaluated to improve the hybrid yield. We have compared conventional HAT selection media with selection media containing azaserine (A) and hypoxanthine (H). Azaserine inhibits *de novo* purine synthesis, while aminopterin inhibits the synthesis of both purines and pyrimidines. As seen in Table 2, AH selection media allowed more hybrids to form under the same conditions than did conventional HAT selection media. These results are supported not only by studies using different hybridoma systems (11), but also using subclones of the WIL-2 cell line as a fusion partner (4,12). By titrating the limiting dose of azaserine that killed the UC-729-6 cell line, it was clear that this inhibition allowed more hybrids to grow than the lowest concentration of aminopterin (36.4% versus 60.0%). Thus, in order to evaluate the true efficacy of selection media, it is important to carefully titrate the inhibitors to the lowest amount necessary to achieve inhibition of growth of the tumor fusion partner.

Generally once hybrids are selected and expanded in culture, subcloning is usually performed for several reasons: (a) to ensure monoclonality of the hybrid cell line, (b) to prevent overgrowth by other possible clones existing in the same initial culture, and (c) to isolate stable subclones that retain the capacity to secrete antibody. The most common method of cloning hybrids is by limiting dilution. Several variations of the limiting dilution procedure have been shown to increase the efficiency of the technique, such as the addition of growth factors and feeder cells. The necessity of these supplements is variable,

Table 2 Comparison of HAT and AH Hybridoma Selection Media

Aminopterin[a] concentration	Parental tumor drug sensitivity	Wells positive for hybrid growth		Azaserine[b] concentration	Parental tumor drug sensitivity	Wells positive for hybrid growth	
		Exp. 1	Exp. 2			Exp. 1	Exp. 2
4.0×10^{-7} M	Dies	10/48	32/96	6.0×10^{-6} M	Dies	0/48	–
2.0×10^{-7} M	Dies	16/48	–	3.0×10^{-6} M	Dies	2/48	–
1.0×10^{-7} M	Dies	10/48	–	1.2×10^{-6} M	Dies	8/48	–
4.0×10^{-8} M	Survives	–	–	6.0×10^{-7} M	Dies	22/48	60/96
				3.0×10^{-7} M	Survives	–	–

Tumor cell line (UC-729-6) was fused with PWM stimulated PBLs (6 days) at a ratio of 1:2 (tumor/PBL) with 50% PEG (MW 3400) and plated in 0.1 ml amounts in RPMI-1640-20% FCS. Wells were screened for hybrid cell growth 3 weeks postfusion

[a]Wells containing aminopterin have 1.6×10^{-5} M thymidine and 10^{-4} M hypoxanthine.

[b]Wells containing azaserine have 10^{-4} M hypoxanthine.

depending on the cloning efficiency of the tumor fusion partner and the growth characteristics of the hybrid to be cloned. The UC-729-6 cell line forms hybrids that are easily cloned, and growth factors or feeder cells are not an essential requirement. This is in direct contrast to the absolute requirement for feeder cells using a different fusion partner (13). However, the addition of irradiated feeder cells in the cloning procedure employed in this study not only increased the cloning efficiency, but also enhanced the growth of the subclones (Table 3). Optimal conditions were obtained by the use of irradiated peripheral blood lymphocytes (PBLs) autologous to the normal lymphocytes used to generate the hybrid.

III. ENHANCEMENT OF ANTIGEN-SPECIFIC CLONES

It is now evident that a few human fusion partners are capable of forming stable immunoglobulin-secreting hybrids. Consequently, the main concern has shifted to isolating a sufficient number of antigen-specific immunoglobulin-secreting lymphocytes to be fused. Unlike the murine hybridoma method in which spleen cells are utilized, the most convenient source of human lymphocytes is circulating blood. Unfortunately, PBLs contain only 10-20% B cells, and form hybrids with lower frequencies than lymphocytes derived from other sources such as lymph node, spleen, and tonsil (2,14,15). Stimulation of PBLs with antigen or mitogen prior to cell fusion has been shown to significantly enhance hybrid formation.

Several mechanisms may account for this enhancement. (a) The increase in hybrid formation coincides with the maximum *in vitro* secretion of immunoglobulin induced by mitogens. It is plausible that membrane changes required to allow an increased vesicle transport and secretion of immunoglobulin could also result in an increased ability of two cells to fuse (16). (b) Mitogen activation has been shown to induce a series of membrane potential changes in lymphocytes that may enhance their fusion potential (17). In support of this proposal, the presence of Ca^{++} in the fusion solution has been shown to increase cell fusion (18,19). Thus, an increase in negative charge by the lymphocyte may allow an ionic "bridge" to form between cells when the fusion solution is added. (c) Enhanced fusion of lymphocytes may be due to a direct ability of mitogens to agglutinate cells. (d) Mitogens may activate lymphocytes to differentiate to a stage necessary for fusion to occur. This differentiation may be due to direct interaction with mitogens or through interaction with lymphokines produced by activated lymphocytes.

As demonstrated in Table 4, lymphocytes fused at a much greater frequency when stimulated with pokeweed mitogen (PWM) prior to fusion as compared with unstimulated lymphocytes. In addition, more immunoglobulin-secreting hybrids were obtained than would have been predicted for the fusion of a hetero-

Table 3 Cloning Efficiency of Human-Human Hybridomas

		Feeder layer					
Exp.	Cells/Well	None	Confluency reached	UC-729-6	Confluency reached	PBLs	Confluency reached
1	50.0	48/48 (100%)	2 wk	96/96 (100%)	2 wk	96/96 (100%)	2 wk
	5.0	16/48 (33%)	2-3 wk	61/96 (64%)	2-3 wk	61/96 (64%)	2 wk
	0.5	6/96 (6%)	3-4 wk	4/96 (4%)	2-3 wk	11/96 (11%)	2-3 wk
2	50.0					96/96 (100%)	1 wk
	5.0					86/96 (90%)	2 wk
	0.5					19/96 (20%)	2-3 wk
3	50.0					96/96 (100%)	1 wk
	5.0					84/96 (88%)	2 wk
	0.5					12/96 (13%)	2-3 wk

Uncloned hybrid cells were diluted in RPMI-1640-20% FCS and plated in 0.1 ml aliquots in 96-well flat-bottomed plates with or without 10^5/well irradiated (4000r) feeder cells. Values represent the average number of viable cell out-growths per number of wells plated.

Table 4 Effect of Lymphocyte Preincubation with Antigen or Mitogen on Recovery of Specific Hybrid Formation

		Unstimulated	Tetanus toxin (TT)	PWM
Subject 1	A	672	672	480
	B	0	0	110
	C	0	0	84
	D	0	0	1
Subject 2	A	576	576	480
	B	20	6	38
	C	16	4	38
	D	0	0	0
Subject 3	A	576	672	672
	B	7	48	152
	C	7	14	94
	D	0	0	0

A = total number of wells plated; B = number of wells containing growing hybridoma cells; C = number of cells containing immunoglobulin (wells scored positive if absorbance at 405 nm was 3 standard deviations higher than average of control wells); D = number of wells containing hybridomas secreting antibody to TT.

PBLs were obtained on days 2, 4, 6, 8, 10, 14, and 21 after immunization and fused fresh or cultured with TT (0.5 LF/ml) or PWM (1:200 dilution) for 6 days. Wells were screened for hybrid growth up to 3 weeks postfusion. Supernatants were tested by ELISA for production of polyclonal anti-TT antibody 3 weeks after fusion.

geneous population of PBLs containing 70% T cells. This implies that B cells preferentially fuse to the B cell lymphoblastoid cell line used in this study or that T-B hybrids are relatively short-lived in culture. Preincubation of PBLs with tetanus toxoid or PWM for 6 days prior to fusion failed to significantly enhance the probability of immune PBLs to form specific hybrids. Although PWM prestimulation markedly increased the total number of hybrids formed, it was not effective enough to efficiently rescue low frequencies of antigen-specific cells from the circulation. In contrast to this study, Butler *et al.* (20) demonstrated that preculturing PBLs with low doses of antigen (5 ng/ml) for 72 hours prior to fusion yielded approximately twice as many antigen-specific hybrids as fusion done without *in vitro* stimulation.

Recently, immune-rosetting with antigen-coupled red blood cells and panning with antigen-coated Petri dishes have been successfully employed to enrich for antigen-specific lymphocytes prior to lymphocyte immortalization (21). The use of these preselection methods will probably become more popular in the near future for creating antigen-specific human hybrids.

IV. PRODUCTION OF BULK QUANTITIES OF HUMAN MONOCLONAL ANTIBODIES

Apart from the technical heroics necessary to isolate stable antigen-specific antibody-producing human hybridomas is the problem of producing bulk quantities of antibodies. The majority of immunoglobulin-secreting human hybridomas are capable of producing only a few micrograms of immunoglobulin per milliliter in spent tissue culture medium. Thus, in order to purify milligram quantities of antibody, it is necessary to generate large volumes of tissue culture supernatant. This problem is easily solved with murine monoclonal antibodies since they may be readily grown *in vivo* as ascites tumors that typically yield immunoglobulin concentrations of 5-10 mg/ml. With human hybridomas, ascites tumors must be grown in immunodeficient mice to avoid xenograft rejection. Abrams *et al.* (22) have recently succeeded in growing mouse-human hybrids in doubly pristane-primed nude mice. In addition, Truitt *et al.* (23) have successfully grown human-human hybrids in nude mice by first passaging the hybridoma as a subcutaneous solid tumor, which then allowed the cells to grow as ascites. As reported in this study (Table 5) and by Truitt *et al.* (23) human-human hybridomas can only be grown as nude mouse ascites if animals received irradiation prior to hybrid inoculation. Nude mouse ascites contains at least 100 times the concentration of antibody that can be developed in tissue culture supernatant from the same hybrid (Figs. 1 and 2). This method of isolating human monoclonal antibodies may be particularly useful for obtaining large quantities of antibody from low secretor hybrids.

V. PROTECTION OF MICE BY ANTI-TT HUMAN MONOCLONAL ANTIBODIES

In conclusion, it has been demonstrated in this study that human monoclonal antibodies can protect mice from a lethal dose of tetanus toxin. As seen in Table 6, 10 μg of antibody can protect mice from over 10 $\times$ the LD_{50} of tetanus toxin in mice. This finding is one of only a few reports (4,24) that have shown protection of mice from tetanus toxin using a human monoclonal antibody. Furthermore, this is the first report of a human monoclonal antibody capable of binding the C fragment of tetanus toxin (Fig. 3). Gigliotti and Insel (24) have generated

Table 5 Production of Human Monoclonal Antibody in Nude Mouse Ascites

Exp.	Pretreatment	Number of mice positive for ascites of those injected with hybrid cells	Time for ascites to develop
1	None	0/2	–
	400r	1/2	3-4 weeks
2	None	0/4	–
	400r	1/4	2 weeks

Nude mice were given 0.5 ml pristane I.P. with or without 400r x-irradiation; 2×10^7 hybrid cells were injected in 0.5 ml of RPMI-1640 without FCS 1 week after pristane and irradiation pretreatment. Mice were observed for ascites production for 6 weeks.

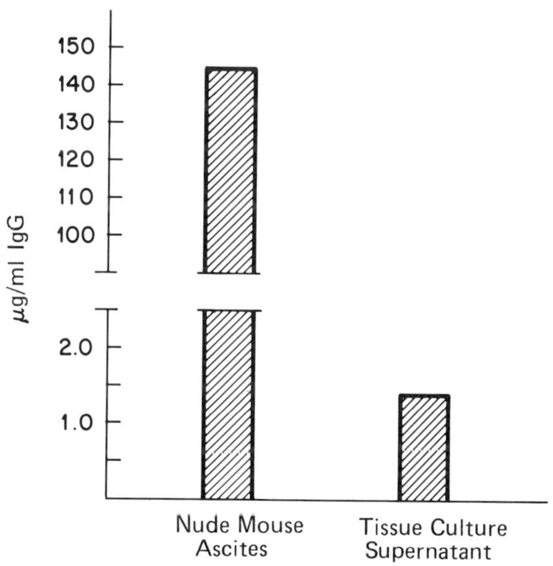

Figure 1 Comparison of immunoglobulin secreted by hybrid BFD-1 in nude mouse ascites versus the tissue culture supernatant. Human IgG was quantitated using the ELISA technique.

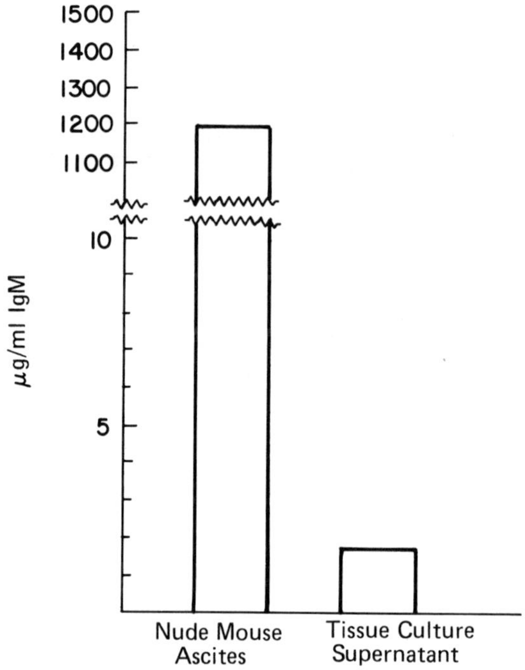

Figure 2 Comparison of immunoglobulin secreted by hybrid 72A11 in nude mouse ascites versus the tissue culture supernatant. Human IgM was quantitated using the ELISA technique.

a mouse-human hybridoma secreting a human monoclonal antibody that recognizes the B fragment of tetanus toxin. Not surprisingly, polyclonal anti-TT antibody purified from the plasma of an individual (subject no. 1) chosen to construct the anti-TT antibody-secreting hybrid had a higher tetanus toxin-neutralizing capacity. This is most likely due to a mixture of affinities and epitope specificities in the polyclonal preparation which maximizes immune complex formation and antigen clearance. Thus, it may be necessary to use several monoclonal antibodies in combination for therapeutic purposes. Although the construction of human hybridomas is still in its infancy, the potential of human monoclonal antibodies as therapeutic reagents is very promising.

Table 6 Neutralization of a Lethal Dose of Tetanus Toxin in Mice with a Human Monoclonal Antibody

Antibody preparation	μg (antibody/mouse)	Number dead/number of total at indicated time (hr) after toxin administration					
		24	48	72	96	120	144
αTT monoclonal antibody	10.0	0/4	0/4	0/4	0/4	0/4	0/4
	1.0	3/4	3/4	3/4	3/4	3/4	3/4
	0.1	4/4	–	–	–	–	–
αTT polyclonal antibody (no. 1)	10.0	0/4	0/4	0/4	0/4	0/4	0/4
	1.0	0/4	0/4	0/4	0/4	0/4	0/4
	0.1	0/4	0/4	0/4	0/4	0/4	0/4
αTT polyclonal antibody (no. 2)	10.0	0/4	0/4	0/4	0/4	0/4	0/4
	1.0	0/4	0/4	0/4	0/4	0/4	0/4
	0.1	0/4	0/4	0/4	0/4	0/4	0/4
Control myeloma protein	10.0	4/4	–	–	–	–	–
PBS	–	4/4	–	–	–	–	–

All animals received 1.0 ng of tetanus toxin with or without test antibody in a total volume of 0.1 ml.

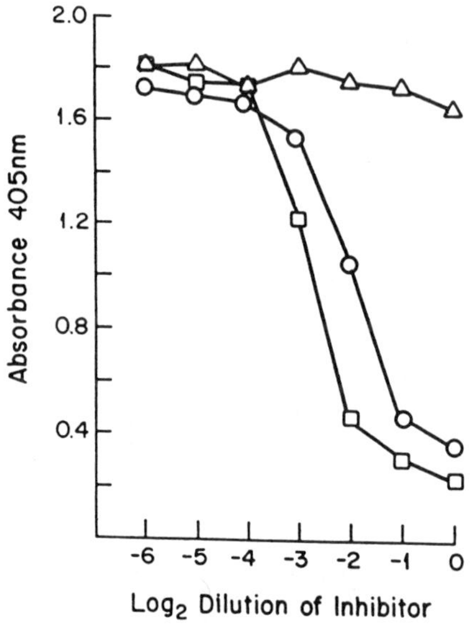

Figure 3 Specificity of a human monoclonal antibody for the C fragment of tetanus toxin. Microtiter plates coated with tetanus toxin were incubated with 1.0 μg of purified antibody in the presence of tetanus toxoid, B or C fragment, or tetanus toxin. Serial twofold dilutions of inhibitors were diluted into constant amounts of antibody (1 μg), with the highest concentration of inhibitor being 10^{-7} M.

ACKNOWLEDGMENTS

This work was supported in part by Grants CA-31080 and CA-5834 from the National Cancer Institute, DHHS.

The data reported in this manuscript were obtained in partial fulfillment of the Ph.D. requirements for Dr. Freimark in the Department of Pathology, State University of New York at Buffalo.

REFERENCES

1. G. Kohler and C. Milstein. Continuous cultures of fused cells secreting antibody of predefined specificity. *Nature, 256*:495 (1975).
2. N. Chiorazzi, R. L. Wasserman, and H. G. Kunkel. Use of Epstein-Barr virus transformed B cell lines for the generation of immunoglobulin-producing human B cell hybridomas. *J. Exp. Med., 156*:930 (1982).

3. L. E. Strike, B. H. Devens, and R. C. Lundak. Production of human-human hybridomas secreting antibody to sheep erythrocytes after *in vitro* immunization. *J. Immunol., 132*:1798 (1984).
4. J. W. Larrich, K. E. Truitt, A. A. Raubitschek, G. Senyk, and J. C. N. Wang. Characterization of human hybridoma secreting antibody to tetanus toxoid. *Proc. Natl. Acad. Sci. (USA), 80*:6376 (1983).
5. D. Emanuel, J. Gold, J. Colacino, C. Lopez, and U. Hammerling. A human monoclonal antibody to cytomegalovirus (CMV). *J. Immunol., 133*:2202 (1984).
6. Y. Shoenfeld, J. Rauch, H. Massicotti, S. K. Datta, J. Andre-Schwartz, B. D. Staller, and R. S. Schwartz. Polyspecificity of monoclonal lupus autoantibodies produced by human-human hybridomas. *N. Engl. J. Med., 308*: 414 (1983).
7. C. M. Crose, A. Linnenbach, W. Hall, Z. Steplewski, and H. Koprowski. Production of human hybridomas secreting antibodies to measles virus. *Nature, 228*:488 (1980).
8. D. Kozbor, A. Lagarde, and J. C. Rodor. Human hybridomas constructed with antigen-specific, EBV-transformed cell lines. *Proc. Natl. Acad. Sci. (USA), 79*:6651 (1982).
9. D. S. Dryer, R. J. Bradley, C. K. Urguhart, and J. F. Kearney. Naturally occurring anti-idiotypic antibodies in myasthenia gravis patients. *Nature, 301*:611 (1983).
10. J. W. Littlefield. Selection of hybrids from matings of fibroblasts *in vitro* and their presumed recombinants. *Science, 145*:709 (1964).
11. G. Buttin, G. LeGuern, L. Phalente, E. C. C. Lin, L. Mediano, and P. A. Cazenave. Production of hybrid lines secreting monoclonal anti-idiotypic antibodies by cell fusion on membrane filters. In F. Melchers, M. Potter, and N. C. Warner (eds.). *Current Topics in Microbiology and Immunology 81*. Springer-Verlag, New York (1978).
12. J. W. Larrich, K. E. Truitt, A. A. Raubitschek, and B. J. Dwyer. An improved method for production of human-human hybrid cells (abstr.). *Hybridoma, 3*:71 (1983).
13. F. Brodin, L. Olsson, and H. O. Sjogren. Cloning of human hybridoma, myeloma and lymphoma cell lines using enriched human monocytes as feeder layers. *J. Immunol. Meth., 60*:1 (1983).
14. M. C. Glassy, H. H. Handley, H. Hagiwara, and I. Royston. UC-729-6, a human lymphoblastoid B-cell line useful for generating antibody-secreting human-human hybridomas. *Proc. Natl. Acad. Sci. (USA), 80*:6327 (1983).
15. J. H. Murray, M. Ho, and M. Sullivan. Evaluation of human fusion parents and optimization of fusion conditions (abstr.). *Hybridoma, 3*:70 (1983).
16. G. E. Woloschak and D. Senitzer. Effect of mitogenic stimulation of murine splenocytes on PEG-induced cell fusion. *Hybridoma, 2*:341 (1983).
17. H. Kiefer, A. J. Bhume, and H. R. Koback. Membrane potential changes during mitogenic stimulation of mouse spleen lymphocytes. *Proc. Natl. Acad. Sci. (USA), 77*:2200 (1980).

18. W. A. Keller and G. Melchers. The effect of high pH and calcium on tobacco leaf protoplast fusion. *Z. Naturforsch. Teil C., 28*:737 (1973).
19. Z. Toister and A. Layter. Ca^{++}-induced fusion of avian erythrocytes. *Biochem. Biophys. Acta, 241*:719 (1971).
20. J. L. Butler, H. C. Lane, and A. S. Fauci. Delineation of optimal conditions for producing mouse-human heterohybridomas from human peripheral blood B cells of immunized subjects. *J. Immunol., 130*:165 (1983).
21. L. Winger, C. Winger, P. Shastry, A. Russell, and M. Longenecker. Efficient generation *in vitro,* from human peripheral blood cells, of monoclonal Epstein-Barr virus transformants producing specific antibody to a variety of antigens without prior deliberate immunization. *Proc. Natl. Acad. Sci. (USA), 80*:4484 (1983).
22. P. G. Abrams, J. J. Ochs, S. L. Giandino, A. C. Morgan, S. B. Wilburn, A. R. Witt, R. K. Oldham, and K. A. Foon. Production of large quantities of human immunoglobulin in the ascites of athymic mice: implications for the development of anti-human idiotype monoclonal antibodies. *J. Immunol., 132*:1611 (1984).
23. K. E. Truitt, J. W. Larrich, A. A. Raubitschek, D. W. Buck, and S. W. Jacobson. Production of human monoclonal antibody in moust ascites. *Hybridoma, 3*:195 (1984).
24. E. Gigliotti and R. A. Insel. Protective human hybridoma antibody to tetanus toxin. *J. Clin. Invest., 70*:1306 (1982)

7

Transfection of Human Cells

An alternative method for the establishment of human hybrid clones

ANTHONY J. STRELKAUSKAS, CATHERINE L. TAYLOR, and MATTHEW R. SMITH*
Medical University of South Carolina, Charleston, South Carolina

PHYLLIS D. BEAR
University of Wyoming, Laramie, Wyoming

The manipulation of genes and genetic material has become almost routine. Considerable evidence using viral-mediated gene transfer has accumulated since calcium phosphate precipitation methods were initially developed (1). Much of this work has pertained to transferred genes coding for identifiable enzymes such as thymidine kinase (2-9), adenine phosphoribosyltransferase (10), hypoxanthine phosphoribosyltransferase (11-13), and dihydrofolate reductase (14). Research in the area of oncogenes relies upon the use of transfection of human and murine cells (15-17). Experiments using Hepatitis B viral plasmids have shown high frequencies of transfection in human cells (18). Mouse/human transfections have also been accomplished in which nonmalignant diploid fibroblasts have been used as recipients for mouse viral DNA in hopes of studying the genetic control of the neoplastic transformation event (19). In addition, studies (20) with cloned mouse genes injected into fertilized eggs have shown that 20-30% of the recipient animals carry the transferred genetic material.

The ability to manipulate specific genes of immunological importance is most aptly demonstrated in experiments where DNA containing the genes responsible for Ig production have been cloned and transfected into specific lymphoid cells (21-25). There is also apparently a cell donor/recipient identity necessary for

**Present affiliation*: Duke University Medical Center, Durham, North Carolina maximum expression of transfected genes (26). In contrast, recent studies (26) have shown that cross-species transfections have successfully been carried out in which murine spleen cells were immortalized by transfecting them with human DNA from the established leukemia cell line Reh. Interestingly, some of these transfectants were genetically diploid and displayed remarkable stability in culture, a trait not usually seen in cross-species cell-cell hybridizations. Several laboratories (27-36) have also been successful in using transfection to bring about the expression of cell MHC surface antigens not present on recipient cells. Recently, human T cell differentiation antigens have also been found on transfected mouse L cells (37).

The information contained in this chapter will describe how transfections of human cells with human DNA can be used to (a), establish human clones producing a desired immunoglobulin, and (b) determine how established cell lines can be used as recipients of hybrid DNA. Detailed phenotypic studies show that transfected DNA is not only taken up, but also transcribed and translated into readily identifiable cell surface proteins. Perhaps most importantly, we present evidence indicating that transfected DNA is taken up and apparently integrated into recipient chromosomes, and that the location of transfected DNA appears to be both random and nonrandom.

I. PROCEDURES

A. Cell Lines

All cell lines used for DNA isolation were maintained in RPMI-1640 medium containing 5% fetal calf serum (FCS), 1% penicillin-streptomycin, 12 ml Hepes buffer, 1.6 ml 7.5% $NaHCO_3$, 50 mg sodium pyruvate, and 584 mg L-glutamine per liter.

B. DNA Purification

DNA was extracted using the method of Bellard *et al.* (38), which involves multiple phenol extractions (Table 1). In these studies, a minimum of two complete extraction procedures were used.

C. Transfection Protocols

Transfection experiments described here were done in three ways. (a) The first involved the immortalization of normal human lymphocytes using DNA obtained from the T cell line JM. Since no functioning immunoglobulin genes should be transferred, a successful experiment could easily be identified if these transfected cells continued to grow indefinitely and continued to produce immunoglobulin. (b) The second set of experiments encompassed the transfection of a T cell line

Table 1 DNA Isolation

1. Lyse cells with proteinase K
2. Phenol extraction no. 1
3. Dialyze
4. Add RNase and T1 RNase
5. Dialyze
6. Add SDS and proteinase K
7. Phenol extraction no. 2
8. Repeat steps 3-6
9. Precipitate DNA with $CaCl_2$
10. Transfect using "glycerol shock"

with DNA from an already established immunoglobulin-producing hybridoma clone. In this case, successful transfection would be indicated by the onset and continuation of the production of immunoglobulin identical to that produced by the donor cells. The success of the transfer is amplified because the DNA-recipient cell line is a T cell that does not synthesize or secrete immunoglobulin. (c) The last series of experiments described here involves the karyotypic examination of normal lymphocytes with ^{3}H-BrdU-labeled DNA from a long-term cell line to determine the genetic events associated with this form of transfection at the chromosomal level. Transfections using unlabeled DNA were done as follows: Peripheral blood lymphocytes (PBLs), PHA stimulated for 3 days were transfected with purified DNA. For each 3×10^6 PBLs, 15 μg of DNA was added. DNA was added to cells suspended in *tris*-buffered saline (TBS) for 40 minutes at 37°C. At this time, 1 ml of media containing 20% FCS was added for 3.5 hours at 37°C. After incubation, the mixture was subjected to 20% glycerol in TBS for 1 minute to complete the transfection procedure.

Experiments using ^{3}H-BrdU-labeled DNA were done in the following way: 100×10^6 Ball-1 cells were labeled with 24 μCi/mmol ^{3}H-BrdU (Amersham). One μl/ml per day of label was added per ml of culture media for 3 days. After 3 days, Ball-1 cells were examined by fluorescence to determine that Ball-1 DNA had been maximally labeled, and DNA was extracted from these cells using the method of Ballard *et al.* (38). The concentration of DNA obtained from Ball-1 cells was 48.6 μg/ml, with an average of 497 cpm.

Peripheral blood lymphocytes, PHA-stimulated for 3 days, were transfected with 15 μg of ^{3}H-BrdU-labeled DNA for each 3×10^6 PBLs. DNA was added to cells suspended in TBS for 40 minutes at 37°C. After this incubation, the PBL-

DNA mixture was divided into two parts. One part was used for examination of radioactivity as well as harvesting for chromosome analysis. The other was subjected to 20% glycerol in TBS for 1 minute to complete the normal transfection procedure. At this time, some cells were also removed for counts and chromosome analysis, while the remaining cells were placed in culture for 24 hours before harvesting and analysis.

D. Cytogenetics

Cells harvested for chromosome analysis were resuspended in 10 ml of RPMI-1640 (Gibco) containing 10% FCS. Colcemid, (Gibco) 100 μl, was added for 1 hour at 37°C. Cells were centrifuged, and 0.075 M KCl was added dropwise to 10 ml for 40 minutes at room temperature. Pelleted cells were then fixed by adding acid fix (three parts methanol to one part acetic acid) dropwise to 10 ml for 30 minutes at room temperature. After three washes using acid-fix, chromosome spreads were prepared by dropping onto slides. All centrifuge steps for both transfection and cytogenetics were performed in a Beckman J6B centrifuge at 1200 rpm.

Slides were scored for BrdU incorporation at each time interval. Duplicate slides were also prepared for autoradiography to be scored for ^{3}H DNA incorporation at a later time.

E. Preparation of Antisera

New Zealand white rabbits were injected with 10×10^6 transfected cells in Freund's complete adjuvant, intramuscularly, and subsequently boosted both intravenously without Freund's and intramuscularly with Freund's incomplete adjuvant. To alleviate the possibility of nonspecific Fc-binding, rabbit immunoglobulins were isolated, pepsin-digested, and chromatographically purified. Briefly, immunoglobulin was precipitated with saturated ammonium sulfate, and dialyzed against 0.1 M NaAc, pH 8.0. The pH of the solution was reduced to 4.3 by the addition of 1 M acetic acid. Pepsin was added (5 mg/ml in 0.1 M NaAc, pH 4.3) to 2% of the total weight of protein and incubated at 37°C overnight. Pepsin-digested fragments were then dialyzed against borate saline buffer (BSB) and purified by Sephadex G-150 chromatography. Total immunoglobulin and $F(ab')_2$ fractions were then dialyzed against normal saline and concentrated to 1 mg/ml.

F. Absorption of Antisera

Rabbit antisera was complement-inactivated at 56°C for 30 minutes, and 0.5 ml volumes were absorbed with 1×10^8 cells. All absorptions were carried out for 2 hours at room temperature with continuous stirring.

G. Binding Assays

Cells were adjusted to 1×10^6 per tube, washed twice in HBSS, and pelleted. The pellet was then sensitized with 50 μl of either rabbit antibody or $F(ab')_2$ raised against the cell type for 45 minutes at 4°C, washed twice with HBSS, and resuspended in 1 ml HBSS. Sensitized cells were then rosetted with 50 μl per tube of goat anti-rabbit Ig-coated human red blood cells (10% by volume in HBSS). The suspension was centrifuged at 600 *g* for 5 minutes, vigorously resuspended, and stained with toluidine blue, and the percentage of rosetted and nonrosetted cells was determined by counting 300 cells with a light microscope.

II. RESULTS

A. Transfection of Normal Lymphocytes with Malignant DNA

In order to determine the effects of this type of transfection, cells from a woman (G.M.) who was a Rhogam donor (i.e., produced anti-Rh antibodies) were transfected with DNA from the T cell line JM. Obviously, continued growth of these cells in culture would indicate successful transfection. This was, indeed, the case with anti-Rh antibody found in the supernatants over a period of several months in culture. Positive wells were subsequently subcloned, tested by enzyme immunoassay for anti-Rh antibody, and also found to be positive. This clone was designated GM-JM-DNA.

1. Cytogenetic Studies

Analyses of GM-JM-DNA transfectants conducted 3 to 4 months after subcloning revealed clones with chromosome numbers varying between diploid and approximately octaploid. Subsequent subclonings to 1 cell/well consistently showed the same variability with respect to chromosomal numbers; however, definitive chromosomal identifications could not be readily determined.

2. Cell Surface Phenotypic Studies

Binding of rabbit antisera prepared against GM-JM-DNA cells was appreciably higher than background levels for both GM-JM-DNA and GM cells, as shown in Figures 1 and 2. Interestingly, this antisera, although prepared against the GM-JM-DNA clone, appears to be more reactive against GM cells. This would be expected because the GM cell was the recipient of the DNA. If this DNA from the JM cell line was in some way incorporated into and used by GM cells, it is possible that surface antigens specific for JM might also appear on the surface of this transfected clone. As can be seen in Figure 3, this is apparently the case because there is definite positive-binding of this antisera to JM cells. The binding to JM cells is apparently specific because similar binding curves are seen with both the total

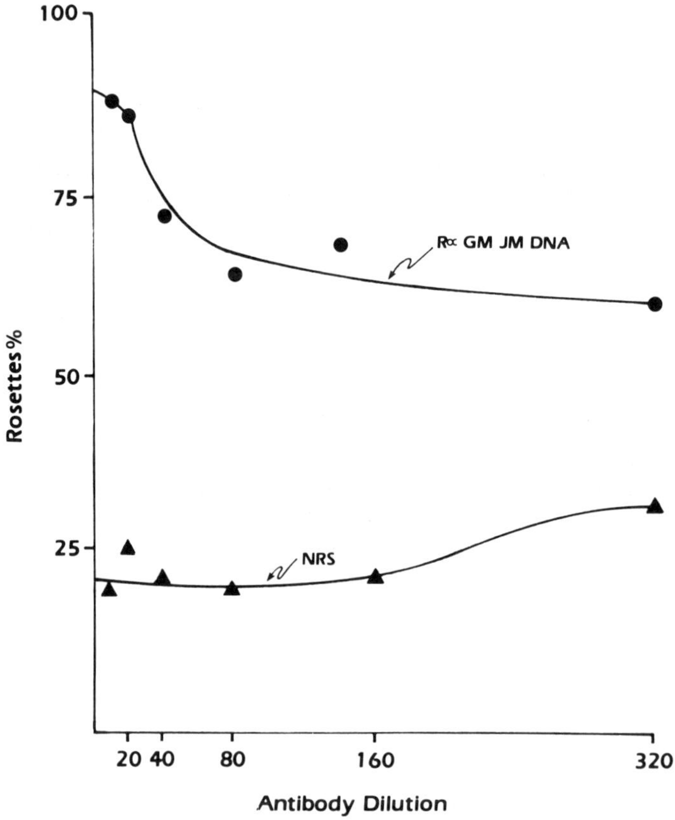

Figure 1 Binding studies of rabbit antisera produced by immunization with the transfected clone GM-JM-DNA. In this case, GM-JM-DNA cells were incubated with rabbit antisera for 1 hour at 4°C. Cells were then washed and rosetted with human red blood cells coupled by the chromium chloride technique with purified goat anti-rabbit $F(ab')_2$. Control values represent the same cell type sensitized with normal rabbit sera (NRS).

rabbit Ig molecules and $F(ab')_2$ fragments (Fig. 4). Comparable $F(ab')_2$ binding was also seen with GM cells (data not shown). Perhaps the most convincing evidence for the presence of both JM and GM surface antigens being present on the clone is shown in Figure 5. After absorption of the rabbit anti-GM-JM-DNA antibody with JM cells, reactivity to JM decreases to approximately background levels. In contrast, however, very little reactivity to GM-JM-DNA cells or GM cells is lost, indicating that the clone has surface antigens associated with both parental cells.

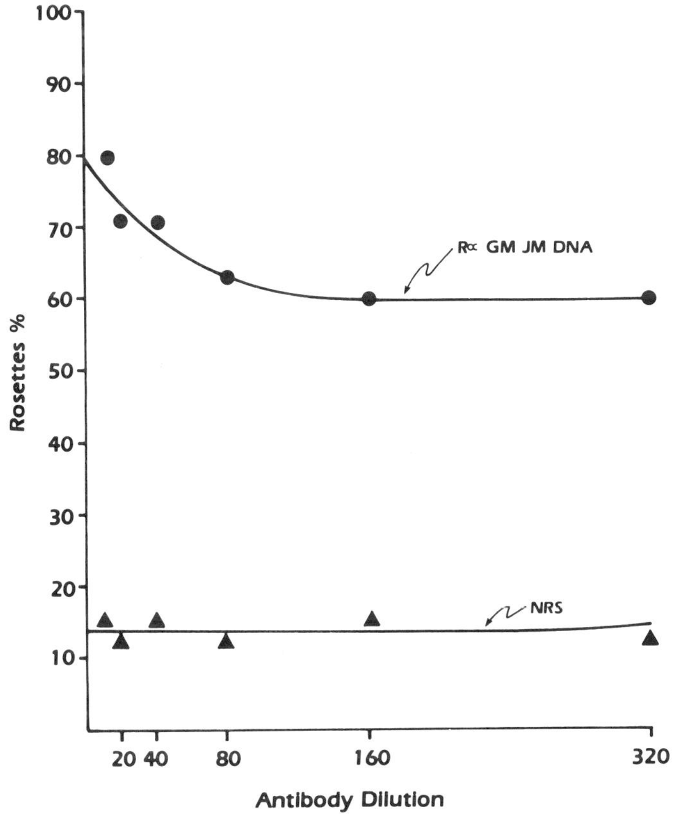

Figure 2 Binding studies of rabbit antisera produced by immunization with the transfected clone GM. In this case, GM cells were incubated with rabbit antisera for 1 hour at 4°C. Cells were then washed and rosetted with human red blood cells coupled by the chromium chloride technique with purified goat anti-rabbit $F(ab')_2$. Control values represent the same cell type sensitized with normal rabbit sera (NRS).

B. Transfection of a T Cell Line with Hybridoma DNA

Since the preceding data indicated that we could construct clones that secreted the appropriate Ig by transfection of normal cells, we endeavored to determine if similar results could be obtained using DNA from already established clones (39, and Chapter 12 of this book). We chose to use as a DNA-recipient, a T cell line which, by definition, is surface Ig-negative and would produce no en-

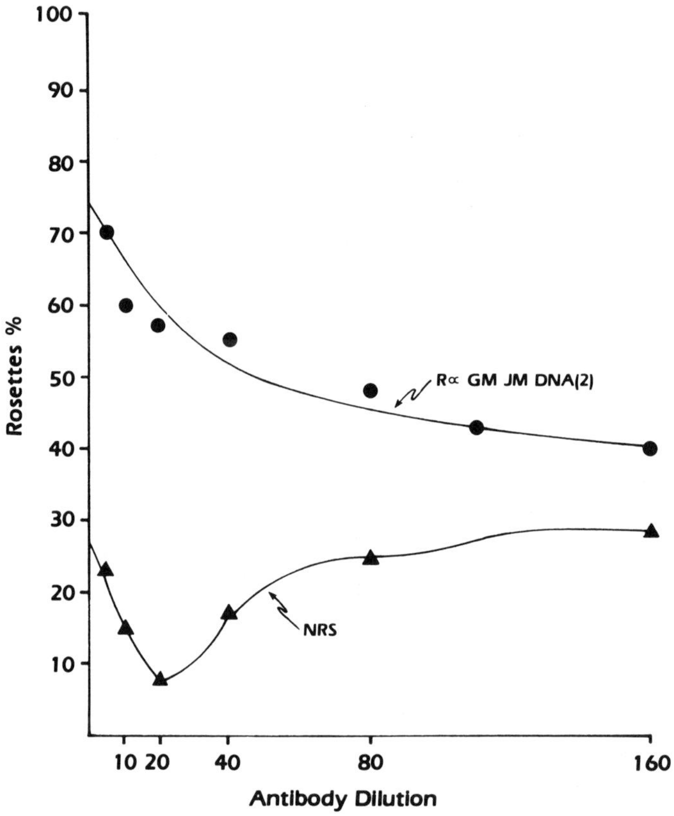

Figure 3 Binding studies of rabbit antisera produced by immunization with the transfected clone JM. In this case, JM cells were incubated with rabbit antisera for 1 hour at 4°C. Cells were then washed and rosetted with human red blood cells coupled by the chromium chloride technique with purified goat anti-rabbit $F(ab')_2$. Control values represent the same cell type sensitized with normal rabbit sera (NRS).

dogenous immunoglobulin. In this way, simple identification of surface or secreted Ig would indicate a successful transfection. Using already established and characterized antibody-producing clones as DNA donors would enable us to determine if specific immunoglobulin genes are transferred during our transfection process.

Transfections were done using 31.5, 21.0, or 10.5 μg/ml of DNA for 2×10^6 JM cells. Transfected cells were placed in culture without any manipulations for

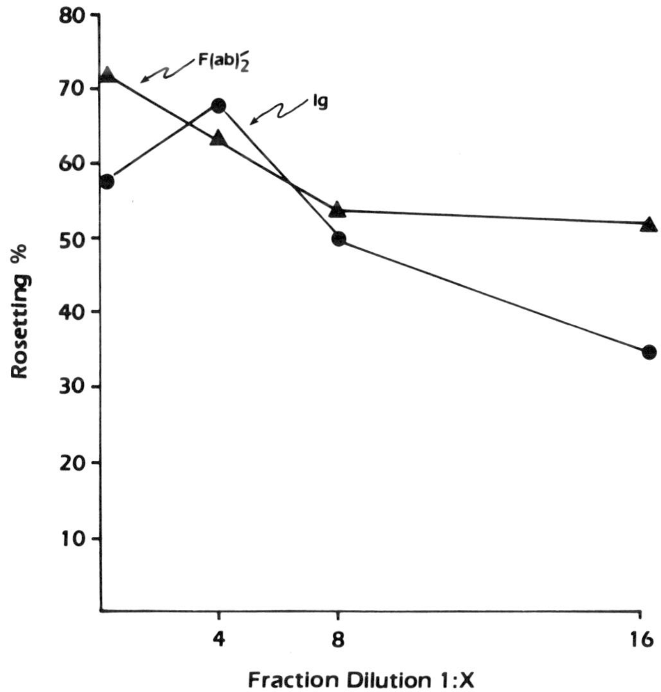

Figure 4 Binding studies were carried out, using both purified total Ig and pepsin-digested purified $F(ab)_2$ fragments of rabbit anti-GM-JM-DNA, to determine whether nonspecific binding due to Fc receptors was giving artifactual results. Once again, the cells were sensitized with either of the antibody preparations at 4°C for 1 hour and washed and rosetted with human red blood cells coupled with goat anti-rabbit $F(ab')_2$.

48 hours. Each putative transfection population was then examined for surface Ig-positive cells on days 2, 4, 6, 12, and 18. Table 2 shows that all of the three populations transfected (designated 6051, 6052, and 6101) had subpopulations of Ig-positive cells, while the control JM cell line did not. Perhaps of greater interest was the observed increase in the size of this Ig-positive subpopulation of cells over time. When supernatants from these populations were tested for binding to SW527, a breast cancer cell line, it was found that values equal to or greater than that of JDB1 (the DNA donor clone) were repeatedly found (Table 3). In order to more precisely examine this reactivity, the 6052 clone was subcloned, and Ig-positive wells were selected and allowed to grow, with the resulting 20 subclones being

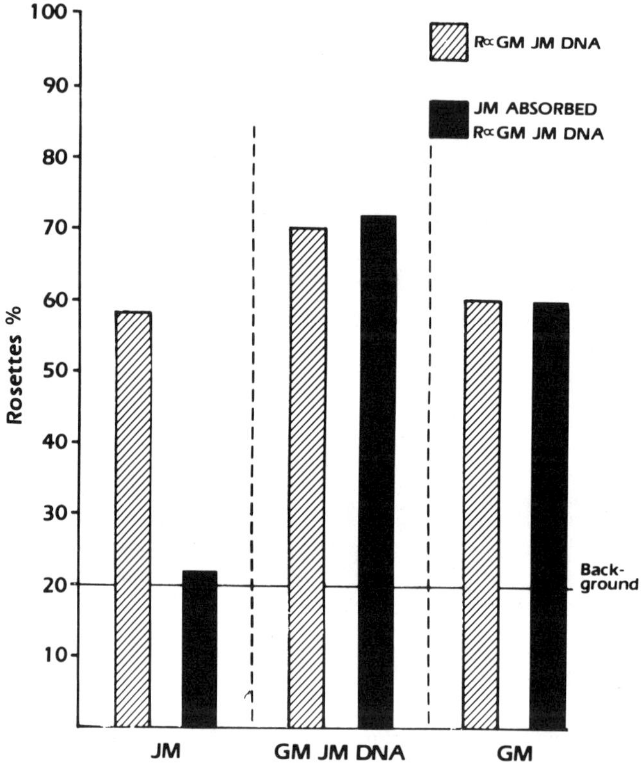

Figure 5 Indirect rosetting was carried out as in Figure 4 to determine the binding of rabbit antisera prepared against GM-JM-DNA before and after absorption with JM cells. Note that the JM cell line used for absorption was the donor of DNA used for absorption was the donor of DNA used to transfect GM cells. Absorptions were carried by incubating 0.5 ml aliquots of complement-inactivated rabbit anti-GM-JM-DNA sera with 0.5 ml packed JM cells for 2 hours at room temperature with continuous stirring. Background levels represent the binding of goat anti-rabbit $F(ab')_2$-coated red cells to cells sensitized with normal rabbit sera.

tested for binding to SW527 (Table 4). Four of these 20 subclones had binding activity equal to or greater than both the original 6052 population and the JDB1 clone from which the DNA was isolated. These four subclones were retained in culture and subsequently retested for binding to SW527 as well as for surface Ig positivity (Table 5). Once again, it was found that three of the four subclones had higher binding percentages with SW527 than did the JDB1 clone from which

Table 2 Surface Ig-Positive Cells After Transfection

Transfected clone	μg/ml DNA used	% Ig-positive cells Day 2	Day 4	Day 6	Day 12	Day 18
6051	31.5	10	32	42	85	16
6052	21.0	15	26	36	78	17
6101	10.5	10	24	36	76	27
JM (control)		3	2	3	0	0

Table 3 Binding of Antibody to SW527 Cells

Clone	% Ig+	% Binding Exp. 1	Exp. 2	Exp. 3
6051	85	76	70	61
6052	78	78	60	42
6101	76	52	50	45
6105	40	32	–	30
JDB1	–	56	52	53

the DNA was isolated. It is also interesting to note there was no apparent correlation with the percentage of Ig-positive cells, amount of Ig produced, or binding levels (Table 5).

1. Cytogenetic Studies

Table 6 shows the karyotypic analysis of each of the subclones compared with the 6052 fusion population from which they originated. In addition, these clones are also compared with JM cells, which were sham transfected with JM-DNA to determine if the transfection process itself could induce cytogenetic alterations. As can be seen, the transfection of JM with JM-DNA does not appear to alter the cells, whereas transfections with clonal DNA show varying kinds of changes with respect to chromosome numbers. Interestingly, some subclones, like SC 27 and SC4, show a variety of cells with varying numbers of chromosomes. In contrast, subclone SC9 is 100% polyploid, with all cells examined containing 90 or more chromosomes. This state of complete polyploidy has not been seen in any of our other experiments with transfection, and the reasons for it are as yet not clear.

Table 4 Binding of Antibody from Subclones of 6052 to SW527 Cells

Subclone (6052)	% Binding on SW527
SC1	24
SC2	6
SC3	22
SC4	73
SC5	32
SC6	26
SC7	22
SC8	36
SC9	52
SC10	54
SC11	10
SC12	20
SC13	24
SC14	12
SC15	30
SC16	36
SC17	6
SC18	56
SC19	26
SC20	8
JDB1	50
Total 6052	48

2. Cell Surface Phenotypic Studies

Although the presence of surface Ig was easily demonstrated (see above), other surface antigens attributable to the transfecting DNA were studied using antisera produced against the transfected subclone (6052 SC10) and absorbed with either the recipient cell line (JM) or the DNA donor line (JDB1). As shown in Figure 6A, the antisera raised against the clone 6052 SC10 is highly reactive with it, even after absorption with JM (the DNA-recipient cell line). As expected, reactivity to the JM cell line can be reduced significantly when absorbed with JM

Table 5 Analysis of Surface Ig Positivity and Antibody Binding to SW527 Cells

Subclone	% Ig	Supernatant Ig conc.	% SW527 binding
SC04	36	1.0 ng/ml	42
SC09	50	3.0 ng/ml	48
SC10	25	5.0 ng/ml	96
SC18	86	7.5 ng/ml	20
JDB1	–	–	58

Ig concentration refers to amount produced over 24-hr period in culture.

Table 6 Analysis of Karyotypes from Transfected Cells

Cell type	JM	JM/JM	6052	SC9	SC10	SC4	SC27
Chromosome no.	46	46	20% 60+	100% 90+	65% 46	85% 46	65% 45
					35% 45	10% 45	25% 46
						5% 90+	5% 44
							5% 90+
Abnormalities	2p-	2p-	2p-	2p-	2p-y-	2p-	2p-

cells (Fig. 6B). In contrast, JM absorption of this sera does not substantially alter the reactivity of this antisera on JDB1 cells (the DNA donor clone) (Fig. 6C). In data not shown, absorption of this antisera with JDB1 cells (the DNA donor clone) shows a dramatic decrease in serum reactivity to JDB1 cells but no diminution of activity toward JM cells. These data indicate that antigens from both the DNA-recipient cells and the DNA donor cells are present on the surface of this transfected clone.

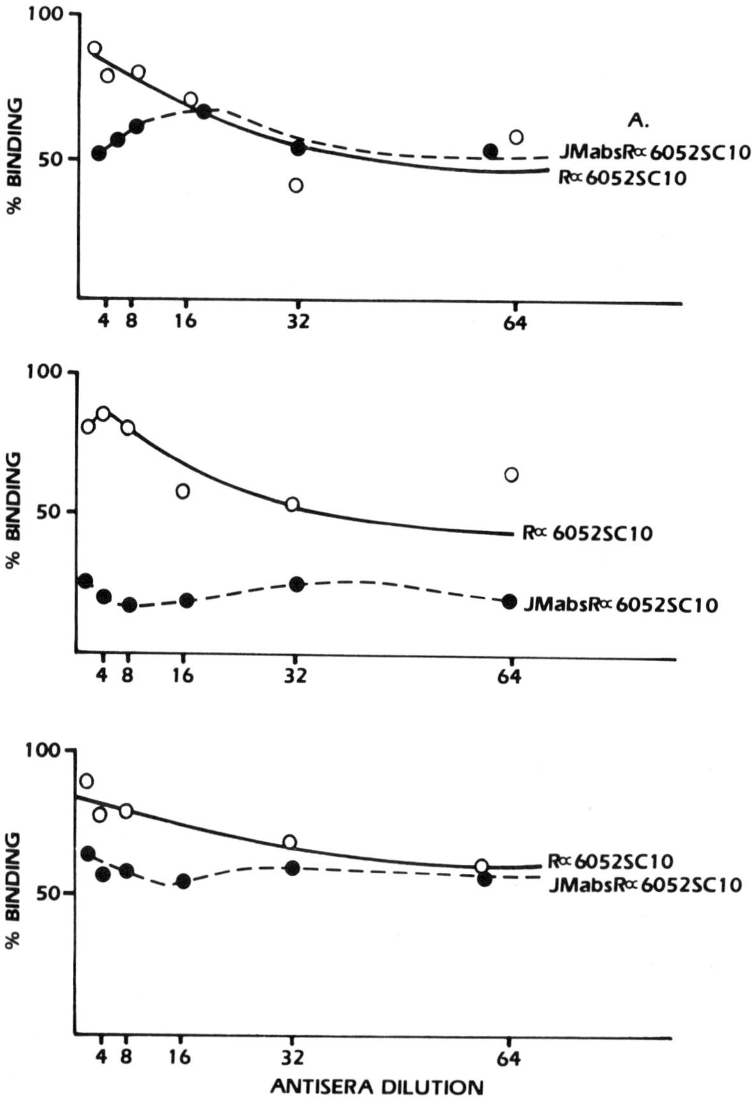

Figure 6 Indirect rosetting as described in Figure 5 was used to determine the binding of rabbit antisera produced against the transfected clone 6052 SC10. (A) The binding of total sera (○) as opposed to sera absorbed, as described in Figure 5, with the cell line JM (●). (B) The binding to the cell line JM of unabsorbed sera (○) as compared with the same sera absorbed with JM cells as described in Figure 5 (●). (C) The binding to JDB1 cells (the hybrid clone used to obtain the DNA used for transfection) of rabbit antisera produced against 6052 SC10 cells and either absorbed (●) or unabsorbed (○) by JM cells.

C. Cytogenetics of Transfection

In order to identify and evaluate the events associated with transfection, ^{3}H-labeled BrdU was incorporated into BALL-1 cells for a period of 48 hours, at which time over 95% of the DNA was labeled. This DNA was then used for transfection of normal human lymphocytes that had been PHA-stimulated. Chromosome spreads from these cells were examined microscopically and by autoradiography at intervals immediately after transfection, but before glycerol shock, immediately after shock, and at 24 hours post-transfection. No uptake of labeled DNA was seen either before or immediately after shock. However, in cells examined after 24 hours, very visible uptake of labeled DNA was seen in chromosomes of the recipient normal PBLs (Fig. 7). Examination of four different chromosome spreads suggested that some chromosomes in the A, C, and E groups may be regularly involved in exogenous DNA uptake (Table 7). However, other chromosomes are apparently not involved in this uptake. In cases where some of the spreads showed involvement of specific chromosomes and some did not, it was assumed that this uptake was random. It should be pointed out that although the examination of only four spreads is not sufficient to reliably prove that these particular chromosomes are routinely susceptible to or involved in the uptake of transfecting DNA, our data suggest this uptake may be more than a series of random events. Interestingly, there is no correlation of chromosomes known to harbor fragile sites with this uptake of transfectant DNA. Unfortunately, transfected cells were not able to be maintained in culture for more than 3 weeks. We feel that this is probably due to the lethal effect of the radioactively labeled DNA used for transfection.

III. CONCLUSIONS

We have clearly shown that it is possible to produce hybrid clones without the necessity for cell-cell fusion. It is obvious that this could facilitate the hybrid construction process since no separation of putative clones and malignant fusion partners is necessary. The DNA used for transfection can easily be kept sterile over chloroform and refrigerated for many months and still be effective for transfection. Additionally, a variety of different DNAs from different cells can be utilized for these strategies. We have shown that the transfection process can be used to transfect normal lymphocytes, thereby producing long-term hybrid cells. In addition, hybrid DNA (i.e., from already established clones) can also be successfully placed into already established long-term cell lines. In view of the consistent problems associated with the construction of stable human hybrid cells, this technology may be of considerable importance in the prolongation of newly developed clones through placement of DNA into established cell lines. We have further illustrated that these types of genetic manipulations result in readily identifiable phenotypic and genotypic changes.

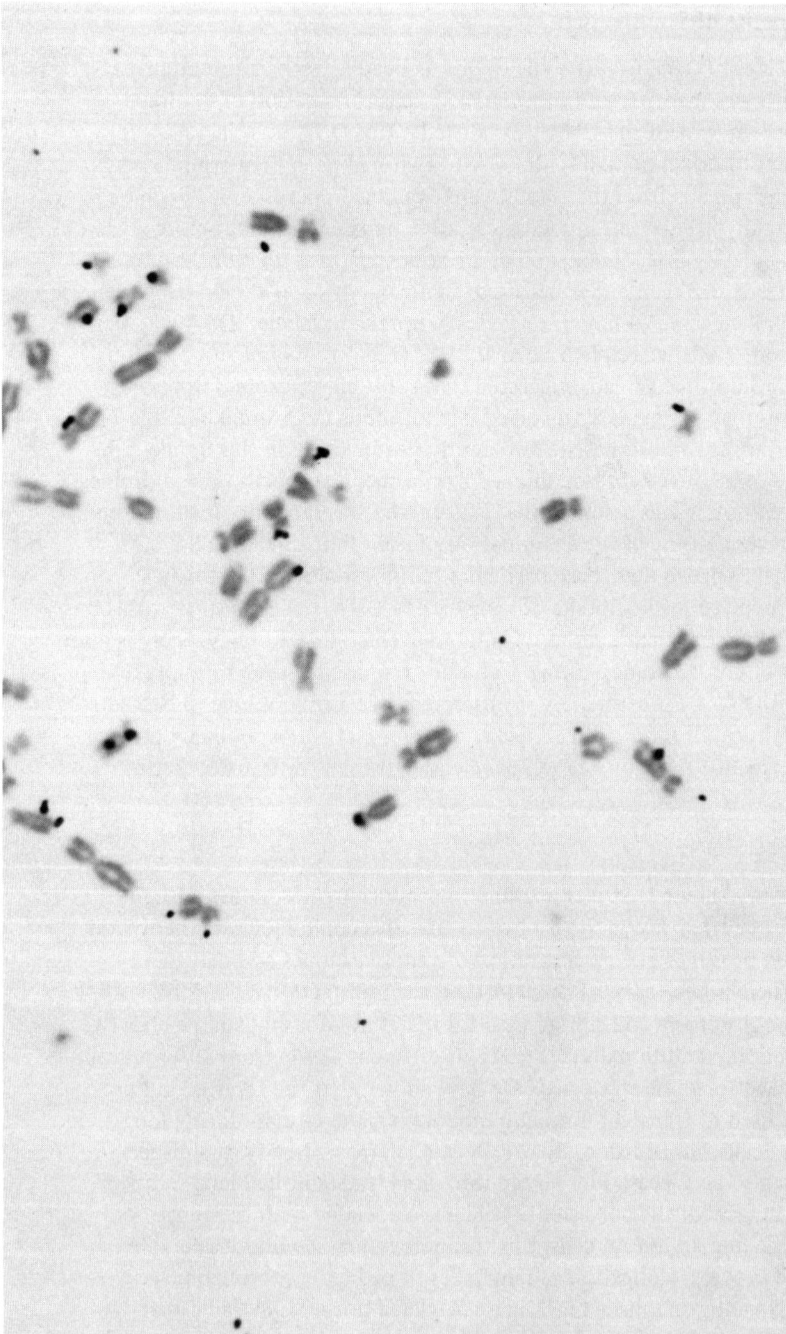

Figure 7 Autoradiographs of chromosome spreads obtained from normal lymphocytes, PHA-stimulated and transfected by Ball-1 DNA-labeled with ^{3}H-Brdu (see text for labeling and transfecting protocols). Autoradiographs were developed for 14 days. Dark circular areas indicate areas of labeled DNA insertions.

Table 7 Uptake of Exogenous DNA After Transfection

Chromosome group		Chromosome spread 1	2	3	4
A	1	+	+	+	+
	2	+	+	+	+
	3	+	+	+	+
B	4	–	–	+	–
	5	–	–	+	+
C	6	+	–	+	–
	7	+	–	–	+
	8	–	–	+	–
	9	+	+	–	–
	10	+	–	+	+
	11	–	+	–	+
	12	+	+	+	+
D	13	–	–	–	–
	14	–	–	+	–
	15	–	–	+	–
E	16	+	–	+	+
	17	+	–	+	+
	18	–	–	–	+
F	19	–	–	–	–
	20	–	–	–	–
G	21	–	–	–	–
	22	–	–	+	+
	X	–	–	+	–
	Y	–	–	–	–

The DNA-mediated transfer of particular traits has been known for quite a long time in mammalian systems, particularly in the case of normal cells transfected with DNA from malignant cells. In this case, the "transformation" of these normal cells could be attributed to a viral of oncogenic event. Several years ago, Wigler *et al.* (10) showed that 20 μg of unfractionated, high molecular weight DNA could be used to successfully transfect APRT-deficient mice.

Other early successful gene transfers into mammalian cells have been reviewed (40). In fact, high-efficiency gene transfer has become almost routine (41).

In many cases, the transfection of cells has been accomplished in systems utilizing enzyme-deficient mutants, such that successful transfection is easily identifiable. However, it has been known for sometime that the transfer of genetic information can lead to phenotypic as well as genotypic changes manifested by the recipient cells (42,43). For instance, it has been demonstrated (28-30) that B lymphoma cells and macrophages can functionally and serologically express proteins coded for by transfecting DNA. The same effect has been well-documented in hamster B cells and L cells induced to express major histocompatibility antigens after transfection (31,32). In many cases, these antigens are serologically indistinguishable from those produced by DNA donor cells (27). This type of experiment with class I MHC antigens has been successful in providing previously unavailable evidence about the identity of molecular domains that are recognized by T cells and alloantibodies (44-47). We have demonstrated the appearance of surface antigens specific for the cells used to obtain DNA on recipient cells through the use of absorbed antisera. These experiments clearly show the presence of surface antigens from both parental cells on transfected cells.

The appearance of antigens specific for DNA donor cells indicates not only cellular uptake, but also transport to and association with nuclear DNA. Further, this exogenous DNA would have to be available in such a form as to be readily transcribed and the resultant RNA translated into identifiable proteins capable of being packaged and transported to the cell surface. In order to understand the events associated with the appearance of these donor phenotypes, it is necessary to envision a series of either translocations or recombinations coupled with highly efficient ligation. This type of high-efficiency ligation and recombination in vertebrate cells has been previously demonstrated by Miller and Temin (48), who showed that transfected cells can mediate ligation and recombination of physically unlinked DNA at nearly 100% efficiency. Further support for transcription, ligation, and recombination events in mammalian systems comes from studies utilizing cloned human 1-antitrypsin genes expressed in hepatoma cells (49), cultured lymphoblasts (50-52), and even pancreatic cells (53) in which transfected genes are readily transcribed. In a recent report, Roth and Wilson (54) defined the relative rates of homologous as well as nonhomologous recombination in transfected DNA.

It should be remembered that most of the current information available concerning the linkage and transcription of transfected DNA concerns experimental designs employing known viral or genetically engineered systems. One of the major drawbacks in defining the relationship between the events associated with gene manipulations and construction of human hybrids is the almost total lack of understanding of the genetic events occurring during cell fusion. This has been further compounded by the tremendous commercial viability of monoclonals, which has, in a sense, caused the scientific and industrial community to bypass fundamental studies in favor of profitability. To date, it remains unclear what genetic events occur when cells are fused. Our data using ^{3}HBrdU indicate that there may be a definite translocation or association of cellular DNA with exogenous transfecting DNA. The requirements for this association are not known, but it may be necessary for the recipient cells to be "receptive." Our experiments using normal cells were all done after cells had been stimulated with PHA. This stimulation could account for the uptake and utilization of exogenous DNA since PHA induces rapid cell division. During these periods of rapid division that require equally rapid DNA synthesis, it may be a simple matter for exogenous DNA to be interjected into forming chromosomes. In a recent report, Reeves *et al.* (55) showed that mammalian cells can rapidly assemble nonintegrated plasmid DNA into "mini-chromosomes." Furthermore, they showed that treatment of transfecting DNA with sodium butyrate can stimulate expression of newly transfected genes by facilitating their assembly into an "active" form. These active forms are apparently associated with nonhistone proteins and are presumed to be more readily transcribed. Our autoradiographs indicate that our transfecting DNA, (which, because of purification, should be relatively histone-free) apparently becomes associated with existing recipient cell chromosomes. This type of association is not currently understood, but the rearrangements of these altered chromosomes coupled with the lack of associated histone proteins in transfected sections may greatly enhance their transcription.

Unquestionably, there is a threshold effect in this transfection procedure because efforts to transfect cells with small amounts of DNA (i.e., $< 5\ \mu g$) have been unsuccessful. There also appears to be an upper limit of approximately 40 μg, above which no increase in transfection is apparent.

Clones produced by transfection appear to be more stable than those obtained in the conventional way. Therefore, because of the ubiquity of DNA, it may be possible to produce stable clones heretofore impossible to construct except through inherently unstable xenogeneic cell fusions.

One of the greatest benefits of transfection in the area of human monoclonals is the potential for increasing the amounts of monoclonal antibody being produced by clones. The paucity of antibody production by human clones has been and continues to be a major problem. If repeated autologous transfections can amplify the number of copies of immunoglobulin genes, the amount of antibody produced by these multiply transfected clones could be greatly enhanced, and recent experiments in our laboratory indicate that this may be the case. More importantly, this type of amplification has been demonstrated and correlated to chromosomal position (56). This type of genetic amplification will also increase the chances of being able to isolate and clone the desired immunoglobulin genes which can then be placed, through vectors, into inexpensive yeast systems, making mass production of these molecules economically feasible.

REFERENCES

1. F. L. Graham and A. J. van der Eb. A new technique for the assay of infectivity of human adenovirus 5 DNA. *Virology, 52*:456 (1973).
2. S. Bacchetti and F. L. Graham. Transfer of the gene for thymidine kinase to thymidine kinase-deficient human cells by purified herpes simplex viral DNA. *Proc. Natl. Acad. Sci. (USA)*, *74*:1590 (1977).
3. K. M. Huttner, G. A. Scangos, and F. J. Ruddle. DNA-mediated gene transfer of a circular plasmid into murine cells. *Proc. Natl. Acad. Sci. (USA)*, *76*: 5820 (1979).
4. N.J. Maitland and J. K. McDougall. Biochemical transformation of mouse cells by fragments of herpes simplex virus DNA. *Cell, 11*:233 (1977).
5. A. C. Minson, P. Wildy, A. Buchan, and G. Darby. Introduction of the herpes simplex virus thymidine kinase gene into mouse cells using virus DNA or transformed cell DNA. *Cell, 13*:581 (1978).
6. L. S. Morse, L. Pereira, B. Roizman, and P. A. Schaffer. Anatomy of herpes simplex virus (HSV) DNA X. Mapping of viral genes by analysis of polypeptides and functions specified by HSV-1 x HSV-2 recombinants. *J. Virol., 26*:389 (1978).
7. R. C. Mulligan and P. Berg. Expression of a bacterial gene in mammalian cells. *Science, 209*:1422 (1980).
8. M. Wigler, S. Silverstein, L. S. Lee, A. Pellicer, Y. C. Cheng, and R. Axel. Transfer of purified herpes virus thymidine kinase gene to cultured mouse cells. *Cell, 11*:23 (1977).
9. M. Wigler, A. Pellicer, S. Silverstein, and R. Axel. Biochemical transfer of single-copy eucaryotic genes using total cellular DNA as donor. *Cell, 14*: 725 (1978).
10. M. Wigler, A. Pellicer, S. Silverstein, R. Axel, G. Urlaub, and L. Chasin. DNA-mediated transfer of the adenine phosphoribosyltransferase locus into mammalian cells. *Proc. Natl. Acad. Sci. (USA)*, *77*:1373 (1979).
11. L. H. Graf, G. Urlaub, and L. Chasin. Transformation of the gene for hypoxanthine phosphoribosyltransferase. *Somatic Cell Genet., 5*:1031 (1979).
12. J. L. Peterson and O. W. McBride. Co-transfer of linked eukaryotic genes and efficient transfer of hypoxanthine phosphoribosyltransferase by DNA-mediated gene transfer. *Proc. Natl. Acad. Sci. (USA)*, *77*:1583 (1980).
13. K. Willecke, M. Klomfass, R. Mierau, and J. Dohmer. Intra-species transfer via total cellular DNA of the gene for hypoxanthine phosphoribosyltransferase into cultured mouse cells. *Mol. Gen. Genet., 170*:179 (1979).
14. M. Wigler, M. Perucho, D. Kurtz, S. Dana, A. Pellicer, R. Axel, and S. Silverstein. Transformation of mammalian cells with an amplifiable dominant-acting gene. *Proc. Natl. Acad. Sci. (USA)*, *77*:3567 (1980).
15. G. H. Yoakum, J. F. Lechner, E. W. Gabrielson, B. E. Korba, L. Malan-Shibley, J. C. Willey, M. G. Valerio, A. M. Shamsuddin, B. F. Trump, and C. C. Harris. Transformation of human bronchial epithelial cells transfected by Harvey ras oncogene. *Science, 227*:1174 (1985).

16. J. M. Bishop. Cellular oncogenes and retroviruses. *Ann. Rev. Biochem., 52*: 301 (1983).
17. D. G. Thomassen, T. M. Gilmer, L. A. Annab, and I. C. Bargett. Evidence for multiple steps in neoplastic transformation of normal and preneoplastic Syrian hamster embryo cells following transfection with Harvey murine sarcoma virus oncogene (V-Ha-ras). *Cancer Res., 45*:726 (1985).
18. G. H. Yoakum, B. E. Korba, J. F. Lechner, T. Tokiwa, A. F. Gazdar, T. Seeley, M. Siegal, L. Leeman, H. Autrup, and C. C. Harris. High-frequency transfection and cytopathology of the hepatitis B virus core antigen gene in human cells. *Science, 222*:385 (1983).
19. J. Doniger, J. A. DiPaolo, and M. C. Popescu. Transformation of Blooms syndrome fibroblasts by DNA transfection. *Science, 222*:1144 (1983).
20. J. L. Marx. Specific expression of transferred genes. *Science, 222*:1001 (1983).
21. A. Ochi, R. G. Hawley, T. Hawley, M. J. Schulman, A. Traunecker, G. Kohler, and N. Hozumi. Functional immunoglobulin M production after transfection of cloned immunoglobulin heavy and light chain genes into lymphoid cells *Proc. Natl. Acad. Sci. (USA), 80*:6351 (1983).
22. D. T. Kurtz. Hormonal inducibility of rat 2 μ globulin genes in transfected mouse cells. *Nature, 291*:629 (1981).
23. D. M. Robins, I. Pack, P. H. Seeburg, and R. Axel. Regulated expression of human growth hormone genes in mouse cells. *Cell, 29*:623 (1982).
24. N. Mantei and C. Weissman. Controlled transcription of a human-interferon gene introduced into mouse L cells. *Nature, 297*:128 (1982).
25. J. Stafford and C. Queen. Cell-type specific expression of a transfected immunoglobulin gene. *Nature, 306*:77 (1983).
26. Z. L. Jonak, V. Braman, and R. F. Kennett. Production of continuous mouse plasma cell lines by transfection with human leukemia DNA. *Hybridoma, 3*: 107 (1984).
27. A. Ben-Nun, E. Choi, K. R. McIntyre, S. A. Leeman, D. J. McKean, J. G. Seidman, and L. H. Glimcher. DNA mediated transfer of major histocompatibility class II I-A^b and I-A^{bm12} genes into B lymphoma cells: molecular and functional analysis of introduced antigens. *J. Immunol., 135*:1456 (1985).
28. A. Ben-Nun, L. H. Glimcher, J. Weis, and J. G. Seidman. Functional expression of a cloned I-A^k gene in B lymphoma cells. *Science, 223*:825 (1984).
29. R. N. Germain, M. A. Norcross, and D. H. Margulies. Functional expression of a transfected murine class II MHC gene. *Nature, 306*:190 (1983).
30. V. Folsom, D. P. Gold, J. White, P. Marrack, J. Kappler, and S. Tonegawa. Functional and inducible expression of a transfected murine class II major histocompatibility complex gene. *Proc. Natl. Acad. Sci. (USA), 81*:2045 (1984).
31. C. Rabourdin-Combe and B. Mach. Expression of HLA-DR antigens at the surface of mouse L-cells co-transfected with cloned human genes. *Nature, 303*:670.
32. B. Malissen, M. Peele Price, J. M. Goverman, M. McMillan, J. White, J. Kap-

pler, P. Marrack, A. Pierres, M. Pierres, and L. Hood. Gene transfer of H-2 class II genes: antigen presentation by mouse fibroblast and hamster B cell lines. *Cell, 36*:319 (1984).

33. H. Golding, J. Bluestone, M. L. Satz, D. Singer, and A. Singer. Generation of primary murine CTL specific for allogeneic and xenogeneic MHC determinants upon stimulation with murine L cells transfected with class I genes. *J. Immunol., 134*:3557 (1985).
34. D. H. Margulies, G. A. Evans, K. Ozato, D. Camerini-Otero, K. Tanak, E. Appella, and J. G. Seidman. Expression of H-2d^{d} and H-2L^{d} mouse major histocompatibility antigen genes in L cells after DNA-mediated gene transfer. *J. Immunol., 130*:463 (1983).
35. B. Malissen, M. Steinmetz, M. McMillan, M. Pierres, and L. Hood. Expression I-A^{k} class II genes in mouse L-cells after DNA-mediated gene transfer. *Nature, 305*:440 (1984).
36. A. L. Mellor, L. Golden, E. Weiss, H. Bullman, J. Hurst, E. Simpson, R. F. L. James, A. R. M. Townsend, P. M. Taylor, W. Schmidt, J. Ferluga, L. Leben, M. Santamaria, G. Atfield, H. Festenstein, and R. A. Flavell. Expression of murine H-2K^{b} histocompatibility antigen in cells transformed with cloned H-2 genes. *Nature, 298*:529 (1982).
37. N. Emi, R. Ueda, and T. Takahashi. Isolation of stable mouse L cell transfectants expressing human T cell differentiation antigen Tp40. *J. Immunol., 134*:2817 (1985).
38. M. Gross-Bellard, P. Dudet, and P. Chambon. Isolation of high-molecular weight DNA from mammalian cells. *Eur. J. Biochem., 36*:32 (1973).
39. A. J. Strelkauskas and C. L. Taylor. Human monoclonal antibody: construction of stable clones reactive with human breast cancer. (In press, *Cancer Immunol. Immunother.*)
40. G. Scangos and F. H. Ruddle. Mechanisms and applications of DNA mediated gene transfer in mammalian cells—a review. *Gene, 14*:1 (1981).
41. C. M. Gorman, D. P. Lane, and P. W. J. Rigby. High efficiency gene transfer into mammalian cells. *Phil. Trans. R. Soc. Lond., B307*:343 (1984).
42. A. Pellicer, D. Robins, B. Wold, R. Sweet, J. Jackson, I. Lowy, J. M. Roberts, G. K. Sim, S. Silverstein, and R. Axel. Altering genotype and phenotype by DNA-mediated gene transfer. *Science, 209*:1414 (1980).
43. J. G. Collard, W. P. van Beck, J. W. G. Janssen, and J. F. Schuven. Transfection by human oncogenes: concomitant induction of tumorigenicity and tumor-associated membrane alterations. *Int. J. Cancer, 35*:207 (1985).
44. K. Ozato, G. A. Evans, G. Shykind, D. H. Margulies, and J. G. Seidman. Hybrid H-2 histocompatibility gene products assigns domains recognized by alloreactive T cells. *Proc. Natl. Acad. Sci. (USA), 80*:2040 (1983).
45. C. S. Reiss, G. A. Evans, D. H. Margulies, J. G. Seidman, and S. J. Burakoff. Allospecific and virus specific cytolytic T lymphocytes are restricted to the N or Cl domaine of H-2 antigens expressed on L cells after DNA-mediated gene transfer. *Proc. Natl. Acad. Sci. (USA), 80*:2709 (1983).
46. M. A. Norcross, D. M. Bentley, D. H. Margulies, and R. M. Germain. Mem-

brane Ia expression and antigen presenting accessory cell function of L-cells transfected with class II MHC genes. *J. Exp. Med., 160*:1316 (1984).
47. B. Arnold, H. G. Burgert, U. Harmann, G. Hammerling, V. Kees, and S. Kvist. Cytolytic T cells recognize the two amino terminal domains $H\text{-}2^k$ antigens in tandem in influenza A infected cells. *Cell, 38*:79 (1984).
48. C. K. Miller and H. M. Temin. High-efficiency ligation and recombination of DNA fragments by vertebrate cells. *Science, 220*:606 (1983).
49. G. Ciliberto, L. Dente, and R. Cortese. Cell specific expression of a transfected human 1-antitrypsin gene. *Cell, 41*:531 (1985).
50. J. Banerji, L. Olson, and W. Schaffner. A lymphocyte-specific cellular enhancer is located downstream of the joining region in immunoglobulin heavy chain genes. *Cell, 33*:729 (1983).
51. S. D. Gillies, S. L. Morrison, V. T. Oi, and S. Tonegawa. A tissue-specific transcription enhancer element is located in the major intron of a rearranged immunoglobulin heavy chain gene. *Cell, 33*:717 (1983).
52. C. Queen and D. Baltimore. Immunoglobulin gene transcription is activated by downstream sequence elements. *Cell, 33*:741 (1983).
53. M. D. Walker, T. Edlund, A. M. Boulet, and M. J. Ruttler. Cell-specific expression controlled by the 5′ flanking region of insulin and chymotrypsin genes. *Nature, 300*:557 (1983).
54. D. B. Roth and J. H. Wilson. Relative rates of homologous and nonhomologous recombination in transfected DNA. *Proc. Natl. Acad. Sci. (USA), 82*: 3355 (1985).
55. R. Reeves, C. M. Gorman, and B. Howard. Mini chromosome assembly of non-integrated plasmid DNA transfected into mammalian cells. *Nuc.Acids Res., 13*:3599 (1985).
56. G. M. Wahl, B. R. deSaint Vincent, and M. L. Derase. Effect of chromosomal position on amplification of transfected genes in animal cells. *Nature, 307*: 516 (1984).

II

SOME APPLICATIONS OF HUMAN MONOCLONAL ANTIBODIES

8

Applications of Human Monoclonal Antibodies in Oncology

LLOYD H. SMITH and NELSON N. H. TENG
Stanford University School of Medicine, Stanford, California

The promise of human hybridomas in the field of oncology has been the production of safe, effective, and highly specific reagents for the diagnosis and treatment of cancer. In addition, detailed dissection of the human immune response to cancer is possible only by using human hybridoma technology. However, technical difficulties in the production of human hybridomas have delayed efforts to produce human monoclonal antibodies (MAbs) with the facility possible using murine systems. Unfortunately, a clear demonstration of specific cancer-associated antigens in human cancer or of specific immune responses to such antigens has been elusive. Finally, a clear advantage of human versus murine MAbs for *in vivo* use in human cancer is still only theoretical. Despite these difficulties, much progress has been made, and in this chapter, we review the current status of human MAbs in oncology by addressing the following questions: (a) What are the technical problems in human hybridoma technology? (b) How specific is the human immune response to cancer? (c) What is the role of human MAbs in cancer diagnosis and therapy?

I. HUMAN HYBRIDOMA TECHNOLOGY: WHAT ARE THE TECHNICAL PROBLEMS?

A. Fusion Partners

1. Malignant Fusion Partners

Mouse Myelomas as Fusion Partners. In contrast to mouse or rat myeloma cell lines, only a few permanent human myeloma cell lines have been established and generally have unfavorable characteristics for use as fusion partners (e.g., slow growing and low yield of hybrids). Consequently, alternative methods have been employed to generate immortalized human immunoglobulin (Ig)-producing cells. The fusion of human lymphocytes with hypoxanthine/aminopterin/thymidine (HAT)-sensitive mouse myeloma cells to create human-mouse hybridomas is easily achieved (1-4), but hybrids are typically unstable and cease production of Ig because of chromosome loss (5,6) or altered gene expression (7). However, exceptions to this phenomenon have been reported (8-10). In parallel but independent work from the same laboratory, Ig secretion by mouse-human clones was found to be as stable as that by human-human clones in one study (10), yet only half as stable after the second subculture in a second study (11). Others (12,13) have reported that stable Ig-secreting mouse-human hybrid clones can be derived by repeated subcloning. The main advantage of employing mouse myeloma fusion partners in the generation of human MAbs appears to be a very high initial yield of hybrid clones, though the ultimate percentage of stable Ig-secreting clones may be inferior to that obtained utilizing some human malignant fusion partners (4).

Human Myeloid or Lymphoblastoid Derivatives as Fusion Partners. A large number of HAT-sensitive malignant fusion partners derived from strictly human sources have been described, many of which are derivatives of human myeloma cell lines (e.g., SKO-007 [14] and RPMI-8226 [15,16]). Others are derivatives of plasma cell leukemia lines (e.g., LICR-LON-HMy2 [17]), lymphoblastoid cell lines (e.g., GM-1500 [18], GM-4672 [19], GK-5 [20], UC729-6/HF2 [21,22], LTR228 [21,23], and H35.1.1 [24]), or B cell lymphoma lines (e.g., RH-L4 [25]). A hybrid line (KR-12), the product of fusion between a lymphoblastoid cell line and a myeloma line (RPMI-8226), has also been described as a fusion partner (26).

Though direct comparison has not been reported for all available fusion partners, variability must exist in fusion frequency, amount of Ig secretion, growth rate, and presence of Epstein-Barr nuclear antigen (EBNA). Reported rates of hybrid formation may be misleading when used to compare fusion partners. Only a few direct comparisons have been published. The median number of clones per 10^7 lymphocytes, given in brackets, has been reported (27) for a number of cell lines as follows: NS-1 [50], LICR-2 [7], SKO-007 [1.5], UC729-6 [12], and GM-4672 [1]. Direct experimental comparison of six human malignant fusion partners (U-266, LICR-LON-HMy2, UC729-6, UC729-6-HF_2, GM4672, and RPMI-8226) and a mouse myeloma line (NS1) for ability to form Ig-secreting clones after fusion of lymphocytes from a patient with leukemia has also been reported (4). The number of hybrid clones formed per 100 wells seeded was highest for NS1 (80%), while UC729-6 (51%) and UC729-6-HF_2 (46%) fused more efficiently than U-266 (38%) or LICR-LON-HMy2 (17%). The percentage of hybrid clones that secreted Ig, however, was highest for LICR-LON-HMy2 (67%). Besides low fusion frequencies, the presence of EBNA in many of these cell lines confers another theoretically unfavorable attribute. Thus, certain cell lines may have both favorable and unfavorable characteristics; the ideal human fusion partner with fusion efficiency rivaling that of mouse myeloma partners, fast growth rate, Ig nonsecreting, and EBNA-negative has not been described.

Interspecies Hybridomas as Fusion Partners. In order to retain some of the favorable characteristics of mouse myeloma fusion partners, and yet allow for secretion of human Ig, interspecies hybrid lines have been produced. Teng *et al.* (28) have reported construction of heteromyelomas for the production of human hybridomas. The heteromyeloma lines were constructed using the human myeloma line FU-266 altered by protoplast transfection of a dominant drug resistance marker (29), followed by fusion with gamma-irradiated mouse myeloma cells. The resultant drug-selected clones have been tested as fusion partners (30). One of the clones, SHM-D33, contained four to five human chromosomes, secreted no measurable Ig, possessed favorable growth characteristics, formed stable Ig-secreting hybrids with high efficiency, and was subsequently employed in the production of several human MAbs recognizing Rhesus (RH_0(D) antigen (31) and gram-negative bacterial endotoxin (32).

Foung *et al.* (33) have described the derivation of cell line SBC-H20, a HAT-sensitive Ig-nonsecreting clone produced after fusion of a mouse myeloma cell line with normal human peripheral blood lymphocytes. The SBC-H20 line was shown to be stable for cell surface expression of human HLA antigens, and was utilized to produce a human MAb recognizing blood group A antigen by fusion with an EBV-transformed cell line secreting the same antibody. The SBC-H20 line was also shown to form hybrid clones with unstimulated or mitogen-stimulated human peripheral blood lymphocytes.

Although some interspecies hybrid lines appear to fuse well and form stable hybridomas secreting human Igs, there are potential disadvantages. For example, theoretically, post-translational modification of human MAbs made in interspecies hybridoma cells could render them immunogenic and, therefore, less useful than human MAbs produced from an entirely human cell.

2. The Human Lymphocyte Partner

The Source of Lymphocytes. The potential sources of lymphocytes from cancer patients for hybridoma study include peripheral blood (PB), lymph nodes (LN), and intratumoral (IT) lymphocytes. Since LN lymphocytes are exposed to many immunogens carried in the afferent lymph, and IT lymphocytes are directly stimulated by the tumor milieu, it is not surprising that lymphocytes from these sources form hybridomas more readily than do PB lymphocytes. Lymph node lymphocytes consistently fuse more efficiently (three- to 50-fold) than do PB lymphocytes when human cell lines are used as fusion partners (10, 22,34,35), though the phenomenon may be less pronounced when mouse myelomas are used as fusion partners (10,27,34). In addition to being more efficient in hybridoma formation than PB lymphocytes, LN and IT lymphocytes should be enriched in B cells sensitized to tumor-associated antigens, and have been reported (36) to yield a larger number of hybrids secreting Ig that react with cancer cells.

Despite the advantage of LN or IT lymphocytes, nodes and tumor are not always available for study, and consequently PB lymphocytes represent the most readily available source of human lymphocytes for hybridoma work. Although the PB lymphocyte pool theoretically contains B cells sensitized to a variety of immunogens, specific B cells are in a low concentration and often in a resting state, incompatible with successful cell fusion. Specific recirculating memory B cells in individuals known to be immune by serologic analysis may be totally absent from the PB lymphocyte pool, but sequestered elsewhere in lymphoid tissue (37). In the most optimistic estimate, the fraction of B cells specific for a given cancer-associated antigen among the total PB B cell population might be comparable with the maximum percentage (approximately 1%) of specific B cells observed after vaccination with specific immunogens (34). However, such a response could be quite transient or affected by individual differences in immune response genotype. Alternatively, because such a response would depend on B-cell proliferation *in vivo,* it could be dramatically reduced or ablated by radiation or chemotherapy. In addition, the yield of B lymphocytes from the PB is low (10^7 per 50 ml) as is the frequency of successful fusion (approximately 10^{-5}), and perhaps even lower for unstimulated resting lymphocytes. Consequently, the chances of deriving desired hybridoma clones from cancer patients using PB lymphocytes is low unless measures are adopted to stimulate and expand the B cell population (e.g., mitogen stimulation, EBV transformation) or enrich it for antigen-specific cells (e.g., *in vitro* sensitization, *in vivo* immunization).

Lymphocyte Stimulation or Enhancement Prior to Fusion.

Mitogen Stimulation. Though prestimulation of PB lymphocytes with pokeweek mitogen (PWM) clearly enhances hybrid formation between human lymphocytes and either mouse or human fusion partners by a factor of two- to 10-fold (23,25,38,39), there are several disadvantages to the use of polyclonal B-cell activators, including the following: (a) although there is stimulation, differentiation, and expansion of the PB B-lymphocytes, there is no enrichment for specific B-cells which may remain rare (34); (b) mitogen-stimulated lymphocytes are not immortal—they cannot be grown continuously to serve as a source for continued experimentation; (c) Ig secretion by mitogen-stimulated lymphocytes may continue for weeks and may be mistaken for secretion by emerging hybrid clones; (d) there is large variation in response to PWM of PB lymphocytes from different individuals, probably based on differences in the populations of T cells that enhance or suppress B-cell proliferation, thereby limiting the reproducibility of the result (40); and (e) PWM also stimulates proliferation of T cells (80% of PB lymphocytes) that may compete during fusion or suppress B-cell proliferation.

Even without mitogen stimulation, removal of T cells has been reported to increase hybrid formation efficiency five- to 20-fold (11). Therefore removal of T cells prior to mitogen stimulation might be expected to enhance B-cell proliferation and hybrid formation. Because PWM activation of B cells is highly T cell-dependent (40,42,43), T cells removed prior to PWM stimulation must be treated with sublethal doses of radiation or mitotic inhibitors to prevent division and then added back to supply the permissive T-cell function. Such treatment also has the advantage of abrogating T-suppressor activity, and may result in high fusion frequencies (23).

Other methods have also been reported for avoiding the potential problems associated with T-cell activation by mitogens and could be useful for human hybridoma work with PB lymphocutes. These include: (a) stimulation of T cell-depleted PB lymphocytes using the T cell-independent polyclonal B-cell mitogen, formalin-fixed *Staphylococcus aureus* Cowan (43); (b) depletion of suppressor T cells from PB lymphocytes by passage over columns of Sephadex (44,45); and (c) inhibition of suppressor T cells by cimetidine (46) or their removal by panning on cimetidine-coated plates (47).

Epstein-Barr Virus (EBV) Transformation. Human MAbs have been derived by production of EBV-transformed human B cell lines secreting antibody to specific antigens (48; for review, see 49). The major technical difficulties that have limited this approach to the production of human MAbs include the small amounts of secreted antibody and instability of the EBV-transformed cell lines. Though some workers have dealt successfully with these problems (49,50) others have reported success in producing human hybridomas using EBV-transformed lymphocytes, resulting in enhanced stability and antibody secretion, as well as increased rates of hybrid recovery when compared with the use of untransformed lymphocytes (for reviews see 51,52). Among many human MAbs now reported to have been produced by the EBV hybridoma technique are human MAbs to tetanus toxoid (53), blood group Rh D antigen (31), lung cancer-associated antigens (36), blood group A antigen (33), *M. leprae* (51), and *Pseudomonas aeruginosa* (52).

Major advantages of the EBV hybridoma technique include the ability to cultivate and preserve mixtures of EBV-transformed lymphocyte cell populations for continued experimentation and the enhanced fusion frequency just mentioned. There are also several potential disadvantages, including the following: (a) Since EBV transformation can elicit a cytotoxic response in T cells from immune individuals, resulting in loss of proliferating EBV-infected B cells, T cells must be removed prior to EBV transformation (49). Incomplete removal of T cells could result in variability of the result. Monocytes in the PB mononuclear cell preparation may act as feeder cells necessary for successful proliferation (49); their loss may also create variability. (b) Successful EBV transformation may be affected by mycoplasma contamination of the EBV stock or other technical variables associated with EBV preparation (49). (c) Only a small fraction (1% or less) of PB B-lymphocytes are transformed into Ig-secreting cell lines by optimal EBV infection (49,50). Consequently, there is a reduction in the probability of producing B cell clones of the desired specificity when compared with methods that activate a larger fraction of the B cell population (e.g., mitogens). However, EBV-transformed lymphocytes appear to be much more efficient as fusion partners than even PWM-stimulated lymphocytes. The overall difference in the probability of recovering a desired B cell clone after fusion of EBV-transformed versus mitogen-stimulated lymphocytes is therefore off-set, though a somewhat larger diversity of B cell specificities would be expected among the mitogen-stimulated clones. (d) Human MAbs derived by the EBV hybridoma method are predominantly of the IgM class. Although IgM antibodies may be less effective *in vivo* than certain IgG subclasses in mediating antibody-directed cytotoxicity, their use as immunoconjugates with cytotoxic agents may avoid such limitations. (e) The *in vivo* use of products produced by EBV-transformed cells may be hazardous due to the presence of virus or transforming DNA. However, the EBV genome has been shown to be lost during hybrid formation in some cases (31). The possibility of HTLV or other retrovirus contamination of products derived from both mouse and human hybridomas must also be assessed prior to *in vivo* utilization.

Preselection of Antigen-Specific Lymphocytes. When the antigen for which a human MAb is desired is available, it can be employed to enrich the B lymphocyte population for antigen-specific cells. A variety of methods have been reported including the following: (a) rosetting with antigen-coated red blood cells (49); (b) panning or adsorption on antigen-coated plates (54); (c) antigen-induced cell capping and subsequent removal of antigen-nonbinding cells (55); (d) fluorescence-activated cell-sorting of cells with fluorescence-labeled antigen (55); (e) antigen-mediated hybridoma formation using pulsed high-voltage electric fields (56); and (f) *in vitro* antigen priming of B lymphocytes by a variety of techniques, resulting in stimulation, proliferation, and differentiation of antigen-specific cells (37,38,49,52,57,58). Such techniques could be useful in deriving human MAbs to cancer-associated antigen which are poor immunogens *in vivo.*

Enhancement by Immunization. Enhancement of B cell immunity specific for certain cancer-associated antigens is theoretically possible by immunization of patients using autologous or allogenic cancer cells or extracts. For example, the majority of melanoma patients vaccinated with irradiated cultured melanoma cells, as part of a controlled trial of adjuvant immunotherapy, showed a boosted serologic response to the melanoma-associated oncofetal antigen, which was separable from a response to alloantigens (59).

In a different approach, Newcastle Diseased Virus lysates of autologous tumor cells have also been administered as vaccines to melanoma patients (60,61). In a phase II study on the effect of Newcastle Disease Virus oncolysate vaccination on stage II melanoma patients, survival was dramatically improved compared with that in a historical control group (62). An augmented B cell response to cancer-associated antigens would be expected in cancer patients vaccinated with autologous viral oncolysates and would, therefore, enhance recovery of hybridomas secreting human MAbs to such antigens. Immunization of cancer patients with autologous viral oncolysate has the potential disadvantage of also augmenting the immune response to nonspecific cellular antigens. However, more specific cancer-associated antigens may become more immunogenic within oncolysates, allowing hybrid formation with "useful" B cell clones that would otherwise be too rare for recovery.

Vaccination of patients following surgery for stage B or C colorectal cancer has recently been reported (63). Viable, dissociated, autologous tumor cells were gamma-irradiated and combined with viable BCG organisms prior to vaccinations. Vaccinated patients not only showed significantly enhanced disease-free survival, but their PB lymphocytes were an efficient source of activated B cells used in the formation of hybridomas secreting human MAbs to colorectal cancer-associated antigens (64).

Immunization with synthetic peptide antigens having sequence homology with certain oncoproteins (65) may be of future benefit in cancer prevention and therapy. Such an approach might also enhance the efficiency of production of desired human MAbs.

B. Screening for Human MAbs to Cancer-Associated Antigens

1. Cell Lines and Tumor Heterogeneity

Cultured cell lines provide an attractive source of target cells for the purpose of screening human hybridoma supernatants for binding activity. Cell lines can often be established from normal and malignant tissue of individual patients. Consequently, there are many cell lines available, and cell suspensions are conveniently employed in a variety of immunoassays for common cancer-associated antigens. Cell lines can be grown in the absence of human Ig, thus avoiding the nonspecific binding as detected by any second antibody techniques. Theoretically, however, screening with cell lines could result in nonidentification of important hybridoma clones secreting MAbs to cancer-associated antigens. Malignant tumors from both human and nonhuman sources are not homogeneous with respect to cellular characteristics (e.g., growth rate, sensitivity to drugs, expression of cellular antigens), but rather are heterogeneous (66-68). Because of this *in vivo* phenotypic diversity, cell lines established *in vitro* may preserve only a segment of the antigen expression present among the tumor cell population *in vivo*. Even cloned lines may exhibit modulation or loss of antigenic expression under certain growth conditions *in vitro* (66,69,70). Although *in vivo* variability in antigenic expression may represent genetically determined variation, other mechanisms are probably also important. For example, subtle changes in glycolipid metabolism may result in changes in the structure of the plasma membrane or glycocalyx, resulting in expression of new antigens, the unmasking of cryptic epitopes, or the loss of other antigenic determinants (71). Regardless of the mechanisms of heterogeneity, the use of cell lines as targets for the screening of hybridomas has the potential short-coming of misrepresenting the range of antigenic phenotypes observed *in vivo*.

2. Tissue Sections and Endogenous Immunoglobulin

Screening hybridoma supernatants for binding to tissue sections of primary or metastatic tumors can be accomplished using immunofluorescent or immunoperoxidase techniques, and has the advantage of allowing demonstration of the *in vivo* heterogeneity of antigen expression (72,73). The use of both parafin-embedded and cryostat sections has been reported, though formaldehyde, parafin, and organic solvents may adversely affect the detection of some cancer-associated antigens (74). A major disadvantage to the use of tissue sections is the presence of endogenous human Ig. Because secondary antibody techniques are usually employed to detect human MAb binding, endogenous human Ig will also be detected, creating a high "background" and possibly obscuring detection of MAb binding to less prominent antigens. Titration of the second antibody has been reported to produce acceptable background (73), but doing this must favor the detection of higher affinity MAbs or MAb binding to more plentiful and, perhaps, polyvalent determinants such as glycolipids (68). This process could result in missing the less abundant but, perhaps, more specific determinants (e.g., univalent peptide epitopes).

Aside from the problem of nonspecific background due to endogenous Ig, the patient's own humoral response may obscure the detection of desired MAbs. If the sites in tissue sections of specific cancer-associated antigens are occupied by high-avidity antibody, such antibody will be detected as part of the endogenous Ig background but will also block MAb binding to the same determinants. MAb binding to the most specific antigens may, therefore, be reduced or go undetected. The use of unlabeled secondary antibody to "block" endogenous human Ig (73) will not improve this hypothetical problem. In fact, membrane-bound Ig may be detected on the tumor cells removed from patients with a variety of malignant diseases (75), though such binding could be nonspecific (e.g., Fc receptors, autoantigens). Although primary tumor cell culture or passage of tumors in nude mice could potentially remove endogenous Ig from tumor cells and tissues prior to use in screening, such treatment carries the risk of distorting *in vivo* antigen expression. To our knowledge, chemical methods that would release endogenous human Ig from tissue sections without altering the integrity of antigen expression have not been reported.

Another problem associated with the use of tissue sections for screening hybridoma supernatants arises because of the heterogeneity of antigen expression. A wide quantitative variation in the expression of target antigen may be present in cancer or normal tissues. Screening with an inadequate MAb concentration may not detect antigen present within some tumors or different cells of the same tumor (76).

3. Cell Surface Versus Cytoplasmic Antigens

Human MAbs to cancer-associated cell surface (CS) antigens may have certain advantages in immunodiagnosis and therapy compared with MAbs directed to internal cellular structures, which may be less available *in vivo*. A variety of techniques of varying sensitivity have been employed to distinguish antibody binding to CS antigens, including indirect immunofluorescence, immunoperoxidase techniques (77), variations of erythrocyte-rosetting assays (78), flow cytometry (79), and immunofiltration (80).

Human MAbs derived from cancer patient lymphocytes have been screened for reactivity to intracellular and CS antigen (10,11). Although human MAbs recognizing intracellular determinants were detected relatively frequently (9% and 3.5% of Ig-secreting clones), MAbs binding antigens restricted to the cell surface were generated much less frequently (< 1%). Possible explanations for this apparent rarity of B cells reactive to CS antigens include the following: (a) abnormal exposure of the immune system of cancer patients to normally sequestered cytoplasmic contents; (b) a wider range of immunogens among cellular contents as opposed to CS molecules; (c) the use of cell lines as targets of screening in these studies, resulting in nondetection of MAbs recognizing CS epitopes only expressed *in vivo*; and (d) a restricted immune response to most cell surface determinants because of immune tolerance mechanisms. Although human MAbs to CS antigens are less frequently derived than those to cellular antigens, even CS antigens may be relatively nonspecific for cancer cells.

II. THE HUMAN IMMUNE RESPONSE TO CANCER: HOW SPECIFIC?

The question of specificity has been a predominant theme in cancer immunology (81). The success of a strategy of immunodiagnosis and immunotherapy based on human MAbs depends on three major assumptions. (a) There are specific antigenic differences between normal and malignant cells that constitute cancer-associated antigens. (b) Cancer-associated antigens exist which are shared by tumors arising in different individuals. (c) Cancer-associated antigens are immunogenic in humans. Evidence characterizing the specificity of such antigens comes from serologic analysis of patients with cancer, as well as data from mouse and human MAbs to cancer-associated antigens.

A. Serologic Data

Reactivity of antibodies or B lymphocytes to cancer cells has been demonstrated with many cancers (e.g., breast, lung, bladder, colon, ovary, uterus) using a variety of techniques including antibody-dependent cytotoxicity, leukocyte migration or adherence inhibition, indirect immunofluorescence, or detection of blocking factor activity; however- the specificity of such reactions has often been difficult to demonstrate (82).

Using a variety of techniques to detect binding of serum antibodies to CS antigens of autologous and allogenic cell lines, the serologic reactivity of cancer patients has been meticulously dissected (for review, see 81). For example, of 75 melanoma patients studied, 56 has serum antibodies to melanoma-associated CS antigens. Further analysis of 30 melanoma sera revealed three specificity classes of reactive antibody and respective antigens. (a) Class I antigens are unique to the autologous tumor and are not expressed on normal autologous cells or any other normal or malignant cells. Four of 30 sera analyzed reacted to this class of antigens, which are unique to individuals and, thus, would have limited applicability in immunodiagnosis and therapy. Using a melanoma patient serum to immunoprecipitate a class I antigen, a 90,000-dalton CS glycoprotein has been identified (83). (b) Class II antigens are expressed on autologous and allogenic cancer cell lines of similar or dissimilar origin, and are not widely detected on normal cells. Class II antigens are shared by allogenic tumor cells. Therefore, MAbs to class II antigens potentially have wide use as reagents for immunodiagnosis and therapy. Five of 30 melanoma sera contained antibodies of this specificity. (c) Class III antigens are distributed widely on many malignant and normal cells of autologous or allogenic origin and, thus, have the least potential for targets of MAb immunodiagnosis or therapy. Of the 30 melanoma sera binding CS antigens on melanoma cells, 21 (70%) were shown to be directed to class III antigens.

Some conclusions can be drawn from these melanoma patient data, which are of importance to the general study of cancer using human MAbs. Though the bulk of the humoral response to the cancer cell surface appears to be nonspecific (class III), shared cancer-associated antigens (class II) exist and are immunogenic. It should, therefore, be possible to isolate human hybridomas secreting MAbs to such antigens. Class II antigens should also be demonstrable using mouse MAbs to cancer-associated antigens.

B. Cancer-Associated Antigens: How Specific?

Table 1 summarizes information on selected examples of a multitude of cancer-associated antigens detected by mouse MAbs and described in the last decade. Many have characteristics of class II antigens, though some have interesting properties not predicted from serologic data.

1. Sensitivity and Heterogeneity

Typically, MAbs to cancer-associated antigens do not react with all tumors of a given histotype, though the examples cited in Table 1 detect a large fraction of each tumor type. This total lack of expression by some tumors may represent the extreme example of tumor heterogeneity, a phenomenon that is also almost uniform among the examples listed. Thus, individual MAbs used for immunodiagnostic reagents would not be highly sensitive for a given tumor histotype, and MAbs used individually in a therapeutic manner would not be expected to be completely efficacious. Groups of MAbs can discriminate a higher fraction of tumors expressing any of a group of antigens (69) and, therefore, a higher fraction of tumor cells within a tumor expressing the same antigens. Multiple MAbs (for example, over 24 MAbs to breast cancer-associated antigens have now been reported [76]) will probably be important in enhancing the efficiency of monoclonal immunodiagnosis and therapy.

2. Specificity

Cancer-associated antigens are often not unique for a given histotype of cancer, but may be expressed also by related or unrelated types of neoplasms. For example, antigen TAG-72, detected by MAb B72.3, is found in 50% of breast carcinomas, but also in 85% of histogenically unrelated adenocarcinomas of the colon (84). The glycolipid GD_3 is shared among malignancies of neuroectodermally derived tissue (melanoma, astrocytoma) (85).

Cancer-associated antigens may have oncofetal expression (e.g., OC125, an antigen present in 85% of serous ovarian neoplasms). OC125 is present also in

Table 1 Examples of Cancer-Associated Antigens Detected with Mouse

Cancer histotype	MAb	Ig class	Antigen designation	Antigen location	Chemical nature	Molecular weight (daltons)
Melanoma	R_{24}	IgG_3	GD_3	Surface	Glycolipid	–
	9.2.27	IgG_{2a}	250K	Membrane core	Proteoglycan glycoprotein	250,000
	4.1	IgG_1	p97	Membrane	Transferin-like sialoprotein	97,000
Breast	B72.3	IgG_1	TAG-72	Cytoplasmic	Glycoprotein complex	220,000 to 400,000
	DF3	IgG_1	–	Benign cell surface; malignant cell cyto-plasm	? glycoprotein	290,000
	3B18	IgG_1	–	Cytoplasmic	ND	ND
Colorectal	17-1A	IgG_{2a}	–	ND	ND	ND
Pancreas	C1-P83	IgG_1	–	Surface and cytoplasmic	Protein or glycoprotein	110,000
	AR2-20	IgG_1	–	Surface	ND	190,000
Lung	TFS-2	IgG_{2b}	–	Surface	ND	39,000
	SM1	IgM	–	Surface	ND	50,000 and 20,000

Monoclonal Antibodies

Degree of expression in cancer tissue and cells	Heterogeneity *in vivo*	Expression in other tumors and cells	Expression in normal tissues or cells	References
Majority malignant melanoma tissues	+	Astrocytomas, some sarcomas	Brain (astrocytes); skin (melanocytes); retina, kidney, intestine	71, 85, 99
Greater than 90% of malignant melanoma tissues	Little	Neuroblastoma cell line	Skin (basal cells, sebaceous glands, hair follicles)	100, 113
Majority malignant melanoma tissues	+	Compound nevi; breast cancer	Sweat gland myoepithelial cells; fetal colon; trace amounts in uterus, colon and other tissues	97, 114
50% breast cancer tissues	+	85% colon cancers	None detected (immunoperoxidase)	84, 115
78% primary, 100% metastatic breast tissues	+	Fibrocystic disease	Normal lactating breast epithelia; other tissues not tested	128
87% breast cancer tissues	+	Fibroadenoma; fibrocystic disease ½ colon cancer	None detected (immunoperoxidase)	116
8/9 colorectal cancer tissues	ND	None detected	None on fibroblast cell lines, peripheral blood or normal colon	117
10/10 pancreatic cancer tissues	+	Breast, colon, adrenal cancer tissues	Tonsil epithelium, fetal colon	118
7/7 pancreatic cancer tissues	+	ND	None detected (indirect immunofluorescence)	119
9/10 lung cancer cell lines	ND	Multiple cancer cell lines, colon, pancreas, uterine	None on blood, spleen, marrow or fibroblast cells	120
6/6 small cell lung cancer tissues	ND	Breast cancer cell lines	None detected (indirect immunofluorescence)	121

(continued)

Table 1 (continued)

Cancer histotype	MAb	Ig class	Antigen designation	Antigen location	Chemical nature	Molecular weight (daltons)
Ovary	OC125	IgG_1	CA 125	Surface	Glycoprotein	>200,000
	MO_V1	IgG_1	–	Surface and cytoplasm	Mucin	High
	3C2	IgM	–	Surface	ND	ND
Renal	S22	IgG_1	gp115	Surface	Glycoprotein	115,000
Terato-carcinoma	Abk21	IgM	K21	Surface	Sulfated glyco-protein (carbo-hydrate deter-minant)	High
Chorio-carcinoma	AbLK26	IgG_{2a}	LK26	Surface	Glycoprotein	35,000

ND = not determined.

fetal peritoneum, amnion, pleura, and mullerian epithelia (86). OC125 also persists in the adult as a differentiation marker for mullerian-derived endometrium and fallopian tube.

Of the cancer-associated antigens detected by the MAbs listed in Table 1, many are expressed in a restricted distribution or in trace amounts in normal tissues. The distribution in normal tissues may follow a pattern suggesting differentiation-related expression, such as OC125. Others appear to have a wider distribution among normal tissues, but are present in only trace amounts. For example, melanoma-associated antigen p97 has been measured by a double-determinant immunoassay to be highly expressed in melanoma tissue (up to 600 ng/mg), but is also present in small amounts in some normal tissues such as uterus (10 ng/mg), colon (2 ng/mg), and skin (0.4 ng/mg) (87). The application of

Degree of expression in cancer tissue and cells	Heterogeneity *in vivo*	Expression in other tumors and cells	Expression in normal tissues or cells	References
85% serous ovarian cancer tissues	+	Benign nonmucinous ovarian tumors; pancreatic, lung, breast, colorectal cancer tissues, melanoma cell lines	Endocervix, endometrium, fallopian tube	86
4/9 nonserous ovarian cancer tissues	ND	Benign mucinous ovarian tumor tissue	Colonic glands	122
Majority serous and endometroid ovarian cancers	ND	None detected (indirect immunofluorescence)	None detected (indirect immunofluorescence)	123
10/20 renal cell cancer tissues	+	Adrenal and bladder cancer tissues; astrocytoma cell line	Normal kidney cell lines; none in tissues (immunoperoxidase)	124
6/9 testicular teratocarcinoma tissues	ND	Renal cancer tissue; renal and colon cancer cell lines	Fetal GI and bronchus; normal kidney cell lines	125
Choriocarcinoma cell lines; 1/1 choriocarcinoma tissue	ND	2/8 teratocarcinoma tissue; renal, colon and breast cancer tissue	Placenta (trophoblast)	126

less sensitive techniques (e.g., indirect immunogluorescence or screening "normal" cell lines) may be responsible for the nondetection of some of the antigens listed in Table 1 among normal tissues and cells, while others may, in fact, be more specific for cancer cells. Cancer-associated antigens related to differentiation determinants might be expected to be present in trace amounts in normal epithelia because of the presence of small numbers of immature reserve cells. However, as the example of p97 demonstrates, antigen expression may be a factor of 100 or more higher in malignant than nonmalignant tissue, possibly permitting more efficient discrimination than is achieved using radiation or chemotherapy. These and other considerations (discussed below) suggest that even cancer-associated antigens with incomplete specificity may be clinically useful.

3. Chemical Nature

Most cancer-associated antigens detected with mouse MAbs that have been characterized contain glycolipid or oligosaccharide antigenic determinants (88). Multiple alterations in glycolipid and oligosaccharide metabolism accompany malignant transformation (71). Glycolipid cancer-associated antigens may appear because of incomplete synthesis with precursor accumulation, such as the appearance of GD_3 in melanoma (71). Activation of abnormal glycosyltransferase enzymes may be responsible for the appearance of other glycolipid cancer-associated antigens. Some of these may be present, but immunologically cryptic, in normal tissues. Examples include the fucogangliosides sialyl Le^a, sialyl Le^x, and sialyl dimeric Le^x, which are expressed in a variety of adenocarcinomas (lung, gastrointestinal, breast), but which are also found in some normal tissues (e.g., pancreas, kidney, granulocytes (71). Some of these glycolipid are shed into the plasma (89). Although shed antigens provide favorable targets for MAbs used in immunodiagnosis, they could by competition, interfere with MAb use in immunotherapy. The inappropriate expression of blood group A antigen in cancers of patients having blood type B or O is an example of "neosynthesis" resulting in a potentially cancer-specific marker since no other tissues in patients with blood type B or O should synthesize blood group A antigen (90). Equally complex metabolic alterations also must affect oligosaccharide structures of glycoproteins, again leading to the expression of aberrant epitopes identifiable by mouse MAbs.

C. The Human Immune Response to Cancer as Demonstrated by Human Monoclonal Antibodies

1. Human MAbs to Glycolipid Determinants

From the examples of mouse MAbs just discussed, a reasonable conclusion is that while no antigenic markers have been discovered as having absolute specificity for any particular cancer, there do exist shared cancer-associated antigens expressed within subsets of malignancies, but which are found only in trace amounts or in a restricted distribution among normal tissues. Although there are examples of antigens to which human MAbs have been produced, but to which mouse MAbs have not (31,39), the prediction that the human immune system might react to more relevant or more specific cancer-associated antigens has yet to be demonstrated. In fact, even from the limited number of human MAbs to cancer-associated antigens characterized at present (Table 2), it appears that the human immune system recognizes as immunogenic types of cancer-associated antigens similar to those that have elicited MAbs in the mouse.

Several glycolipids are cancer-associated, as demonstrated by mouse MAbs. The melanoma-associated antigen OFA-I-2 has been shown to be the ganglioside

GD_2 (91), and is immunogenic in the context of human neuroectodermal malignancy. Human MAbs to GD_2 have been derived from a EBV-transformed melanoma patient lymphocyte cell line.

2. Human MAbs to Antigens in Normal Tissues and Cells

One of the disadvantages in the production of mouse MAbs to cancer cells or extracts is the large number of hybridoma clones producing antibody reactive to nonspecific cellular antigens. However, since the serologic data reviewed above suggest that many cancer patients produce antibodies of low specificity, human MAbs reactive to nontumor-specific cellular antigens are also expected. For example, human MAbs directed to different cytoskeletal proteins of the intermediate filament family have been produced using cancer patient lymphocytes (27). The specificity of other human MAbs derived from cancer patient lymphocytes suggests a restriction to certain differentiated cell types. Human MAb M54 recognizes intracellular determinants on cultured cells of epithelial origin, while MAb M304 recognizes antigens restricted to cultured cells of neuroectodermal origin (27). Human MAb RI37, derived from LN lymphocytes from a breast cancer patient, interacts with an antigen on the surface of normal human B lymphocytes (27). Whether immune responses to nonspecific and differentiation antigens are, indeed, cancer-induced or whether they are found to some degree as part of the immunologic repertoire among normal individuals is an interesting question that deserves further study.

3. Human MAbs to Shared Cancer-Associated Antigens

As shown in Table 1, mouse MAbs can discriminate cancer-associated antigens often expressed in a heterogenous manner, which are shared among malignancies of similar and often dissimilar histogenesis. Furthermore, their presence in normal tissue is characterized by a trace or restricted distribution. As illustrated in Table 2, cancer-associated antigens detected by *human* MAbs have similar characteristics. For example, human MAb MBE6, an IgM derived from axillary LN lymphocytes of a breast cancer patient, reacted with a determinant present, but heterogeneously expressed, in the vast majority of malignant breast tumors. The antigenic determinant was also present in some fibroadenomas and some nonbreast cancer tissues (lung, colon, thyroid); its distribution in non-neoplastic tissues was restricted to weak binding in areas of fibrocystic disease and normal breast epithelium (8,92). Human MAb CA 27 (25) is an example of several human MAbs to breast cancer-associated antigens having similar specificity (73). MAb CA 27 (25) also reacts heterogeneously with the majority of malignant breast tumors, with some fibroadenomas and nonbreast cancer tissues, and with the normal epithelia of renal collecting tubules and sebaceous glands.

In addition to those listed in Table 2, human MAbs to cancer-associated antigens have been reported for vulvar (35), cervical (35), Wilms (35), brain (93), and

Table 2 Examples of Cancer-Associated Antigens Detected with Human Monoclonal Antibodies

Cancer histotype	MAb	Ig class	Malignant fusion partner	Source of lymphocytes	Antigen designation	Antigen location	Chemical nature
Melanoma	L72	IgM	None (product of EBV transformed line)	PB	OFA-I-2	Membrane	Ganglioside GD_2
	Ma4	IgM	Human LICR-2	LN	—	Surface	Lipid
Breast	MBE6	IgM	Mouse NS-1	LN	—	Cytoplasmic	ND
	CA27(25)	IgG	Mouse M5	LN	—	Cytoplasmic	ND
Leukemia	aml-18	IgG	Human RH-L4B	PB	—	Surface and cytoplasmic	Protein
Prostate	MHG7	IgM	Mouse NS-1	LN	—	Surface and cytoplasmic	ND
Cervix	CL NH11	IgG	Human UC729-6	LN + PB	—	Surface and cytoplasmic	ND

Table 2 (continued)

Cancer histotype (MAb)	Degree of expression in cancer tissues and cells	Heterogeneity *in vivo*	Expression in other tumors and cells	Expression in normal tissues and cells	References
Melanoma (L72)	65% melanoma cell lines	ND	Glioma, neuroblastoma, retinoblastoma, chondrosarcoma cell line	Adult brain and spinal cord; fetal brain	91
(Ma4)	1/4 melanoma cell lines	ND	Multiple cancer cell lines (breast, colon, lung, and others)	None detected (normal cell lines)	10, 27
Breast (MBE6)	81% primary, 100% metastatic breast cancer tissues	+	2/6 fibroadenomas; lung, colon, thyroid cancer tissues	Breast epithelium; areas of fibrocystic disease	8, 92
(CA27[25])	76% primary, 100% metastatic breast cancer tissues	+	2/3 fibroadenoma; gastric colon and lung cancer tissues	Normal breast adjacent to cancer; kidney, skin	73
Leukemia (aml-8)	41% acute myelogenous leukemia cells	+	Other types of leukemia cells	Weak reaction to normal bone marrow cells	39
Prostate (MHG7)	4/5 prostate cancer tissues; 3/4 prostate cancer cell lines	+	2/3 benign prostatic hypertrophy; lung and colon cancer cell lines	None in skin or kidney (indirect immunofluorescence)	74
Cervix (CL NH11)	2/2 cervical cancer tissues; 3/3 cervical cancer cell lines	ND	Multiple cancer cell lines (prostate, melanoma, colon, hepatoma	Fibroblast cell lines	127

LN = lymph node; ND = not determined; PB = peripheral blood.

lung (36,94) tumors, though their characterization is less complete than those listed in Table 2. Further investigation is obviously needed to more completely characterize the range of human B lymphocyte specificities directed toward cancer tissues from healthy individuals and cancer patients.

III. HUMAN MAbs IN CANCER DIAGNOSIS AND THERAPY: WHAT IS THEIR ROLE?

A. Clinical Use of MAbs: Specificity Requirements

Given the fact that most MAbs to cancer-associated antigens, which have been extensively characterized, are not completely specific for any given malignancy, how specific must a MAb be to be useful clinically? MAbs to less specific cancer-associated antigens may still be useful for *in vitro* applications, such as detection of circulating antigen for diagnosis or patient management or for histopathologic determination of tumor type or prognosis. For example, though the glycolipids sialyl Le^a and sialyl Le^x are present in a number of normal tissues (71), they are normally not present in serum. However, one or the other is present in the majority of cancer patient sera, allowing for the serologic diagnosis of cancers expressing these glycolipids (89). MAbs identifying the most consistently and least heterogeneously expressed antigens would be of most use, regardless of source. Similarly, less specific MAbs (mouse or human) could be useful in *ex vivo* removal or killing of tumor cells prior to autologous bone marrow grafting in cancer patients treated with supralethal radiation or chemotherapy, as long as the MAbs lacked specificity for normal bone marrow cells.

In vivo human applications of MAbs include administration for both diagnostic (e.g., radionuclide imaging) and therapeutic uses. For both purposes, it would seem that success might require a higher degree of MAb specificity than would be necessary for some *in vitro* applications. However, mouse MAbs to epithelial membrane antigen of the human milk fat globule provides an example to the contrary. Although epithelial membrane antigen is widely distributed in normal secretory epithelia (e.g., kidney, breast, uterus, sebaceous glands), its absence in normal ovary, coupled to the favorable radionuclide-imaging characteristics of the ovary (separable from major blood pool), has allowed efficient imaging of primary ovarian cancers (95). Such a technique could be useful, despite the apparent nonspecificity of the antigen, in screening asymptomatic women for ovarian cancer, who have no detectable mass but who are at high risk for developing ovarian cancer on the basis of epidemiologic factors.

MAbs recognizing cancer-associated antigens also expressed in some normal tissues might be expected to have toxic effects on those normal tissues when the MAbs are administered *in vivo,* limiting their usefulness. For example, if a MAb or its potent immunoconjugate cross-reacted with normal epithelia of vital organs (e.g., kidney, gastrointestinal tract, brain), serious side-effects might occur. However, there are several reasons why less specific MAbs could be useful for *in vivo* applications, including the following: (a) The accessibility of the target antigen in normal tissue may be far less than in tumor tissue, permitting the less specific MAb to have a salutory effect without undue toxicity. For example, even though the glycolipid antigen SSEA-1 is highly expressed in normal mouse kidney, radiolabeled MAbs to SSEA-1 injected into mice do not accumulate significantly in kidney, but rather are selectively sequestered by teratocarcinomas growing in such mice (96). (b) MAbs cross-reacting with antigens in some normal tissues (e.g., hair follicles, breast epithelia) may have physiologically less important consequences. Other normal tissues that cross-react may have been removed during primary surgical therapy (e.g., uterus, fallopian tubes). (c) The quantitative expression of target antigen in normal tissues may be far less than in tumor tissues, permitting adequate discrimination at optimal MAb doses. An example is melanoma-associated antigen p97, which may be present in melanoma tissues 50 to 100 times its concentration in normal tissues (97).

In summary, the degree of usefulness of mouse or human MAbs to cancer-associated antigens also cross-reacting with antigens in some normal tissues could be underestimated. The possible *in vivo* effects of even the most specific MAbs are unknown until tested *in vivo.* Observations of great importance to the future *in vivo* use of human MAbs have accumulated from clinical trials of mouse MAbs in human cancer patients.

B. Therapeutic Use of MAbs: Mouse MAbs and Human Cancer

A number of clinical trials of mouse MAbs to leukemia and lymphoma-associated antigens have been reported (for review, see 98), and several reports of phase 1 clinical trials of mouse MAbs to solid cancer-associated antigens have now appeared (99-101). Information regarding tumor dynamics following MAb treatment, therapeutic and toxic effects, and the human immune response to mouse MAbs has been gained.

1. Tumor Dynamics Following MAb Treatment

The dramatic cancer cell killing associated with passive administration of MAbs in animal model systems (102) is dependent on cellular effectors (e.g., natural killer cells, macrophages) and on the Fc portion of the Ig molecule. IgM MAbs have been ineffective in some animal model systems, with IgG_{2a} and IgG_3 being the most effective subclasses (98). Consequently, these subclasses have been used in clinical trials to date, though IgM MAbs or IgG MAbs of other subclasses have not been shown to be ineffective in humans. In fact, IgM MAbs may be effective in killing some tumors in nude mice, such as melanoma cells expressing GD_2 (41).

Although some examples of dramatic improvement have been reported after

MAb therapy, a transient or insignificant response occurs in most patients. Possible mechanisms of tumor cell escape from mouse MAb killing include the following: (a) In the presence of the antibody, a reversible redistribution of cell curface antigen may occur, resulting in the loss of surface antigen expression through modulation. (b) Genetic variants that do not express the target antigen are spared by MAb therapy. (c) Free target antigen may saturate incoming MAb, preventing cell killing. (d) Loss of mouse MAb-mediated cell killing may occur as a result of an anti-mouse Ig response. (e) An insufficient number of effector cells or their inhibition as a result of immune complex or blocking factor formation may reduce tumor cell killing. Examples of these mechanisms thought to be responsible for failure of MAb therapy of patients with leukemia and lymphomas have included rapid antigenic modulation, saturation by circulating antigen, blocking of MAb effect by anti-mouse antibody, and shortage of effector cells (98). The emergence of genetic variants of B-cell lymphoma idiotypes has also been observed, and may result in tumor escape in patients treated with anti-idiotype MAbs (103,104).

2. Therapeutic Effects

In general, therapeutic effects of mouse MAbs have been transient or lacking, but this is perhaps expected considering the massive tumor burdens possessed by patients selected for phase 1 study, and also considering the uncertainty over the optimum or maximum doses of passively administered mouse MAb. Some beneficial responses have been observed in some leukemia and lymphoma patients. A number of leukemia patients had transient reductions in circulating leukemia cells and some had partial remissions; a lymphocytic lymphoma patient treated with a mouse anti-idiotype MAb had a complete remission lasting longer than 1 year (98).

Mouse MAb phase 1 trials in patients with solid cancers have included 29 patients with metastatic gastrointestinal cancer using mouse MAb 17-1A (101, 105), eight patients with metastatic melanoma using mouse MAb 9.2.27 (100), and 12 patients with metastatic melanoma using mouse MAb R_{24} (99). Remission of disease has been reported among five patients with metastatic gastrointestinal cancer treated with MAb 17-1A, and may have correlated with the presence of an anti-idiotype antibody response to the mouse MAb (105). Demonstrable benefit was achieved in three patients with melanoma treated with mouse MAb R_{24} to ganglioside GD_3 (99). MAb R_{24} elicited an inflammatory response around sites of tumors, and tumors which progressed despite MAb R_{24} therapy remained strongly GD_3-positive, implicating escape mechanisms other than antigenic modulation. Among the melanoma patients treated with MAb 9.2.27, no measurable decrease in the size of metastatic tumors was observed, even though there was localization of the mouse MAb in biopsied tumor specimens (106).

3. Toxic Effects

Toxicity has been absent or minimal in the majority of patients treated with purified mouse MAbs. In studies in patients with leukemia and lymphoma, fever, chills, flushing, nausea, vomiting, transient coagolopathy, and anaphylactic reactions were observed in some patients treated with lower doses, while one patient had renal impairment after administration of 1500 mg of mouse MAb (98). Fever was uniformly observed among melanoma patients given up to 200 mg mouse MAb 9.2.27, and one patient manifested signs of serum sickness syndrome which resolved with treatment (100). Although several patients developed rashes, no generalized dermatologic phenomena occurred despite the presence of the MAb 9.2.27 target antigen in sebaceous glands, hair follicles, and basal epithelial cells. Pruritis and urticarial skin lesions, especially in skin surrounding tumor sites, were common among melanoma patients treated with up to 528 mg mouse MAb R_{24} (99). The severity of the skin reactions decreased with a decreased MAb infusion rate. Six patients developed urticarial lesions over the face, trunk, and limbs, and one patient developed wheezing after rapid MAb infusion. Despite the occurrence of transient skin reactions and despite the presence of the target antigen GD_3 in melanocytes of normal skin, no lasting dermatologic changes, including skin pigment changes, were observed over a 9 month follow-up period. Similarly, there were no neurologic, ophthamologic, or renal changes despite the presence of GD_3 in normal brain, retina, and kidney.

4. The Immune Response to Mouse MAbs

Antiglobulins. Humoral responses to administered mouse MAbs in the form of human anti-mouse Ig (antiglobulin) have been detected in the majority of MAb-treated leukemia and lymphoma patients (98). In some patients, the emergence of antiglobulin activity was correlated with a decrease in the decrement of circulating tumor cells achieved after administration of successive MAb doses. Antiglobulin activity has also been reported among a large fraction of patients with gastrointestinal cancer given mouse MAb 17-1A (107), especially those receiving less than 200 mg of MAb and melanoma patients given mouse MAb R_{24} (99).

The antiglobulin response has been studied in detail among leukemia patients given MAb T101 and melanoma patients given MAb 9.2.27 (108). Sera from healthy individuals and pretreatment cancer patient sera were shown to contain small amounts of pre-existing IgG and IgM antiglobulins. Antiglobulin levels increased significantly in three of nine patients with melanoma, four of four patients with cutaneous T cell lymphoma, and none of 11 patients with chronic lymphocytic leukemia. The increases observed were highest for IgG antiglobulin, suggesting a secondary immune response. Antiglobulins were directed toward common mouse determinants on the F_c region, and occasionally cross-reacted with rabbit IgG. Antiglobulin responses in the three patients with melanoma (one with antiglobulin as high as 175 mg/ml) did not inhibit localization of MAb 9.2.27 in biopsied tumor tissues. No toxicity was attributed to the antiglobulin responses.

Anti-idiotype Antibodies. Antibodies with anti-idiotype specificity represent a minor component of the antiglobulin activity elicited in pateints by mouse MAbs (98,105,108), though there are examples of apparent MAb blocking *in vivo* by anti-idiotype antibodies (98). It has been suggested that remission of metastatic gastrointestinal cancer in five patients following single injections of mouse MAb 17-1A were related to the presence of an anti-idiotypic antibody response (105). Presumably, the presence of the anti-idiotypic antibody, because of an "internal image" of the MAb 17-1A target antigen, results in a beneficial enhancement of the patients' immune response towards the antigen and, thus, tumor regression. The rate of occurrence of such anti-idiotypic antibodies among patients who did not experience remission was not reported.

C. Therapeutic Use of Human MAbs: Expected Problems and Possible Solutions

Although some examples of the administration of human MAbs to cancer patients have appeared (93,109), and despite the experience with *in vivo* use of mouse MAbs, many unknowns associated with *in vivo* use of MAbs remain to be characterized. Table 3 lists some of these sources of variability. Characterization of some of these phenomena has been possible in patients treated with mouse MAbs; others are beginning to be explored experimentally in tumor model systems.

1. Patient Variables

Although the majority of patients treated with mouse MAbs apparently manifested no toxic effects, individual variability in the tolerance to the toxic effects of MAbs is expected. Many of the dermatologic and respiratory reactions appear to be related to the dosage rate of MAb administration, while other reactions, such as serum sickness or anaphylactic reaction, were sporadic. A similar range of toxic effects may occur when treating patients with human MAbs.

An antiglobulin response has been observed in many patients treated with mouse MAbs, and may have resulted in therapeutic failure in some. However, despite the antiglobulin response, melanoma patients given mouse MAb 9.2.27 continued to have localization of MAb in tumor tissue (106). Gastrointestinal cancer patients given larger doses (>200 mg) of mouse MAb 17-1A had a much lower rate of antiglobulin response than did those treated with lower doses (105). Consequently, the ultimate effects of antiglobulin response on therapeutic efficacy using optimized regimens may not preclude the usefulness of mouse MAbs *in vivo*.

Table 3 Variables in the *In Vivo* Use of MAbs

Patient variables
- Toxicity
  - Individual variability
  - Rate of administration
- Immune response
  - Non-idiotype determinants (e.g., allotype determinants, xenogenic determinants)
  - Idiotype determinants
  - ? Beneficial effects of anti-idiotype antibodies

Tumor variables
- Tumor burden
- Tumor vascularity
- Histopathologic factors
  - Tumor grade, presence of inflammation or necrosis

Antigenic variables
- Intensity of antigen expression
  - Tumor tissue vs. normal tissues
- Heterogeneity of antigen expression
  - Effects of biological response modifiers
- Modulation in the presence of MAb
- Antigen nonexpressing genetic variants
- Antigen secretion or shedding
- Chemical nature, location, and accessibility of target antigen
- Mediation of successful internalization of MAb conjugates

MAb variables
- MAb distribution in tumor and normal tissues
  - MAb specificity, avidity
  - Optimal dosage; rate and route of administration
  - $F(ab')_2$ vs. intact MAb
  - Effects of conjugation on distribution
  - MAb clearance mechanisms
  - Persistence in tissues

(continued)

Table 3 continued)

MAb variables (continued)
- Unconjugated MAbs–tumor effects
  - Ig isotype, subclass
  - Availability of effector cells, C′
- MAb-immunoconjugate variables
  - Effects of conjugation on MAb specificity and avidity
  - Type and stability of chemical linkage
  - Toxic consequences of unconjugation
  - Toxin or drug internalization requirements
  - Radionuclide type
    - Radius of killing
    - Particle type
    - t-½

The hypothesis that human MAbs would be less immunogenic than mouse MAbs and, therefore, more useful has not been adequately tested. Though human serum products are safe compared with animal serum products, immune responses may occur even to human MAbs. Allotypic determinants (e.g., Gm allotypes of IgG) may be immunogenic in some individuals. Anti-idiotype responses are to be expected in some patients by extrapolations from the mouse MAb data. In addition, human MAbs derived from mouse-human hybridomas or heteromyelomas could conceivably be subject to post-translational modifications (e.g., glycosylation) characteristic of mouse cellular products, rendering them immunogenic in humans. The use of $F(ab')_2$ fragments could avoid some of these problems. Toxic immunoconjugates of MAbs might reduce the immune response to the MAb by binding and killing B cells recognizing the Mab as antigenic. Unestablished at present are the possible beneficial effects of anti-idiotypic antibodies or the possible adverse effects of blocking factor formation as a result of MAb administration.

2. Tumor Variables

Though many of the cancer patients treated with mouse MAbs in phase 1 trials had large metastatic tumor burdens, the probability of success with any form of immunotherapy will be inversely proportional to the tumor mass. The tumor grade, vascularity, and the presence of inflammation or necrosis are also important variables what may affect the outcome of MAb therapy.

3. Antigenic Variables

Variables of target antigen expression, including intensity of expression, heterogeneity, and modulation, are obviously of key importance since they are almost ubiquitous phenomena. The approach of administration of multiple MAbs directed at different antigens has been mentioned. MAb conjugates with alpha- or beta-emitting radionuclides might be able to achieve killing of many nearby antigen-nonexpressing cancer cells. Alternatively, biological response modifiers (e.g., interferon), which enhance CS antigen expression by nonexpressor cells, could be administered in conjunction with MAbs to enhance their efficacy (75). The emergence of antigen-nonexpressing genetic variants or blocking of administered MAbs by secreted or shed antigens are problems not solved by the above manipulations.

4. MAb Variables

The optimal MAb doses, dosage rates, and routes of administration are unknown, and the mechanisms of MAb clearance are complex phenomena. Variation in the specificity and avidity of MAbs or their use as Ig fragments or immunoconjugates add to this complexity. As has been the case for mouse MAbs, unconjugated human MAbs may be cytotoxic to tumor cells *in vivo.* The importance of Ig isotype and subclass for human MAb-mediated cytotoxicity has not been established. Though animal data have suggested that IgG_{2a} and IgG_3 are much more effective in directing cellular cytotoxicity, a human IgM directed to ganglioside GD_2 has been shown to suppress the growth of human melanoma cells in nude mice (41). This is an important finding prior to the use of unconjugated human MAbs in phase 1 trials since many are IgM (see Table 2).

One of the potential advantages of MAb conjugates (110) with drugs, toxins, or radionuclides is that tumor cell killing would be Ig isotype- or subclass-independent. The use of immunoconjugates is, however, associated with a number of other uncertainties. First, conjugation may interfere chemically or sterically with MAb binding. The MAb conjugate may unconjugate *in vivo,* leading to reduced efficacy and potential toxicity. MAb conjugates with drugs and toxins must enter the cell for toxic effect. A major problem is that not all cell surface antigen targets mediate successful internalization of the MAb conjugate (111). For ricin A chain MAb conjugates, some target antigens may mediate internalization by routes that render the toxin ineffective; a reversible type of chemical linkage, rather than irreversible, also appears to be important (111). Target antigens that are shed or secreted may be ineffective targets for MAb toxin conjugates (112).

MAb radionuclide conjugates do not need to be internalized to achieve toxicity and, therefore, have a potential advantage over MAb drug or toxin conjugates. However, radiolabeled MAbs can accumulate in normal tissues, especially in the liver and the spleen, leading to unwanted toxicity. Liver and spleen binding of MAbs is probably mediated by Fc receptors and could, in theory, be blocked by administration of aggregated Ig. Another possible solution is utilization of $F(ab')_2$-radiolabeled MAb fragments, which have been shown to significantly reduce accumulation of ^{131}I-labeled MAbs in the liver and spleen of patients with melanoma (46). Yet another advantage of radionuclide-MAb conjugates is the killing of nearby tumor cells that do not express the target antigen. Though administration of biological response modifiers (e.g., interferon) to enhance antigen expression may improve tumor cell killing, nearby normal cells are also exposed to radiation, leading to toxic effects.

IV. SUMMARY AND PROSPECTS

Progress and remaining areas of difficulty in the application of human MAbs to human cancer diagnosis, management, and therapy can be summarized as follows: (a) Many technical aspects of the construction of human hybridomas have been solved, though the optimum malignant fusion partner for human MAb production is probably yet to be derived. (b) The problem of poor availability of stimulated B cells is not adequately solved by the use of EBV-transformed or mitogen-stimulated PB lymphocytes. *In vitro* methods of enhancement and immunization of cancer patients with autologous tumor cells or oncolysates may allow more rapid progress. (c) Screening human hybridomas for MAbs to relatively specific cancer-associated antigens remains a point of difficulty. Current methods probably select for the most immunogenic but perhaps not the most specific antigens. (d) Tumor heterogeneity remains an important impediment to the application of MAbs for cancer diagnosis and therapy. Although one solution is to employ multiple MAbs to different cancer-associated antigens, the search for more specific and less heterogeneously expressed antigens continues. (e) Although therapeutic trials with mouse MAbs suggest acceptable levels of toxicity, trials of human MAbs are yet to be reported. Theoretically, human monoclonal technology has opened the door for meticulous analysis of the human immune response not previously possible with mouse methods. (f) Many questions remain concerning the optimum form of MAb immunoconjugates to be used in cancer immunotherapy.

The fascinating prospect of modulating the immune response of cancer patients by administration of anti-idiotypic antibodies displaying antigen-like structures (105) deserves further investigation. Cancer patients treated with either mouse or human MAbs to cancer-associated antigens may have an anti-idiotypic response, which could be preserved in human hybridomas secreting monoclonal anti-idiotype antibodies. Such human monoclonal anti-idiotype antibodies would contain an "internal image" of the target antigen (105), the effects of which, when administered to cancer patients, would be of great interest.

In the future, genetic engineering techniques may allow for more reliable and permanent preservation of MAb production (57). As more specific and less heterogeneously expressed cancer-associated antigens are characterized, the power of MAb immunodiagnosis and therapy will be enhanced. The characterization of optimal target antigens by MAbs and their subsequent isolation may allow identification of specific T cell clones. The availability of human T cell clones or hybridomas specifically sensitized to target cancer-associated antigens and now capable of specific tumor cell killing could further magnify the power of cancer immunotherapy.

ACKNOWLEDGMENT

This work was supported in part by Grant CA 36422 from the National Cancer Institute and the Robert L. Seidner Research Fund.

REFERENCES

1. R. Levy and J. Dilley. Rescue of immunoglobulin secretion from human neoplastic lymphoid cells by somatic cell hybridization. *Proc. Natl. Acad. Sci. (USA)*, *76*:2411 (1978).
2. J. Schwaber and E. P. Cohen. Human x mouse somatic cell hybrid clone secreting immunoglobulins of both parental types. *Nature, 244*:44 (1973).
3. J. Schwaber. Immunoglobulin production by a human-mouse somatic cell hybrid. *Exp. Cell. Res., 93*:343 (1979).
4. P. G. Abrams, J. A. Knost, G. Clarke, S. Wilburn, R. K. Oldham, and K. A. Foon. Determination of the optimal human cell lines for development of human hybridomas. *J. Immunol., 131*:1201 (1983).
5. M. C. Weiss and H. Green. Human-mouse hybrid cell lines containing partial complements of human chromosomes and functioning human genes. *Proc. Natl. Acad. Sci. (USA)*, *58*:1104 (1967).
6. M. Nabholz, V. Miggiano, and W. Bodmer. Genetic analysis with human-mouse somatic cell hybrids. *Nature, 223*:358 (1969).
7. R. L. Raison, K. Z. Walker, C. R. E. Halnan, D. Briscor, and A. Basten. Loss of secretion of mouse-human hybrids need not be due to the loss of a structural gene. *J. Exp. Med., 156*:1380 (1982).
8. J. Schlom, D. Wunderlich, and Y. A. Teramoto. Generation of human monoclonal antibodies reactive with human mammary carcinoma cells. *Proc. Natl. Acad. Sci. (USA)*, *77*:6841 (1980).
9. H. C. Lane, J. H. Mostowski, and A. S. Fauci. Human monoclonal anti-keyhole limpet hemocyanin antibody-secreting hybridoma produced from peripheral blood B lymphocytes of a keyhole limpet cyanin-immune individual. *J. Exp. Med., 155*:333 (1982).
10. R. J. Cote, D. M. Morrissey, A. M. Houghton, E. J. Beattie, Jr., H. F. Oettgen,

and L. J. Old. Generation of human monoclonal antigodies reactive with cellular antigens. *Proc. Natl. Acad. Sci. (USA), 80*:2026 (1983).

11. A. N. Houghton, H. Brooks, R. J. Cote, M. C. Taormina, J. F. Oettgen, and L. J. Old. Detection of cell surface and intracellular antigens by human monoclonal antibodies. Hybrid cell lines derived from lymphocytes of patients with malignant melanoma. *J. Exp. Med., 158*:53 (1983).
12. D. Wunderlich, Y. A. Teramoto, C. Alford, and J. Schlom. The use of lymphocytes from axillary lymph nodes of mastectomy patients to generate human monoclonal antibodies. *Eup. J. Cancer Clin. Oncol., 17*:719 (1981).
13. A. Imam, M. M. Drushella, C. R. Taylor, and Z. A. Tokes. Generation and immunohistological characterization of human monoclonal antibodies to mammary carcinoma cells. *Cancer Res., 45*:263 (1985).
14. L. Olsson and H. S. Kaplan. Human-human hybridomas producing monoclonal antibodies of predefined antigenic specificity. *Proc. Natl. Acad. Sci. (USA), 77*:5429 (1980).
15. Y. Matsuoko, G. E. Moore, Y. Yagi, and D. Pressman. Production of free light chains of immunoglobulin by a hematopoietic cell line derived from a patient with multiple myeloma. *Proc. Soc. Exp. Biol. Med., 125*:1246 (1967).
16. J. W. Pickering and F. B. Gelder. A human myeloma cell line that does not express immunoglobulin but yields a high frequency of antibody-secreting hybridomas. *J. Immunol., 129*:406 (1982).
17. P. A. W. Edwards, C. M. Smith, A. M. Neville, and M. J. O'Hare. A human-human hybridoma system based on a fast-growing mutant of the ARH-77 plasma cell leukemia-derived line. *Eur. J. Immunol., 12*:641 (1982).
18. C. M. Croce, A. Linnenbach, W. Hall, Z. Steplewski, and J. Koprowski. Production of human hybridomas secreting antibody to measels virus. *Nature, 288*:488 (1980).
19. Y. Shoenfeld, S. C. Hsn-Lin, J. Gabriels, L. E. Silberstein, B. C. Furie, B. Furie, B. D. Stollar, and R. S. Schwartz. Production of autoantibodies by human-human hybridomas. *J. Clin. Invest., 70*:205 (1982).
20. D. S. Dwyer, R. J. Bradley, C. K. Urguhart, and J. F. Kearny. Naturally occurring anti-idiotypic antibodies in myasthenia gravis patients. *Nature, 301*: 611 (1983).
21. J. A. Levy, V. Viroloinen, and V. Defeudi. Human lymphoblastoid lines from lymph node and spleen. *Cancer, 22*:517 (1968).
22. M. C. Glassy, H. H. Handley, H. Hagiwara, and I. Royston. UC 729-6, a human lymphoblastoid B-cell line useful for generating antibody-secreting human-human hybridomas. *Proc. Natl. Acad. Sci. (USA), 80*:6327 (1983).
23. J. W. Larrick, K. E. Truitt, A. A. Raubitschek, G. Senyk, and J. Wang. Characterization of human hybridomas secreting antibody to tetanus toxoid. *Proc. Natl. Acad. Sci. (USA), 80*:6376 (1983).
24. N. Choirazzi, R. L. Wasserman, and H. G. Kinkel. Use of Epstein-Barr virus-transformed B-cell lines for the generation of immunoglobulin-producing human B-cell hybridomas. *J. Exp. Med., 156*:930 (1982).

25. L. Olsson, H. Kronstrøm, A. Cambon-De Mouzon, C. Honsik, T. Brodin, and B. Jacobsen. Antibody producing human-human hybridomas. I. Technical aspects. *J. Immunol. Meth., 61*:17 (1983).
26. D. Kozbor, P. Tripputi, J. C. Roder, and C. M. Croce. A human hybrid myeloma for production of human monoclonal antibodies. *J. Immunol. Meth., 133*:3001 (1984).
27. R. J. Cote and A. N. Houghton. The generation of human monoclonal antibodies and their use in the analysis of the humoral immune response to cancer. In E. G. Engleman, S. K. H. Foung, J. Larrick, and A. A. Raubitschek (eds.). *Human Hybridomas and Monoclonal Antibodies.* Plenum Press, New York (1985).
28. N. N. H. Teng, L. S. Lam, F. Calvo Riera, and J. S. Kaplan. Construction and testing of mouse-human heteromyelomas for human monoclonal antibody production. *Proc. Natl. Acad. Sci. (USA), 80*:7308 (1983).
29. F. Riera Calvo, S. B. Blam, N. N. H. Teng, and H. S. Kaplan. Somatic cell hybrid selection with a transfectable dominant marker. *Som. Cell. Mol. Genet., 10*:123 (1984).
30. N. N. H. Teng and M. Bieber. The use of heteromyelomas in the enhancement of human monoclonal antibody production. In A. H. Bartal and Y. Hirshaut (eds.). *Hybridoma Formation.* Humana Press, New York (in press).
31. D. Bron, M. B. Feinberg, N. N. H. Teng, and H. S. Kaplan. Production of human monoclonal IgG antibodies against Rhesus (D) antigen. *Proc. Natl. Acad. Sci. (USA), 81*:3214 (1984).
32. N. N. H. Teng, H. S. Kaplan, J. M. Herbert, C. Moore, H. Douglas, A. Wunderlich, and A. I. Braude. Protection against gram-negative bacteremia and endotoxemia with monoclonal IgM antibodies. *Proc. Natl. Acad. Sci. (USA), 82*: 1790 (1985).
33. S. K. H. Foung, S. Perkins, A. Rabitschek, J. Larrick, G. Lizak, D. Fishwild, E. G. Englman, and F. C. Grumet. Rescue of human monoclonal antibody production from an EBV-transformed B-cell line by fusion to a human-mouse hybridoma. *J. Immunol. Meth., 70*:83 (1984).
34. K. G. Burnett, J. P. Leund, and J. Martinis. Human monoclonal antibodies to defined antigens. In E. G. Engleman, S. K. H. Foung, J. Larrick, and A. A. Raubitschek (eds.). *Human Hybridomas and Monoclonal Antibodies.* Plenum Press, New York (1985).
35. M. C. Glassy, H. H. Handley, and I. Royston. Design and production of human monoclonal antibodies to human cancers. In E. G. Engleman, S. K. H. Foung, J. Larrick, and A. A. Raubitschek (eds.). *Human Hybridomas and Monoclonal Antibodies.* Plenum Press, New York (1985).
36. S. P. Cole, B. G. Campling, I. H. Louwman, D. Kozbor, and J. Roder. A strategy for the production of human monoclonal antibodies reactive with lung tumor cell lines. *Cancer Res., 44*:2750 (1984).
37. R. E. Callard, G. W. McCaughan, J. Babbage, and R. L. Souhami. Specific *in vitro* antibody responses by human blood lymphocytes: apparent nonresponsiveness of PBL is due to a lack of recirculating memory B-cells. *J. Immunol., 129*:153 (1982).

38. G. C. B. Astaldi, E. P. Wricht, C. Willems, W. P. Zeijemaker, and M. C. Janssen. Increase of hybridoma formation by human lymphocytes after stimulation *in vitro*: effect of antigen, endothelial cells and PWM. *J. Immunol., 128*: 2539 (1982).
39. L. Olsson, R. B. Andreasen, B. Christensen, and P. Biberfeld. Antibody producing human-human hybridomas. II. Derivation and characterization of an antibody specific for human leukemia cells. *J. Exp. Med., 159*:537 (1984).
40. R. G. Keightley, M. D. Cooper, and A. R. Lawton. The T cell dependence of B cell differentiation induced by pokeweed mitogen. *J. Immunol., 117*:1538 (1976).
41. M. Katano and R. F. Irie. Human monoclonal antibody to tumor-associated ganglioside GD_2: suppressed growth of human melanoma in nude mice. *Immunol. Lett., 8*:169 (1984).
42. F. Gmelig-Meylig, A. G. C. M. Uytde Haag, and R. E. Ballieux. Human B-cell activation *in vitro*. T-cell dependent pokeweed mitogen-induced differentiation of blood B lymphocytes. *Cell. Immunol., 33*:156 (1977).
43. J. Pryjma, J. Munoz, R. M. Galbraith, H. H. Fudenberg, and G. Virella. Induction and suppression of immunoglobulin synthesis in cultures of human lymphocytes: effects of pokeweed mitogen and *Staphylococcus aureus* Cowan I. *J. Immunol., 124*:656 (1980).
44. I. A. Ly and R. I. Mishell. Separation of mouse spleen cells by passage through columns of Sephadex-G-10. *J. Immunol. Meth., 5*:239 (1974).
45. M. K. Hoffmann, S. Pollack, S. E. Krown, and R. S. Mittler. Deletion of active human suppressor T-lymphocytes from peripheral blood by Sephadex G-10 filtration. *J. Immunol. Meth., 55*:327 (1982).
46. G. L. Buraggi, L. Callegaro, G. Mariani, A. Turrin, N. Bascinelli, A. Attili, E. Bombardieri, G. Terno, G. Plassio, M. Dovis, M. Mazzuca, P. G. Natali, G. A. Scassellati, U. Rosa, and S. Ferrone. Imaging with ^{131}I-labeled monoclonal antibodies to a high-molecular weight melanoma-associated antigen in patients with melanoma: efficacy of whole immunoglobulin and its $F(ab')_2$ fragments. *Cancer Res., 45*:3378 (1985).
47. I. S. Barsoum, H. S. S. Dahawi, F. M. Gamil, M. Habib, M. A. E. L. Alamy, and D. G. Colley. Immune responses and immunoregulation in relation to human schistosomiasis in Egypt. II. Cimetidine reversal of histamine-mediated suppression of antigen-induced blastogenesis. *J. Immunol., 133*:1576 (1984).
48. M. Steinitz, G. Klein, S. Koskimies, and O. Makela. EB virus induced B lymphocyte cell lines producing specific antibody. *Nature, 269*:420 (1977).
49. D. H. Crawford. Production of human monoclonal antibodies using Epstein-Barr virus. In E. G. Engleman, S. K. H. Foung, J. Larrick, and A. A. Raubitschek (eds.). *Human Hybridomas and Monoclonal Antibodies*. Plenum Press, New York (1985).
50. A. W. Siadak and M. E. Lostrom. Cell-driven viral transformation. In E. G. Engleman, S. K. H. Foung, J. Larrick, and A. A. Raubitschek (eds.). *Human Hybridomas and Monoclonal Antibodies*. Plenum Press, New York (1985).
51. J. C. Roder, D. Kozbor, S. P. C. Cole, T. Atlaw, B. C. Campling, R. C. McGarry,

and D. Kozbor. The Epstein-Barr virus–hybridoma technique. In E. G. Engleman, S. K. H. Foung, J. Larrick, and A. A. Raubitschek (eds.). *Human Hybridomas and Monoclonal Antibodies.* Plenum Press, New York (1985).

52. J. Larrick, A. A. Raubitschek, B. Dyer, G. S. Hart, D. Lippman, D. Hohnsen, M. Wang, and H. Weintraub. *In vitro* expansion of human B-cells for the production of human monoclonal antibodies. In E. G. Engleman, S. K. H. Foung, J. Larrick, and A. A. Raubitschek (eds.). *Human Hybridomas and Monoclonal Antibodies.* Plenum Press, New York (1985).
53. D. Kozbor and J. C. Roder. *In vitro* stimulated lymphocytes as a source of human hybridomas. *Eur. J. Immunol., 14*:23 (1984).
54. L. Winger, C. Winger, P. Shastry, A. Russel, and M. Longnecker. Efficient generation *in vitro* of monoclonal Epstein-Barr virus–transformants producing specific antibody to a variety of antigens, without prior deliberate immunisation. *Proc. Natl. Acad. Sci. (USA), 80*:4484 (1983).
55. D. Kozbor and J. C. Roder. Requirements for the establishment of high-titered human monoclonal antibodies against tetanus toxoid using the Epstein-Barr virus technique. *J. Immunol. 127*:1275 (1981).
56. M. M. S. Lo, S. M. Strittmatter, L. D. Hester, S. H. Snyder, T. Y. Tsong, and M. K. Conrad. Monoclonal antibody production by receptor-mediated electrically induced cell fusion. *Nature, 310*:792 (1984).
57. N. N. Teng, G. R. Reyes, M. Bieber, K. E. Fry, K. S. Lam, and J. M. Hebert. Strategies for stable human monoclonal antibody production: construction of heteromyelomas, *in vitro* sensitization, and molecular cloning of human immunoglobuli genes. In E. G. Engleman, S. K. H. Foung, J. Larrick, and A. A. Raubitschek (eds.). *Human Hybridomas and Monoclonal Antibodies.* Plenum Press, New York (1985).
58. M. K. Hoffman and J. A. Hirst. Principles of *in vitro* immunization of human B lymphocytes. In E. G. Engleman, S. K. H. Foung, J. Larrick, and A. A. Raubitschek (eds.). *Human Hybridomas and Monoclonal Antibodies.* Plenum Press, New York (1985).
59. R. F. Irie, A. E. Giullano, and D. L. Morton. Oncofetal antigen: tumor-associated fetal antigen immunogenic in man. *JNCI 63*:367 (1979).
60. W. A. Cassel, D. R. Murray, A. H. Rorbin, Z. L. Olkowski, and M. E. Moore. Viral oncolysate in the management of malignant melanoma. I. Preparation of the oncolysate and measurement of immunological responses. *Cancer, 40*: 672 (1977).
61. D. R. Murray, W. A. Cassel, A. H. Torbin, Z. L. Olkowski, and M. E. Moore. Viral oncolysate in the management of malignant melanoma. II. Clinical studies. *Cancer, 40*:680 (1977).
62. W. A. Cassel, D. R. Murray, and H. S. Phillips. A phase II study of the post-surgical management of stage II malignant melanoma with a Newcastle disease virus oncolysate. *Cancer, 52*:856 (1983).
63. H. C. Hoover, Jr., N. G. Surdyke, R. B. Dangel, L. C. Peters, and M. G. Hanna, Jr. Prospectively randomized trial of adjuvant active-specific immunotherapy for human colorectal cancer. *Cancer, 55*:1236 (1985).

64. M. V. Haspell, H. C. Hoover, R. P. McCabe, N. Pomato, and M. G. Hanna, Jr. Human colon cancer generation of tumor-specific human monoclonal antibodies. *Proc. Am. Assoc. Cancer Res., 25*:236 (1984).
65. T. Tanaka, D. J. Slamon, and M. J. Cline. Efficient generation of antibodies to oncoproteins by using synthetic peptide antigens. *Proc. Natl. Acad. Sci. (USA), 82*:3400 (1985).
66. G. H. Heppner. Tumor heterogeneity. *Cancer Res., 44*:2259 (1984).
67. R. S. Kerbel. Possible impact of tumor heterogeneity on tumor marker studies. *Prog. Cancer Res. Ther., 29*:197 (1984).
68. P. A. W. Edwards. Heterogeneous expression of cell-surface antigens in normal epithelia and their tumors revealed by monoclonal antibodies. *Br. J. Cancer, 51*:149 (1985).
69. P. H. Hand, M. Nuti, D. Colcher, and J. Schlom. Definition of antigenic heterogeneity and modulation among human mammary carcinoma cell populations using monoclonal antibodies to tumor-association antigens. *Cancer Res., 43*:728 (1983).
70. P. H. Hand, D. Colcher, D. Salomon, J. Ridge, P. Noguchi, and J. Schlom. Influence of spacial configuration of carcinoma cell populations on the expression of a tumor associated glycoproetin. *Cancer Res., 45*:833 (1985).
71. S. Hakomori. Aberrant glycosylation in cancer cell membranes as focused on glycolipids: overview and perspectives. *Cancer Res., 45*:2405 (1985).
72. Y. A. Teramoto, R. Mariani, D. Wunderlich, and J. Schlom. The immunohistochemical reactivity of a human monoclonal antibody with tissue sections of human mammary tumors. *Cancer, 50*:241 (1982).
73. A. Imam, M. M. Drushella, C. R. Taylor, and Z. A. Tökes. Generation and immunohistological characterization of human monoclonal antibodies to mammary carcinoma cells. *Cancer Res., 45*:263 (1985).
74. D. H. Lowe, H. H. Handley, J. Schmidt, I. Royston, and M. C. Glassy. A human monoclonal antibody reactive with human prostate. *J. Urol., 132*:780 (1984).
75. D. Sulitzeanu, B. Bercorici, Y. Gorsky, and I. S. Levij. Membrane-bound immunoglobulin on cells in effusions from patients with malignant disease. *Israel J. Med. Sci., 12*:1329 (1976).
76. J. Schlom, D. Colcher, P. H. Hand, J. Greiner, D. Wunderlich, M. Weeks, P. B. Fisher, P. Noguchi, S. Pestka, and D. Kufe. Monoclonal antibodies reactive with breast tumor-associated antigens. *Adv. Cancer Res., 43*:143 (1985).
77. A. Imam and Z. A. Tökes. Immunoperoxidase localization of a glycoprotein on plasma membrane of secretory epithelium from human breast. *J. Histochem. Cytochem., 29*:581 (1981).
78. R. Ueda, H. Shiku, M. Pfreundschuh, T. Takahashi, L. T. C. Li, W. R. Whitmore, H. F. Oettgen, and L. J. Old. Cell surface antigens of human renal cancer defined by autologous typing. *J. Exp. Med., 150*:564 (1979).
79. R. C. Bast, Jr., M. Feeny, H. Lazarus, L. M. Nadler, R. B. Colvin, and R. C. Knapp. Reactivity of a monoclonal antibody with human ovarian carcinoma. *J. Clin. Invest., 68*:1331 (1981).

80. M. C. Glassy, H. H. Handley, P. H. Cleveland, and I. Royston. An enzyme immunofiltration assay useful for detecting human monoclonal antibody. *J. Immunol. Meth., 58*:119 (1983).
81. L. J. Old. Cancer immunology: the search for specificity–G.H.A. Clowes memorial lecture. *Cancer Res., 41*:361 (1981).
82. J. C. Hager and G. H. Heppner. Evaluation of specific immune reactivity in human patients with solid cancers. In H. Walters (ed.). *The Handbook of Cancer Immunology, Volume 4. Immune Status in Cancer Treatment and Prognosis.* Garland Press, New York (1978).
83. F. X. Real, M. J. Mattes, A. N. Houghton, H. F. Oettgen, K. O. Lloyd, and L. J. Old. Class I (unique) tumor antigens of human melanoma. Identification of a 90,000 dalton cell surface glycoprotein by autologous antibody. *J. Exp. Med., 160*:1219 (1984).
84. D. Stragnmignoni, R. Bowen, B. Atkinson, and J. Schlom. Differential reactivity of monoclonal antibodies with human colon adenocarcinomas and adenomas. *Int. J. Cancer, 31*:543 (1983).
85. F. Graus, C. Cordon-Cardo, A. M. Houghton, M. R. MeLamed, and L. J. Old. Distribution of the ganglioside GD_3 in the human nervous system detected by R24 mouse monoclonal antibody. *Brain Res., 324*:190 (1984).
86. S. E. Kabawat, R. C. Bast, Jr., W. R. Welch, R. C. Knapp, and R. B. Colvin. Immunopathologic characterization of a monoclonal antibody that recognizes common surface antigens of human ovarian tumors of serous, endometroid and clear cell types. *Am. J. Clin. Pathol., 79*:98 (1983).
87. J. P. Brown, R. G. Woodbury, C. E. Hart, I. Hellstrom, and K. E. Hellstrom. Quantitative analysis of melanoma-associated antigen p97 in normal and neoplastic tissues. *Proc. Natl. Acad. Sci. (USA), 78*:539 (1981).
88. T. Feizi. Demonstration by monoclonal antibodies that carbohydrate structures of glycoproteins and glycolipids are onco-developmental antigens. *Nature, 314*:53 (1985).
89. D. Chia, P. I. Terasaki, J. Galton, N. Suyama, M. Hirota, and D. Katz. Use of monoclonal antibodies to sialated Lewis^x and sialated Lewis^a for serological tests for cancer. *Cancer Res., 45*:435 (1985).
90. S. Hakamori. Glycosphingolipids as tumor-associated and differentiation markers. *JNCI, 71*:231 (1984).
91. L. D. Cahan, R. F. Irie, R. Singh, A. Cassadenti, and J. C. Paulson. Identification of human neuroectodermal tumor antigen (OFA-I-2) as ganglioside GD_2. *Proc. Natl. Acad. Sci. (USA), 79*:7629 (1982).
92. Y. A. Teramoto, R. Mariani, D. Wunderlich, and J. Schlom. The immunohistochemical reactivity of a human monoclonal antibody with tissue sections of human mammary tumors. *Cancer, 50*:241 (1982).
93. J. Phillips, K. Sikora, and J. V. Watson. Localization of glioma by a human monoclonal antibody. *Lancet, ii*:1214 (1982).
94. K. Sikora and R. Wright. Human monoclonal antibodies to lung cancer antigens. *J. Cancer, 43*:696 (1981).
95. A. A. Epenetos, S. Mather, M. Granowska, C. C. Nimmon, L. R. Hawkins,

K. E. Britton, J. Shepherd, J. Taylor-Papdimitrion, H. Durbin, and J. S. Malpas. Targeting of iodine-123-labeled tumor-associated monoclonal antibodies to ovarian, breast, and gastrointestinal tumors. *Lancet, ii*:999 (1982).

96. B. Ballou, R. Jaffe, R. J. Taylor, D. Solter, and T. R. Hakala. Tumor radioimmunolocation: differential antibody retention by antigenic normal tissue and tumor. *J. Immunol., 132*:2111 (1984).
97. J. P. Brown, R. G. Woodbury, C. E. Hart, I. Hellstrom, and K. E. Hellstrom. Quantitative analysis of melanoma-associated antigen p97 in normal and neoplastic tissues. *Proc. Natl. Acad. Sci.* (*USA*), *78*:539 (1981).
98. R. Levy and R. A. Miller. Tumor therapy with monoclonal antibodies. *Fed. Proc. 42*:2650 (1983).
99. A. M. Houghton, D. Mintzer, C. Cordon-Cardo, S. Weltz, B. Fliegel, S. Vadhan, E. Corswell, M. R. MeLamed, J. F. Oettgen, and L. J. Old. Mouse monoclonal IgG_3 antibody detecting GD_3 ganglioside: a phase I trial in patients with malignant melanoma. *Proc. Natl. Acad. Sci.* (*USA*), *82*:1242 (1985).
100. R. K. Oldham, K. A. Foon, A. C. Morgan, Jr., C. S. Woodhouse, R. W. Schroff, P. G. Abrams, M. Fer, C. S. Schoenbergee, M. Farrell, E. Kimball, and S. A. Sherwin. Monoclonal antibody therapy of malignant melanoma: *in vivo* localization in cutaneous metastasis after intravenous administration. *J. Clin. Oncol., 2*:1235 (1984).
101. H. F. Sears, J. Mattis, D. Herlyn, P. Hayry, B. Atkinson, C. Ernss, Z. Steplewski, and H. Koprowski. Phase-1 clinical trail of monoclonal antibody in treatment of gastrointestinal tumors. *Lancet, i*:762 (1982).
102. J. D. Berstein, M. R. Tam, and R. L. Nowinski. Mouse leukemia: therapy with monoclonal antibodies against a thymus differentiation antigen. *Science, 207*:68 (1980).
103. T. Meeker, J. Lowder, M. L. Cleary, S. Stewart, R. Warnke, J. Sklar, and R. Levy. Emergence of idiotype variants during treatment of B-cell lymphoma with anti-idiotype antibodies. *N. Engl. J. Med., 312*:1658 (1985).
104. M. Raffeld, L. Neckers, D. L. Longo, and J. Cossman. Spontaneous alteration of idiotype in a monoclonal B-cell lymphoma. Escape from detection by anti-idiotype. *N. Engl. J. Med., 312*:1653 (1985).
105. H. Koprowski, D. Herlyn, M. Lubeck, E. DeFreitas, and J. F. Sears. Human anti-idiotype antibodies in cancer patients: is the modultation of the immune response beneficial for the patient? *Proc. Natl. Acad. Sci.* (*USA*), *81*:216 (1984).
106. R. W. Schroff, C. S. Woodhouse, K. A. Foon, R. K. Oldham, M. M. Farrell, R. A. Klein, and A. C. Morgan, Jr. Intratumor localization of monoclonal antibody in patients with melanoma treated with antibody to a 250,000 dalton melanoma-associated antigen. *JNCI, 74*:299 (1985).
107. H. F. Sears, D. Herlyn, Z. Steplewski, and H. Koprowski. Effects of monoclonal antibody immunotherapy on patients with gastrointestinal adenocarcinoma. *J. Biol. Resp. Modifiers, 3*:138 (1984).
108. R. W. Schroff, K. A. Foon, S. M. Beatty, R. K. Oldham, and A. C. Morgan,

Jr. Human antimurine immunoglobulin responses in patients receiving monoclonal antibody therapy. *Cancer Res., 45*:879 (1985).

109. K. Sikora, T. Alserson, and H. Smedley. The clinical potential of human monoclonal antibodies in oncology. In B. D. Boss, R. Langman, I. Trowbridge, and R. Dulbecco (eds.). *Monoclonal Antibodies and Cancer.* Academic Press, New York (1983).

110. E. S. Vitetta, K. A. Krolick, M. Miyama-Inaba, W. Cushley, and J. W. Uhr. A new approach to cancer therapy. *Science, 219*:664 (1983).

111. M. J. Bjorn, D. Ring, and A. Frankel. Evaluation of monoclonal antibodies for the development of breast cancer immunotoxin. *Cancer Res., 45*:1214 (1985).

112. K. Tsukazaki, E. G. Hayman, and E. Rouslahti. Effects of ricin A chain conjugates of monoclonal antibodies to human alpha-fetoprotein and placental alkaline phosphatase on antigen-producing tumor cells in culture. *Cancer Res., 45*:1834 (1985).

113. A. C. Morgan, Jr., D. R. Galloway, and R. A. Reisfeld. Production and characterization of monoclonal antibody to melanoma-specific glycoprotein. *Hybridoma, 1*:27 (1981).

114. R. G. Woodbury, J. P. Brown, M. Yeh, I. Hellstrom, and K. E. Hellstrom. Identification of a cell surface protein p97 in human melanomas and certain other neoplasms. *Proc. Natl. Acad. Sci. (USA), 77*:2183 (1980).

115. D. Colcher, P. H. Hand, M. Nuti, and J. Schlom. A spectrum of monoclonal antibodies reactive with human mammary tumor cells. *Proc. Natl. Acad. Sci. (USA), 78*:3199 (1981).

116. C. A. White, R. Dulbecco, R. Allen, M. Bowman, and B. Armstrong. Two monoclonal antibodies selective for human mammary carcinoma. *Cancer Res., 45*:1337 (1985).

117. M. Herlyn, Z. Steplewski, D. Herlyn, and H. Koprowski. Colorectal carcinoma-specific antigen: detection by means of monoclonal antibody. *Proc. Natl. Acad. Sci. (USA), 76*:1438 (1979).

118. N. H. Schmiegel, H. Kalthoff, R. Arndt, J. Gieseking, H. Greten, G. Kloppel, C. Kreiker, A. Ladak, V. Lampe, and S. Ulrich. Monoclonal antibody defined human pancreatic cancer-associated antigens. *Cancer Res., 45*:1402 (1985).

119. J. Chin and F. Miller. Identification and localization of human pancreatic tumor-associated antigens by monoclonal antibodies to RWP-1 and RWP-2 cells. *Cancer Res., 45*:1723 (1985).

120. T. Okabe, T. Kaizu, M. Fujisawa, J. Watanabe, K. Kajima, J. Yamashita, and F. Takaku. Monoclonal antibodies to surface antigens of small cell carcinoma of the lung. *Cancer Res., 44*:5273 (1984).

121. S. D. Bernal and J. A. Speak. Membrane antigen in small cell carcinomas of the lung defined by monoclonal antibody SM1. *Cancer Res., 44*:265 (1984).

122. S. Miotti, S. Aquanno, S. Canevari, A. Diotti, R. Orlandi, S. Sonnie, and M I. Colnaghi. Biochemical analysis of human ovarian cancer associated

antigens defined by murine monoclonal antibodies. *Cancer Res., 45*:826 (1985).

123. Y. Tsuji, T. Suzuki, H. Nishiura, T. Takemura, and S. Isajima. Identification of two different surfact epitopes of human ovarian epithelial carcinomas by monoclonal antibodies. *Cancer Res., 45*:2358 (1985).
124. C. L. Finstad, C. Cordon-Cardo, N. H. Bander, W. F. Whitmore, M. R. MeLamed, and L. J. Old. Specificity analysis of mouse monoclonal antibodies defining cell surface antigens of human renal cancer. *Proc. Natl Acad. Sci. (USA), 82*:2955 (1985).
125. W. J. Rettig, C. Cordon-Cardo, J. C. S. Ng, H. F. Oettgen, L. J. Old, and K. O. Lloyd. High molecular weight glycoproteins of human teratocarcinoma defined by monoclonal antibodies to carbohydrate determinants. *Cancer Res., 45*:815 (1985).
126. W. J. Rettig, C. Cordon-Cardo, J. P. Koulos, J. L. Lewis, Jr., J. F. Oettgen, and L. J. Old. Cell surface antigens of human trophoblast and choriocarcinoma defined by monoclonal antibodies. *Int. J. Cancer, 35*:469 (1985).
127. H. Hagiwara and G. H. Sato. Human x human hybridoma producing monoclonal antibody against autologous cervical carcinoma. *Mol. Biol. Med., 1*: 245.
128. D. Kufe, G. Inghirami, M. Abe, D. Hayes, H. Justi-Wheller, and J. Shlom. Differential reactivity of a novel monoclonal antibody (DF3) in human malignant versus benign breast tumors. *Hybridoma, 3*:223 (1984).

9

Human Monoclonal Antibodies to Cancer Cells

KAROL SIKORA
Royal Postgraduate Medical School, London, England

Monoclonal antibodies (MAbs) allow the precise definition of the individual molecular components in complex structures such as the cell surface, cytoskeleton, and nucleus. Over the last decade, millions of hybridoma supernatants have been screened for potentially useful antibody activity. Mouse and rat MAbs raised against human antigens have identified epitopes on a variety of molecules of clinical interest. Indeed, such antibodies are already of clinical use in the diagnosis of cancer by providing markers of tumor load and for the radioimmunolocalization of tumor deposits (1,2). Promising preliminary results in therapeutic trials with such antibodies in patients with colorectal cancer (3), lymphoma (4), and glioma (5) have recently been reported. A major problem with such antibodies has been their lack of specificity. Although the target antigens recognized may often be expressed in increased quantities on tumor cells, most MAbs derived so far show no absolute tumor specificity. The same antigens are present in small quantities on stem cells in normal tissue and only in increased abundance on tumor cells. The xenogeneic immunization schedules used for preparing these monoclonal antibodies emphasize certain components of the cell surface. These include the blood group glycoproteins and histocompatibility antigens that are shared by normal and neoplastic cells. Herein lies the first potential advantage of human MAbs. By not crossing a species barrier, the relatively weak tumor antigens can be emphasized.

A second advantage of human monoclonal antibodies is that they allow us to evaluate the human immune system and how it interacts with a malignant tumor.

There are many diseases mediated through the immune response, including autoimmunity, graft versus host disease, various forms of immunosuppression, and almost certainly part of the control process of cancer (6). The complex network of the immune system has often precluded a detailed analysis of the pathogenesis of immunological disorders. By dissecting out the function of antibodies produced by different lymphocytes, we can piece together the way in which a patient's humoral immune response is working so as to discover and characterize the antigens eliciting these responses.

The third advantage of human MAbs concerns their administration to patients. Clearly, the administration of rat or mouse protein can result in problems (i.e., the abrogation of the antibody's effect and the secondary consequences of circulating immune complexes with the possibility of serum sickness). It is surprising, perhaps, that mouse and rat antibodies have caused no serious clinical troubles to date, even after long-term administration to patients (7).

I. DO TUMOR ANTIGENS EXIST?

There is considerable evidence that the immune system is able to recognize tumor cells. Almost nothing is known about the molecular nature and genetic specificity of the components on the cancer cell surface involved in this recognition. Although we have learned much about the role of the histocompatibility antigen complex in control of immune response, we have not yet identified the nature of the antigens that make a cancer cell recognizable. A variety of immunological assays have been used to examine components on the cell surface. Several groups of antigens can be detected on tumor cells, some of which are shared with normal cells (Table 1).

Normal transplantation antigens can be detected serologically and by cell-mediated lympholysis *in vitro* (8). These histocompatibility antigens are important in studying the immune response to cancer for two reasons. The first is that unless syngeneic systems are used in any animal experimentation, there will be confusion in the detection of antigens specific for transformed cells and not on normal counterparts (9). The second is that some tumor-specific transplantation antigens may, in fact, be modified forms of histocompatibility antigens (10). In a variety of animal systems, tumor-specific transplantation antigens (TSTAs) have been detected. These are defined by a rejection assay which involves the immunization of groups of syngeneic animals, either by excision of the growing tumor or by repeated injections of tumor cells made inactive by irradiation or other means (11). After a suitable interval, the animals are challenged by viable tumor cells, and the growth of the resultant tumors is compared with those in a group of unimmunized animals. Several observations have been made from such studies. There appears to be a considerable range of immunogenicities among different

Table 1 Surface Antigens on Cancer Cells

1. Normal histocompatibility antigens
2. Tumor-specific transplantation antigens
3. Virus antigens
4. Embryonic antigens
5. Differentiation antigens
6. Transformation-specific antigens

experimental tumors (12). Chemically induced tumors often possess specific rejection antigens (i.e., the immunization with one tumor confirms immunity only to itself and not to others, even when induced by the same carcinogen in another location in the same animal) (13). Clearly, such assays are not possible with human tumors, so we do not know if human TSTAs exist. Considerable work has gone into the construction of MAbs against rodent TSTAs to identify their molecular nature. To date, no conclusive evidence of the successful construction of a MAb to TSTAs in a rodent system is available (14).

In virally induced experimental tumors, the surface antigen characteristic of the transforming virus can, under certain circumstances, act as a transplantation antigen (15). Embryonic antigens are defined by antisera and cytotoxic lymphocytes prepared in syngeneic animals by injection of preparations of embryonic tissue (16). Such sera detect antigens on a wide variety of tumor cells, which may well represent products expressed during the rapid growth of cells both in embryogenesis and tumorigenesis. Normal tissue antigens that appear during differentiation can be expressed in neoplastic cells. Under certain circumstances, such antigens may appear tumor-specific. The most extreme example is the idiotype of the immunoglobulin expressed on neoplastic B lymphocytes in certain lymphomas (17). Conventional monoclonal antibodies have revealed new antigenic systems, often in glycoproteins or glycolipids. The sharing of specificities between these molecules often can make it difficult to classify fully the epitopes recognized by individual antibodies. The dominance of xenogeneic determinants has also confused the issue.

The evidence for a serological response to surface antigens in patients with several cancer types is now good. Rigorous testing of sera for antibody-binding activity to tumor cells derived from the same individual has demonstrated three classes of antigen (18). The first class of antigens includes the individually unique tumor antigens seen only on a single tumor. The second consists of shared tumor antigens present on autologous and some allogeneic tumor cells. The third includes normal cell surface antigens widely distributed on both normal and tumor cells. Although melanoma has been the most carefully examined serological response in glioma, patients with renal cell, breast, colon, or lung cancer have been identified by several techniques. Human monoclonal antibodies may, therefore, have great potential for discriminating human tumor cells from their normal counterparts.

II. HUMAN MONOCLONAL ANTIBODY PRODUCTION

A. Lymphocyte Source

Tremendous technical problems surround the production of human MAbs. The first problem is the source of lymphocytes. Few studies have used immunized patients as a source of stimulated B cells for antitumor antibodies. Model systems in which volunteers are hyperimmunized with tetanus toxin or the Rhesus D blood group antigen (19) have also been used. Recently studies (20) have indicated that immunization with autologous colorectal tumor cells as part of an immunotherapy program has resulted in a high yield of human MAbs of the correct specificity. Peripheral blood cells are notorious for fusing poorly. Although 100 ml of human peripheral blood produces, at best, 10^8 lymphocytes, only about 30% are B lymphocytes with fusion potential. Lymphocytes from the lymph nodes surrounding tumors can be obtained easily in diseases such as breast, lung, and colorectal cancer. Lymphocytes can also be extracted from tumors directly, chopping the tumor finely in suitable buffer and separating lymphocytes by Ficoll or other sedimentation. More sophisticated approaches using a cell sorter can also extract the appropriate cell population. In our attempts to raise monoclonal antibodies against a variety of tumor types, we have used predominantly regional lymph nodes that have been teased apart, and high yields of viable lymphocytes have been extracted. Samples have been collected from several hospitals, often from great distances. Lymphocytes extracted from lymph nodes placed directly into tissue culture media appear to preserve their viability for longer than 12 hours.

B. Fusion

One of the major hurdles in reliably producing human hybridomas is the existence of a suitable myeloma partner. Considerable time and effort have been spent on this problem by many groups throughout the world (Table 2). The basic problem is that human myelomas do not grow well in culture. This may be a reflection of the general problem that human tumors, on the whole, grow poorly *in vitro*. Many investigators (21,22) have used interspecies fusions with mouse or rat myelomas. These fusion products have gone on to secrete human immunoglobulin, but unfortunately the human chromosomes are preferentially shed after prolonged

Table 2 Successful Human Fusion Partners

Species	Cell	Selection	Ig H	Ig L	μg/ml	Antibody	Reference
Mouse	NS1	6TG	-	k	50	TAA	22
	NS0	6TG	-	-	50	TAA	23
Rat	Y3	6TG	-	k	100	TAA	29
	Y0	6TG	-	-	100	TAA	29
Human	GM-1500	6TG	k	g	—	Measles	21
	HMy2	6TG	k	g	10	TAA	29
	SK007	8AG	l	e	10	DNCB	43
	RPMI-8226	—	l	g	—	—	44
	UC729-6	6TG	k	m	9	TAA	45
	HFB-1	6TG	-	-	—	H. inf.	46
	LTR228	6TG	k	m	5	TT	47
	WI-L2-HF2	6TG	k	-	30	—	24

growth in culture. Although cloning and recloning at every step seem to result in some stability, ultimately it is only by using human lines that successful stable hybridizations can be obtained.

The major problems of existing lines are slow growth rate, low hybridization frequency, and the continued secretion of immunoglobulin coded for by genes of the parental myeloma (Table 3). This results in the formation of mixed immunoglobulins, thereby diluting the activity of any antibody that is produced. Furthermore, the amount of antibody secreted by human hybridomas is less than 10 μg/ml. We have used predominantly two lines, the LICR LON-HMy2 (23) and the WI L2-729HF-2 (24) line, which are both resistant to 8-azaguanine and die on

Table 3 Problems with Human Hybridomas

1. Slow growth rate
2. Low hybridization frequency
3. Low cloning efficiency
4. Mixed Ig production
5. Low Ig production

medium supplemented with hypoxanthine, aminopterin, and thymidine (HAT). Cell fusion has been induced by polyethylene glycol (25). We have no experience with electrofusion and know of no experimental evidence of its potential advantages.

For fusion, 5×10^7 HMy2 or HF2 cells and approximately the same number of lymphocytes isolated from lymph nodes associated with a tumor were suspended in serum-free Dulbecco's modified eagles medium (DMEM), mixed and centrifuged at 1500 rpm for 10 minutes in a 50 ml conical-bottomed plastic centrifuge tube. The supernatant was drained off completely, and 0.5 ml of polyethylene glycol (PEG), molecular weight 1500, 41.7% WV, with 15% dimethylsulphoxide (DMSO) in serum-free DMEM was added to the pellet and the cells were gently resuspended using the tip of a 1-ml pipette. After 1 minute, 4.5 ml of PEG 1500, 33% WV, in serum-free medium (but without DMSO) was added and the mixture was gently stirred for 3 minutes. Next, 4 ml of DMEM with 10% fetal calf serum (FCS) was added dropwise, and the mixture was rocked for a further 4 minutes. This was then either centrifuged if large aggregates were present or directly resuspended by slowly adding 45 ml of DMEM with 10% FCS. The mixture was taken up carefully with a wide-bore 25-ml pipette and dispensed equally into each of 96 wells of a Linbro plate. After 24 hours, the medium was partly replaced by DMEM containing HAT with 20% FCS. Selective medium was renewed daily for at least 7 days. Hybrid cells appeared in the wells from the third week onwards. New hybrids ceased appearing by the seventh week. Supernatants from wells containing hybrids were taken for testing, supplemented with 10 mM Hepes and 0.1% azide, and stored at 4°C. Bulk supernatants from cloned hybrids growing in roller bottles were in Iscoves serum-free medium, supplemented with 5 μg/ml of insulin. Bulk supernatants were harvested and concentrated using a Millipore CX10 (10,000 daltons exclusion) ulfiltration unit (Fig. 1).

C. *In Vitro* Immunization

Immunization of lymphocytes can be carried out *in vitro* to increase the yield of antigen-stimulated cells. Lymphocytes harvested from human samples in the normal way are isolated, and dead cells are removed by Ficoll separation. The stimulant effect of added antigen can be increased by depleting a subpopulation of T cells. Suppressor T lymphocytes, which bear histamine H-2 receptors, were removed by layering the purified lymphocyte suspension on a human serum albumin/cimetidine-coated petri dish (Cel-ect H-2 plates, SG7002 dish kit, Serogen Inc., Boston, MA) (25). The lymphocyte suspension was incubated for 1 hour at 37°C in a gassed incubator. The dish was gently washed, with the panning buffer supplied with the kit and nonadherent H2R cells recovered. Such cells were washed and resuspended at 2×10^6 cell/ml in RPMI-1640 media containing 10% heat-inactivated human serum autologous with that of the lympho-

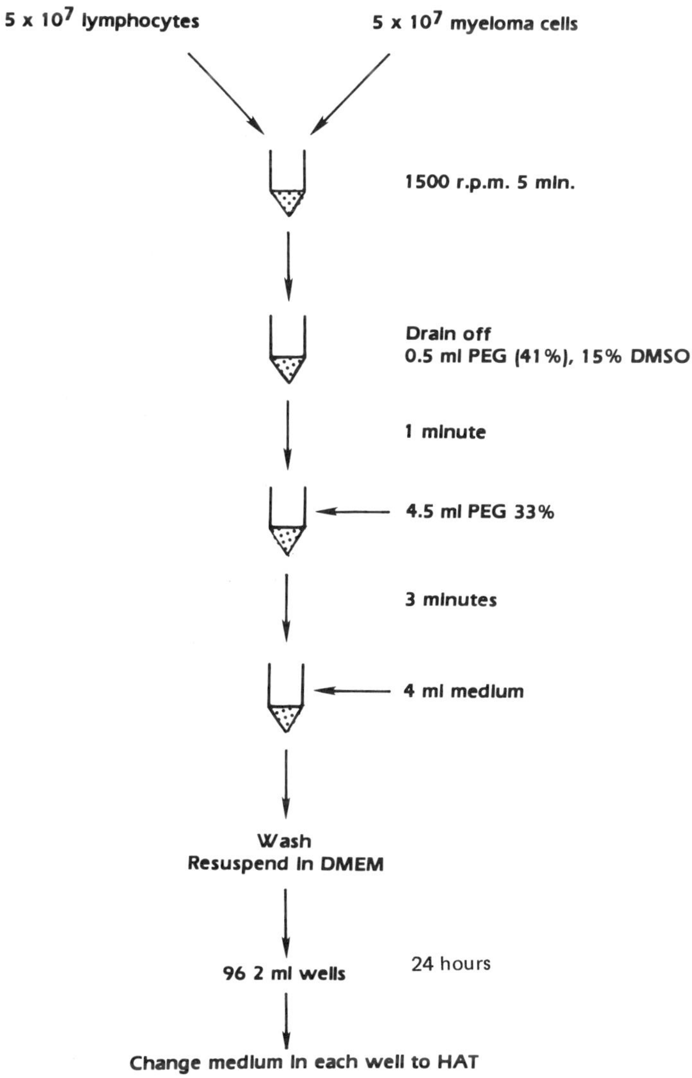

Figure 1 Polvethylene glycol (PEG) fusion protocol currently in use for HMy2 and HF-2 myeloma lines.

cyte sample. Cells were placed in 25 ml conical tissue-culture flasks in a final volume of 15 ml. Then 5 ml of spent mixed lymphocyte culture supernatant in RPMI-1640 was added as a nonspecific activator containing the necessary growth factors such as B-cell growth factor (BCGF). The desired antigen was also added at concentrations of 1-50 μg/ml. The cells were cultured for 7 days before radioimmunoassay to screen for specific antibody directed against the immunizing antigen. Lymphocytes from positive flasks were washed after this time and fused in the normal way to either HMy2 or HF2 to produce hybridomas. Evidence of a higher yield of specific antibody against albumin, sheep erythrocytes, Rhesus D positive human erythrocytes, tetanus toxins, and, more recently, peptide fragments has now been obtained (26). An example of the construction MAbs to synthetic peptide fragments of the c-*myc* oncogene product is shown in Figure 2. Other methods for enriching for the relevant lymphocytes prior to fusion are listed in Table 4.

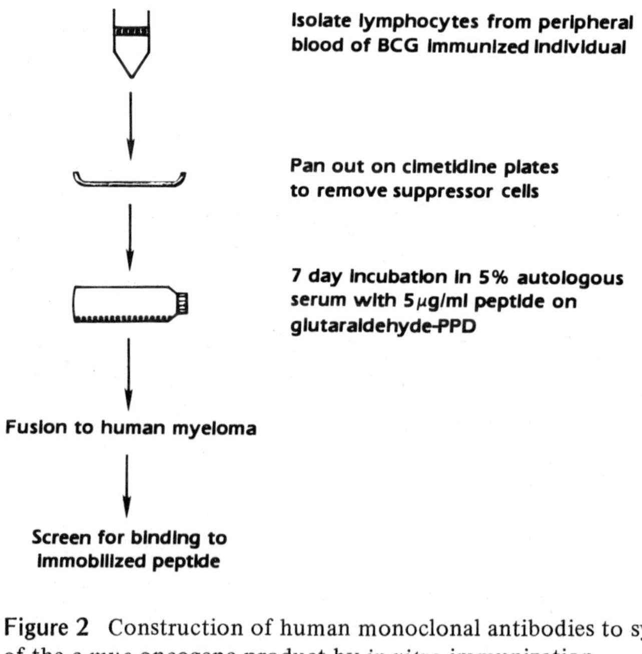

Figure 2 Construction of human monoclonal antibodies to synthetic fragments of the c-*myc* oncogene product by *in vitro* immunization.

Table 4 Selection of Lymphocytes Prior to Fusion

1. Clinical immunization
2. *In vitro* immunization
3. Suppressor cell deletion
4. Timing of *in vitro* stimulation
5. Antigen-specific enrichment

III. HYBRIDOMA AND SUPERNATANT CHARACTERIZATION

Normal lymphocytes, when plated out under the conditions used after hybridization, will continue to secrete immunoglobulin for up to 6 weeks. No clones are seen to emerge, but the continued secretion of human immunoglobulin provides a trap for the optimist. Furthermore, if Epstein Barr virus is present, it is possible for lymphoblastoid lines to emerge. There are several ways to obtain evidence of hybridization (Table 5).

The first is to type the immunoglobulins (see section III.A). Surface immunoglobulins can also be characterized using immunofluorescence techniques. Another method to identify hybrids rapidly is to use a flow cytometer to analyze their DNA content. A suspension of putative hybridoma cells is washed and, after pelleting, resuspended in a solution of ethidium bromide. This intercalates within base pairs of nucleotides in the DNA of the cell, and a flow cytometer can be used to measure the DNA content in each cell. Hybridomas were cultured in 25-ml tissue-culture flasks in the log phase. Cells were washed in EBSS containing 1% bovine serum albumin and adjusted to 10^6 cells/ml. Cells were pelleted and resuspended in ethidium bromide, 0.05% mg/ml in hypotonic (0.1%) sodium citrate. DNA histograms were obtained using a flow cytometer which incorporated an argon laser. Hybrids showed a consistent and stable increase in their DNA content.

Morphological changes also occur after hybridization. Although undetect-

Table 5 Evidence for Hybridoma Formation

1. Morphology
2. DNA content
3. Karyotype
4. New Ig chain production
5. HLA typing

able by light microscopy, stereo scanning or conventional electron microscopy shows an increase in the number of pseudopodia in hybrid cells compared with the myeloma or unfused lymphocytes.

A. Immunoglobulin Assay

The detection of low concentrations of specific immunoglobulins is a prerequisite for the development of human hybridoma systems. The assays currently available for human immunoglobulins include radial immunodiffusion, electroimmunoassay, antibody-coupled red cell lysis, and double-antibody inhibition radioimmunoassay. Not all these assays are sensitive in the microgram range, and they often show loss of specificity when the concentration of immunoglobulin is low. Therefore, we developed a rapid solid-phase radioimmunoassay that is chain-specific at concentrations of immunoglobulin less than 20 ng/ml (27). Furthermore, commercially available polyclonal and monoclonal antibodies are used making the assay readily available for any laboratory. Figure 3 illustrates the principle whereby an adsorbed rabbit anti-human immunoglobulin first binds to any human immunoglobulins in the supernatant; bound Ig chains are then characterized by a second antibody that is a mouse chain-specific monoclonal against human immunoglobulin. The rabbit anti-human immunoglobulin is produced by immunizing rabbits with purified human immunoglobulins.

The antiserum was diluted in phosphate-buffered saline (PBS) to 1:1000. Then 50 λ aliquots were added to a round-bottomed 96-well vinyl plastic plates and incubated overnight at 4°C. These plates were subsequently washed in medium containing Earles-buffered salt solution, 1% bovine serum albumin, and 0.01% sodium azide adjusted to pH 7.4 by 1 M sodium hydroxide. After washing four times by flicking the contents of the wells into a sink and replacing them with 50 μl of medium, the plates, containing 50 μl of medium in each well, were left for 1 hour at room temperature. This ensured complete saturation of the plastic binding sites by bovine serum albumin in the complete medium. Sensitivity of the technique was determined by titrating human serum containing known amounts of different immunoglobulin, starting at 50 μg/ml in 50 μl.

After incubating for 1 hour at room temperature, the plates were washed in the manner previously described, and 50 μl of chain-specific mouse monoclonal anti-human immunoglobulin was added. Monoclonal antibodies were used at a concentration of 1:5000 (approximately 1 ng/ml of mouse immunoglobulin). After 1 hour of incubation with the relevant monoclonal antibodies, the plates were washed and rat anti-mouse immunoglobulin coupled with ^{125}I by the chloramine-T method was added. After a final incubation of 1 hour and four subsequent washes in complete medium, the plates were air-dried and the wells were cut with a hot wire and counted in a gamma-counter. The concentrations of immunoglobulin secreted by bybrids from one fusion is shown in Figure 4. It

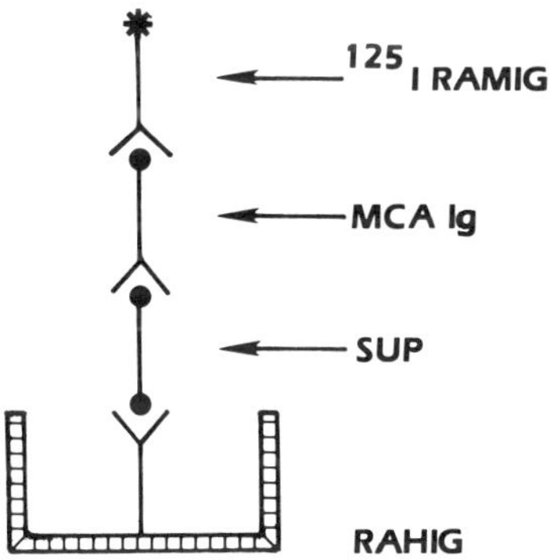

Figure 3 Chain typing of immunoglobulins in human hybridoma supernatants.

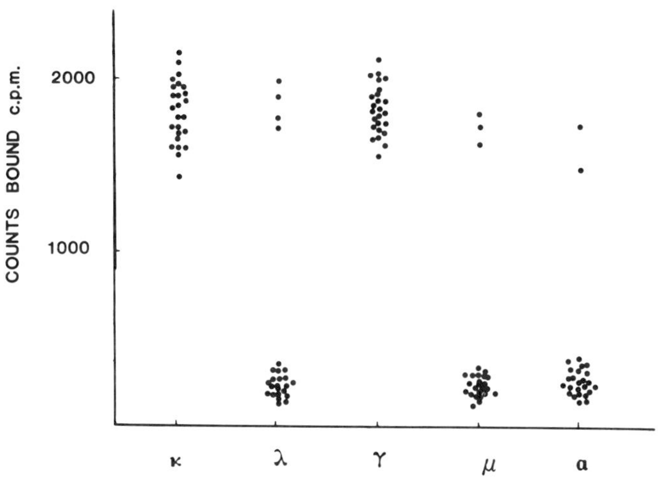

Figure 4 Results of chain typing assay in 35 human hybridomas produced from a patient with malignant glioma.

can be seen that for all the hybrids produced with human, kappa, and gamma chains, the chain is produced by the parent HMy2 myeloma. In addition, over 30% produce new immunoglobulins. These immunoglobulins are coded for by genes from the donor lymphocytes. This sensitive immunoassay is able to detect specific chains at concentrations of less than 100 ng/ml. Microliter quantities of test fluid can be handled and large numbers of samples can be dealt with in one batch.

B. Antibody Production

In the final analysis, it is the production of useful monoclonal antibodies of defined specificity that must justify the technique used (28). Human MAbs have now been made against a variety of tumors, measles virus, various haptens, and bacterial antigens (Table 2). In order to assay for anti-tumor activity, we used a variety of human tumor cell lines. These were grown, usually as monolayers, freshly trypsinized, and washed. They were suspended in assay medium identical to that used for immunoglobulin typing. Viable cells were counted by trypan-blue exclusion and adjusted to a concentration of 2×10^6/ml. Next, 50 μl of cell suspension was placed into each well of a round-bottomed microtiter plate that had previously been incubated overnight with 50 μl of poly-L-lysine and phosphate-buffered saline at 37°C. Cells were fixed for 1 hour in 0.25% glutaraldehyde and washed three times in medium. Fifty microliters of supernatant was added and incubated at room temperature for 1 hour. After washing three times, 50 μl of mouse anti-human light-chain antibody at a dilution of 1:5000 was added and incubated for 1 hour. The final stage of the assay was the addition of 50 μl radioiodinated rabbit anti-mouse immunoglobulin. After a further hour, the cells were washed and counted in a gamma-counter.

Table 6 Human Hybridoma Production from Cancer Patients

Tumor	Samples	Fusions	Patient hybrids	Total hybrids	MAbs
Lung	25	15	9	43	4
Breast	37	17	9	32	2
Colon	46	13	4	15	0
Glioma	42	23	14	104	8
Kidney	4	0	0	0	0
Sarcoma	3	0	0	0	0
Melanoma	4	2	2	6	1
Uterus	15	6	3	7	0
Stomach	17	8	3	9	0
Bladder	21	0	0	0	0
Burkitts	5	3	3	5	0
Total	219	87	44	221	15

The results of lymphocytes fusion from 219 cancer patients are shown in Table 6. Antibodies were initially screened for binding activity against a cell line most appropriate to the source of the donor lymphocyte. Despite the sensitivity of the binding assay, the counts were low. After concentration, however, reasonable titration curves were obtained. The specificity of binding was determined by using several tumor and normal cell lines (Table 7). So far, all the antibodies isolated, with or without *in vitro* immunization, show a similar distribution of binding activity. No individual tumor or tissue specificity was detected (29).

Our screening technique for these antibodies involved binding to the cell surface of immobilized cell lines. This technique precludes the detection of antibodies that bind to nonmembrane components such as those of the cytoskeleton. Other workers (30,31) have shown clearly that many human monoclonal antibodies are against such structures. Therefore, we analyzed the antibodies that gave tumor binding for their ability to bind to a cytoskeletal preparation of the relevant cell line. No evidence of cytoskeletal binding was found.

Table 7 Binding of Human Hybridoma Supernatants to Various Human Cell Lines Peripheral Lymphocytes and Red Cells

Supernatant	G/CCM	HT29	MOR	CALU1	MCF7	MRC5	PBL	RBC
Glioma								
LGL1-1C3	+++	++	+	-	+++	-	-	-
LGL1-1C6	+++	++	+	-	++	-	-	-
LGL1-1D6	+++	+	++	+	+	-	±	-
LGL1-2C1	++	++	+	+	-	-	-	±
LGL7-1A2	++	+	+	-	+	±	-	±
LGL7-3A2	++	+	+	++	-	-	-	-
LGL10-3BS	++	+	+	-	++	-	-	-
LGL22-4D6	++	+	++	+	+	-	-	+
Lung								
LLU1-3D1	++	++	++	++	+	-	-	±
LLU6-1A1	++	+	++	++	+	±	-	±
LLU6-2A4	+++	+	+	+	-	-	-	-
LLU6-3D4	++	+	++	++	+	-	-	-

IV. IMPROVING HUMAN HYBRIDOMA PRODUCTION

We have demonstrated that lymphocytes from patients with several tumor types can be successfully fused with human myeloma lines to produce stable hybridomas. Immunoglobulins are secreted, several of which have been shown to have weak binding to tumor cell lines by an indirect immunoassay. Evidence for hybridization, rather than outgrowth of lymphoblastoid lines from the patients lymphocytes, was provided by the continued secretion of HMy2 Ig as well as the new Ig chains in the supernatants of cloned hybridomas. Flow cytometric DNA analysis showed the stably increased DNA content characteristic of hybrids. More detailed karyotypic analysis has now been performed on some of these hybridomas, confirming a stably increased chromosome number.

Many problems still remain. The low fusion frequency results in a large workload to produce small numbers of hybrids. Several methods have now been used to attempt to increase this frequency. These have included the provision of feeder cells and secondary *in vitro* stimulation by either antigen (tumor cells) or pokeweed mitogen. No overall increase in fusion frequency was observed. A second problem is the continued secretion of the HMy2 kappa- and gamma-immunoglobulin chains by the hybridomas. The true assessment of the numbers of hybrids secreting Ig coded for by genes of the donor lymphocytes is thus difficult. Furthermore, mixed antibody molecules comprised of chains coded by both myeloma or lymphocyte genes will occur. Such molecules will have a reduced antibody activity. A third problem is the low antibody secretion of between 1 and 5 μg/ml. Large amounts of tissue-culture supernatant must be concentrated in order to increase signal to noise ratio in the radioimmunoassay. The poorly developed endoplasmic reticulum in all hybrids examined by electron microscopy suggests that the rate of protein synthesis may be the limiting factor. The initial screen for anti-tumor antibody activity may be unable to detect the small amounts of weak antibodies. Finally, the low anti-tumor binding activity hinders the analysis of the specificity of the resulting antibodies. A combination of low secretion rate, mixed Ig chain molecules and low affinity can all contribute to this low binding.

V. CLINICAL USE

A. Radioimmunolocalization

The detection and localization of metastatic spread are a major problem in managing patients with cancer. The presence of metastases affects the choice of therapy for individual patients. Recent developments, such as CT scanning and ultrasound imaging, have improved the accuracy of staging. A significant proportion of patients still have metastatic disease that remains undetected at the time of therapy. Over the last decade, antibodies raised by immunizing animals with human tumors have been used after coupling to a radioisotope to detect neoplasms (32). Antisera with the required specificity to discriminate between normal and malignant tissue are difficult to produce. The development of the monoclonal antibody technology yields unlimited quantities of pure reagents of defined specificity. There are now several reports on the use of mouse or rat monoclonal antibodies for the localization of colorectal cancer (33), breast cancer (34), melanoma (35), and ovarian cancer (36). The major advantage of a human antibody is lack of response to it by the recipient's immune system.

We studied two antibodies for their clinical potential in tumor localization. One (LGL1-1D6) was derived from intratumoral lymphocytes from a patient with glioma (37). The other (LLU6-2A4) was from a patient with carcinoma of the bronchus (38).

Serum-free supernatants from the two cloned hybridomas were collected, and ammonium sulphate was added to a final concentration of 50%. The precipitate was spun at 15,000 *g* for 20 minutes, and the pellet was redissolved in PBS. After two successive precipitations, the pellet was finally taken up in PBS and loaded onto a protein-A sepharose-4B affinity column and eluted using a glycine HCl buffer, pH 2.8. After dialysis against PBS, the purified antibody was iodinated with ^{131}I using a modified chloramine-T technique. Efficacy of both antibodies was screened by using xenografts of both lung and glioma cell lines established in nude mice. Twelve patients with malignant glioma and 15 patients with intrathoracic tumors were studied. One milligram of labeled antibody was administered by slow intravenous injection in 10 ml of normal saline solution, 12 hours after the patients had received 120 mg of potassium iodide by mouth to block thyroid uptake of free radioiodine. Forty-four hours later, 0.05 mCi of technetium-99m (Tc^{99m})-labeled human serum albumin was injected intravenously in order to outline the blood pool. Scans were obtained 30 minutes after the second injection. Images were obtained using a gamma-camera. The data were recorded on a Varian V77 computer, which simultaneously recorded the ^{131}I and Tc^{99m} distribution.

Good images of glioma were seen in eight of 12 patients. For this tumor, clear images could be seen without resorting to subtraction techniques. With the human anti-lung tumor, good MAb localization was seen in nine patients; an additional patient, who was initially thought to have carcinoma of the bronchus but was subsequently found to have a malignant thymoma, gave no image with this antibody. This antibody does not bind to lymphoma cells *in vitro*. examples of scans are shown in Figures 5 and 6.

Despite the relatively low affinity for their target antigen, the quality of the images obtained was very similar to those seen with conventional rat or mouse immunoglobulins. Not all patients gave tumor images. There are several reasons for this, including variation in target antigen expression on tumors, differences in radiolabeled antibody handling kinetics, and vascular access to tumor. Clearly,

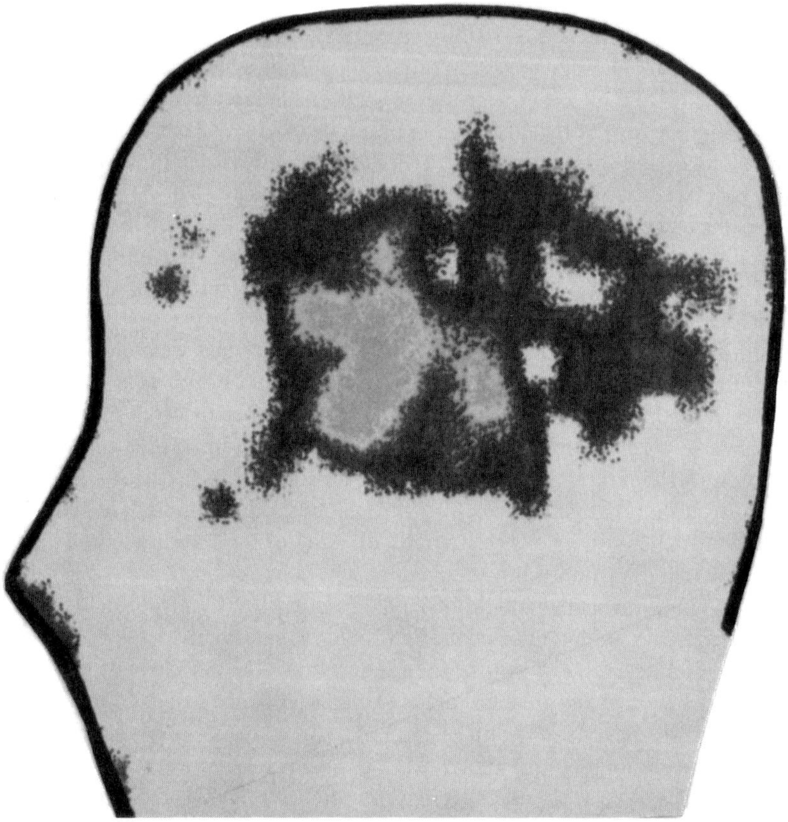

Figure 5 Human MAb scan in a patient with malignant glioma.

human MAbs have considerable potential for the development of clinically useful detectors of cancer.

B. Therapeutic Potential

To study the feasibility of continuous administration of human monoclonal antibodies directed against glioma, we designed a chamber that enables hybridoma cells to be cultured in the subcutaneous tissue (39). This chamber allows antibodies to diffuse out, and nutrients and oxygen (necessary for continued cell viability) to diffuse in. Because cells are unable to traverse the membrane pores of the device, there is no risk that malignant cells put in the chamber can metas-

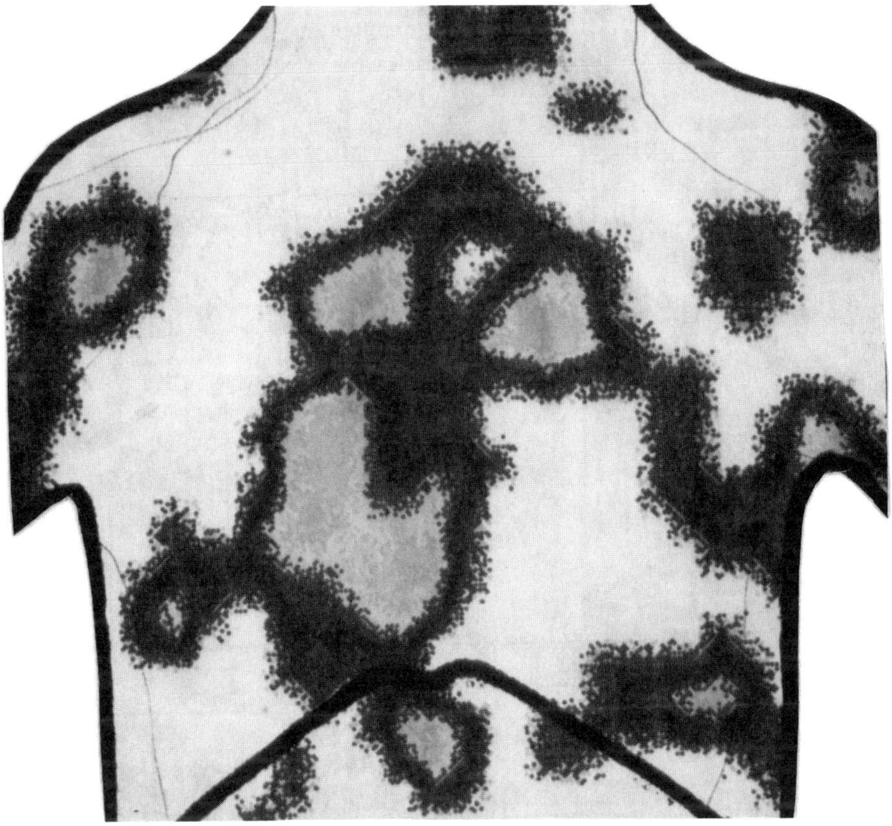

Figure 6 Human MAb scan in a patient with bronchial carcinoma.

tasize. The chamber has now been inserted into three patients with recurrent glioma, in whom the kinetics of internally labeled antibody release has been monitored.

The chamber consists of a cylindrical diffusion cavity constructed of Delrin, a synthetic homopolymer. The upper section contains an outlet and inlet hole to which there 21 gauge needles are inserted. This assembly screws into the lower cylindrical section, which has an internal and external flange at the base. The internal flange holds a 3-cm diameter injection Millipore filter. The external flange enables the chamber to be immobilized in the subcutaneous tissue. The filter allows the free diffusion of large molecules, but not of cells, between the chamber and the patient's extracellular fluid (Fig. 7).

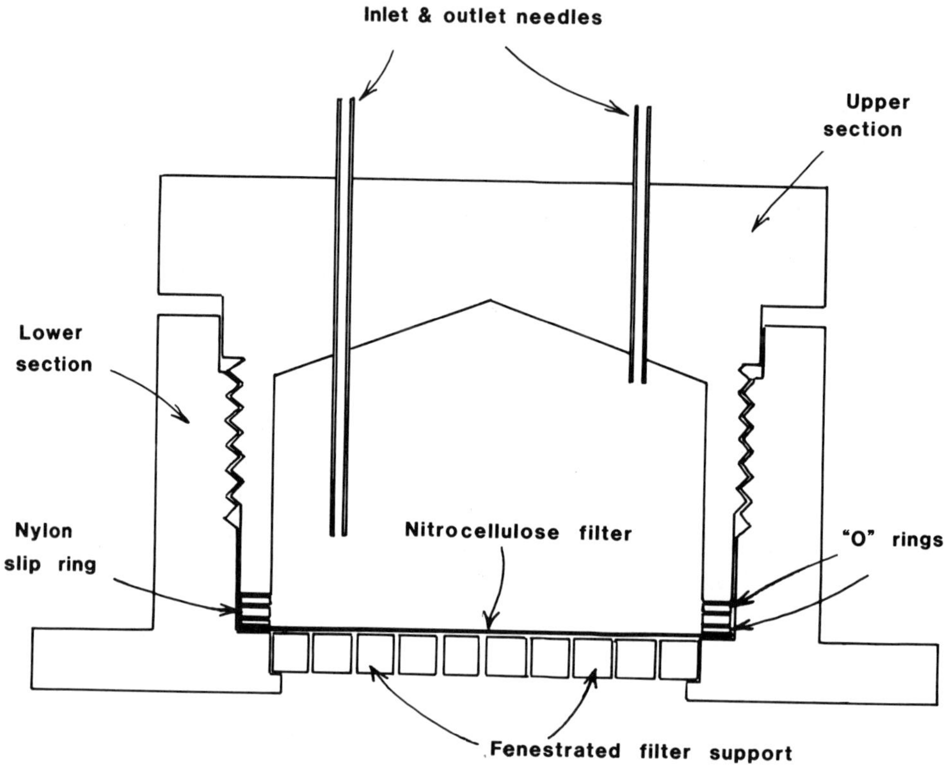

Figure 7 A diffusion chamber for the *in vivo* production of human MAbs from hybridoma.

A total of 10^7 hybridoma cells were pulse-labeled with 100 μCi of tritiated lysine monohydrochloride and placed in the chamber. Serum samples were collected from the patient at regular intervals after the insertion of the chamber. Trichloroacetic acid precipitable to H3 counts was determined by scintillation counting. Release of tritiated monoclonal antibody from the chamber into the blood stream occurred within the 3 days after injection of pulse-labeled cells into the chamber. The device has remained *in situ* for up to 3 months and caused no problems. There is no evidence of infection or of inflammatory response around the chamber, and no evidence of spread of hybridoma cells outside the chamber. There has been no change in the patient's serum Epstein-Barr virus titer. We believe that this device can be used to study the long-term effects of MAbs produced *in vivo*.

VI. THE FUTURE

The stumbling block in the human monoclonal antibody field has been the vagaries of their production. When one considers the number of conventional rodent hybridomas screened to produce a panel of useful reagents, it is not surprising that success with human systems has not been so rapid. Most current advancements center around the development of more successful hybridomas production (Table 8). New myelomas and fusion techniques, such as electrofusion, have so far failed to make significant impact. It is too early to assess the merits of the new immortalizing vectors or transfection systems (40). However, as we learn more about the *in vitro* requirements for successful B-lymphocyte propagation, it is likely that the number of clones lines will increase. Some form of prefusion selection procedure is clearly necessary to reduce the sheer volume of work required at the screening stage. For well-defined antigens, such as purified proteins or synthetic peptides, the selection of the relevant subset of B lymphocytes is now feasible. Where the antigens are largely undefined (e.g., the elusive tumor-specific antigens) such preselection is impossible.

Considerable progress has occurred in our ability to manipulate the gene products of the immunoglobulin loci in secreting plasma cell lines. Chimeric anti-

Table 8 Human MCA—The Future

1. New hybridoma techniques
    - New myelomas
    - Peptide immunization
    - Prefusion selection
    - Electrofusion
    - Growth factors
    - Combined EBV-fusion systems
2. Immortality transfer
    - Transfection
    - Gene insertion
3. Protein engineering
    - Chimeric molecules (mouse V, human C)
    - Recombinant proteins
    - Antibody design
4. Clinical peptide immunization
5. Clinical application

bodies with mouse variable-regions and human constant-regions have now been produced (41). This allows the conversion of almost any mouse antibody into one that has at least the secondary characteristics of a human antibody, which may well be adequate to confer all the advantages of human reagents discussed above. Recombinant proteins from antibody-secreting lines are also available. In a particularly intriguing study (42), the c-*myc* oncogene was tagged onto a mouse immunoglobulin gene and resulted in the synthesis of a protein coded for by both genes. The same group is now coupling the ricin gene to that of an anti-tumor antibody in order to construct an intact powerful immunotoxin. Computer-modeling techniques are becoming increasingly more sophisticated, allowing the three-dimensional structure of protein-protein interactions to be clearly analyzed. This may soon result in the computer-assisted design of antibodies for specific epitopes. The combining of these elegant technologies will almost certainly yield highly specific human MAbs for clinical use in the near future.

REFERENCES

1. K. Sikora, H. Smedley, and P. Thorpe. Tumour imaging and drug targeting. *Br. Med. Bull., 40*:240 (1984).
2. H. M. Smedley, P. Finan, E. Lennox, A. Ritson, F. Takei, P. Wraight, and K. Sikora. Localisation of metastatic carcinoma by a radiolabelled monoclonal antibody. *Br. J. Cancer, 47*:253 (1983).
3. H. F. Sears, B. Atkinson, J. Mattis, C. Ernst, D. Herlyn, Z. Steplewski, P. Hayry, and H. Koprowski. Phase-I clinical trial of monoclonal antibody in treatment of gastrointestinal tumours. *Lancet I*:762 (1982).
4. R. A. Miller, D. G. Maloney, J. McKillop, and R. Levy. *In vivo* effects of murine hybridoma monoclonal antibody in a patient with T-cell leukaemia. *Blooc, 58*:78 (1981).
5. A. A. Epenetos, N. Courtenay Luck, D. Pickering, G. Hooker, H. Durbin, J. P. Lavender, and C. G. McKenzie. Antibody guided irradiation of brain glioma by arterial infusion of radioactive monoclonal antibody against epidermal growth factor receptor and blood group A antigen. *Br. Med. J., 290*: 1463 (1985).
6. G. A. Currie, *Cancer and the Immune Response.* Arnold, London (1974).
7. J. Ritz, J. M. Pesando, S. E. Sallan, L. A. Clavell, J. Notis-McConarty, P. Rosenthal, and S. F. Schlossman. Serotherapy of acute lymphoblastic leukaemia with monoclonal antibody. *Blood, 58*:361 (1981).
8. E. S. Lennox and K. Sikora. Definition of human tumour antigens. In A. J. McMichael and J. W. Fabre (eds.). *Monoclonal Antibodies in Clinical Medicine.* Academic Press, London (1982).
9. K. Sikora and E. Lennox. Tumour antigens. In P. Lachmann and D. K. Peters (eds.). *Clinical Aspects of Immunology. Blackwell, Oxford (1982).*

10. G. Invernizzi and G. Parmiami. Tumour associated transplantation antigens of chemically induced sarcoma cross reacting with allogeneic histocompatibility antigens. *Nature, 254*:713 (1975).
11. K. Sikora, G. Koch, S. Brenner, and E. Lennox. Partial purification of TSTA from methylcholanthrene induced murine sarcomas by immobilised lectins. *Br. J. Cancer, 40*:831 (1979).
12. T. Pearson, K. Sikora, and E. Lennox. Measurement of H-2 antigen and immunogenicity of methylcholanthrene induced murine sarcomas. *Br. J. Cancer, 37*:530 (1978).
13. R. W. Baldwin. Immunological aspects of chemical carcinogens. *Adv. Cancer Res., 18*:1 (1973).
14. E. Lennox and K. Sikora. Definition of human tumour antigens. In A. J. McMichael and J. W. Fabre (eds.). *Monoclonal Antibodies in Clinical Medicine.* Academic Press, London (1982).
15. R. Kurth. Tumour virus proteins at the cell surface. *Nature, 256*:613 (1975).
16. S. E. Chism, S. Wallis, P. C. Burton, and N. L. Warner. Analysis of murine oncofetal antigens as tumor associated transplantation antigens. *J. Immunol., 117*:1870 (1976).
17. R. A. Miller, D. G. Maloney, R. Warnke, and R. Levy. Treatment of B cell lymphoma with monoclonal anti-idiotype antibody. *N. Engl. J. Med., 306*: 517 (1982).
18. L. J. Old. Cancer immunology: the search for specificity. *Cancer Res., 41*: 361 (1981).
19. D. Kozbor and J. C. Roder. Requirements for the establishment of high-titered human monoclonal antibodies against tetanus toxoid using the Epstein-Barr virus technique. *J. Immunol., 127*:1275 (1981).
20. M. V. Haspel, R. P. McCabe, N. Pomato, N. J. Jenesch, J. V. Knowlton, L. C. Peters, H. Hoover, and M. G. Hanna. Generation of tumour cell reactive human monoclonal antibodies using peripheral blood lymphocytes from actively immunised colorectal carcinoma patients. *Cancer Res., 45*:3951 (1985).
21. C. M; Croce, A. Linnenbach, W. Hall, Z. Steplewski, and H. Koprowski. Production of human hybridomas secreting antibodies to measles virus. *Nature, 288*:488 (1980).
22. R. J. Cote, D. M. Morrissey, A. N. Houghton, E. J. Beattie, Jr., H. F. Oettgen, and L. J. Old. Generation of human monoclonal antibodies reactive with cellular antigens. *Proc. Natl. Acad. Sci.* (*USA*), *80*:2026 (1983).
23. P. A. W. Edwards, C. M. Smith, A. M. Neville, and M. J. O'Hare. A human-human hybridoma system based on a fast growing mutant of the ARH-77 plasma cell leukemia-derived line. *Eur. J. Immunol., 12*:641 (1982).
24. J. G. Heitzmann and M. Cohn. The WI-L2-729-HF_2 human hybridoma system. *Mol. Biol. Med., 1*:235 (1983).
25. J. Cavagnaro and M. Osband. Successful *in vitro* primary immunisation of human peripheral blood mononuclear cells. *Bio Techniques 3*:30 (1983).
26. S. Kar, T. Alderson, and K. Sikora. Human monoclonal antibodies to the c-*myc* oncogene product. (submitted.)

27. K. Sikora, T. Alderson, and J. Ellis. A sensitive chain specific radioimmunoassay for human immunoglobulins using monoclonal antibodies. *J. Immunol. Meth., 57*:151 (1983).
28. D. Kozbor and J. C. Roder. The production of monoclonal antibodies from human lymphocytes. *Immunol. Today, 4*:72 (1983).
29. K. Sikora, T. Alderson, J. Ellis, J. Phillips, and J. Watson. Human hybridomas from patients with malignant glioma. *Br. J. Cancer, 47*:135 (1983).
30. L. Olsson, H. Kronstrom, A. C-D. Mouzon, L. Honsik, T. Brodin, and B. Jacobsen. Antibody producing human-human hybridomas. I. Technical aspects. *J. Immunol. Meth., 61*:17 (1983).
31. J. Satoh, B. S. Prabhakar, M. V. Haspel, F. Ginsberg-Fellner, and A. L. Notkins. Human monoclonal autoantibodies that react with multiple endocrine organs. *N. Engl. J. Med., 309*:217 (1983).
32. D. M. Goldenberg, E. E. Kim, F. H. Deland, S. Bennett, and F. J. Primus. Radioimmunodetection of cancer with radioactive antibodies to carcinoembryonic antigen. *Cancer Res., 40*:2984 (1980).
33. J-P. Mach, F. Buchegger, M. Forni, J. Ritschard, C. Berchie, J-D. Lumbroso, M. Schreyer, C. Giradet, R. S. Accolla, and S. Carrel. Use of radiolabelled monoclonal anti-CEA antibodies for the detection of human carcinomas by external photoscanning and tomoscintiscanning. *Immunol. Today, 2*:239 (1981).
34. A. A. Epenetos, S. Mathew, and M. Granowska. Targeting of iodine 123 labelled monoclonal antibodies to ovarian, breast and gastrointestinal tumours. *Lancet, ii*:999 (1982).
35. S. Larsson, J. P. Brown, P. W. Wright, I. Hellstrom, and K. E. Hellstrom. Imaging of melanoma with ^{131}I-labelled monoclonal antibodies. *J. Nucl. Med., 24*:123 (1983).
36. T. F. Primus, F. H. Deland, and D. M. Goldenberg. Monoclonal antibodies for radioimmunodetection of cancer. In G. L. Wright (ed.). *Monoclonal Antibodies and Cancer.* Marcel Dekker, New York (1984).
37. K. Sikora, T. Alderson, J. Phillips, and J. V. Watson. Human hybridomas from malignant gliomas. *Lancet, i*:11 (1982).
38. K. Sikora, A. Nethersell, A. Ritson, and H. Smedley. Tumour localisation by human monoclonal antibodies. *Med. Oncol. Tumor Pharmacother., 2*:77 (1985).
39. J. V. Watson, T. Alderson, K. Sikora, and J. Phillips. Subcutaneous culture chamber for continuous infusion of monoclonal antibodies. *Lancet, i*:99 (1983).
40. K. Sikora and T. Alderson. Eucaryotic vectors for lymphocyte immortalization. (submitted.)
41. A. Ochi, R. G. Hanley, T. Hawley, M. Shulman, A. Traunecker, G. Kohler, and N. Hozumi. Functional immunoglobulin M production after transcription of cloned immunoglobulin heavy and light chain genes into lymphoid cells. *Proc. Natl. Acad. Sci. (USA), 80*:6351 (1983).

42. M. S. Neuburger, G. T. Williams, and R. O. Fox. Recombinant antibodies possessing novel effector functions. *Nature, 312*:604 (1984).
43. L. Olsson and H. S. Kaplan. Human-human hybridomas producing monoclonal antibodies of predefined antigenic specificity. *Proc. Natl. Acad. Sci.* (*USA*), *77*:5429 (1980).
44. S. A. Clark, N. H. Stimson, A. R. Williamson, and H. M. Dick. Human hybridoma cell lines; a novel method of production. *J. Supramol. Struct. 40*: 100 (1981).
45. M. C. Glassy, H. H. Handley, H. Hagiwara, and I. Royston. UC-729-6—a human lymphoblastoid line useful for generating antibody secreting human-human hybridomas. *Proc. Natl. Acad. Sci.* (*USA*), *80*:6327 (1983).
46. K. W. Hunter, G. W. Fischer, V. G. Hemming, S. R. Wilson, R. J. Hartzman, and J. M. Woody. Antibacterial activity of a human monoclonal antibody to haemophilus influenzae type B capsular polysaccharide. *Lancet, ii*:798 (1982).
47. J. W. Larrick, K. E. Truitt, A. Raubitschek, G. Senyk, and J. Wang. Characterization of human hybridomas secreting antibody to tetanus toxoid. *Proc. Natl. Acad. Sci.* (*USA*), *80*:6367 (1983).

10

Human Monoclonal Antibodies in the Management of Acute Leukemia

RINETTE B. ANDREASEN and LENNART OLSSON
State University Hospital, Rigshospitalet, Copenhagen, Denmark

Immunological analysis of human leukemic cells began in the early 1970s, and the development of monoclonal antibodies (MAbs) against cell surface antigens on leukemic cells and their normal counterparts has recently been used in diagnosis and classification of leukemias. In 1975 Kohler and Milstein (1) developed the murine monoclonal antibody technology. Five years later, two independent groups (2,3) reported on human-human hybridomas and the promise of human monoclonal antibodies. A number of technical obstacles have delayed the establishment of human-human hybridoma technology as a routine procedure comparable with rodent hybridoma production. The majority of these technical difficulties and their impact on the efficiency of procedures for establishment of antibody-secreting human-human hybridomas were reviewed recently (4,5). Inadequacies were found for both of the partners used for the fusion. The access to optimally antigen-primed human B lymphocytes, which for obvious reasons in most cases has to be done outside the human body, has been low compared with splenocytes of a hyperimmunized mouse. In addition, the available human myeloma lines have been disappointing in regard to hybrid formation, antibody secretion, and stability in comparison with their murine counterparts. However, peripheral blood lymphocytes (PBL) have been used as B lymphocyte source for producing mouse-human hybridomas (6) as well as human-human hybridomas (7) which secrete antibodies against relevant antigens. Lymphocytes from spleen (7), lymph nodes, and bone marrow have also been used successfully (8,9).

In the last few years, technological improvements have facilitated human-human hybridoma technology. Several *in vitro* antigen-priming systems have been described (10,11). Some of the problems in the *in vitro* priming systems have been the highly variable efficiency and the need for a large amount of antigen. Moreover, *in vitro* antigen-priming systems usually result only in IgM-producing B lymphocytes. Some investigators (12,13) claim that the tumor-suppressive effect of IgM antibodies is weak, and that IgG antibodies may be more effective because they can recruit killer cells for antibody-dependent cellular cytotoxicity. It is a major obstacle to the generation of specific IgG-producing B lymphocytes by *in vitro* antigen-priming procedures that the currently used culture conditions only permit B-lymphocyte propagation in culture for approximately 10 days, which is a too short period to result in specific IgG-producing B lymphocytes. The *in vitro* antigen-priming system developed by van Ness *et al.* (14) has the advantage that it only requires low amounts of antigen ($< 1\ \mu g/10^7$ immune cells). Such amounts of antigen can often be obtained by simple elution from SDS gels and, therefore, obtained in rather purified forms as compared with a total cell extract. However, the use of denatured proteins as antigenic material excludes an immune response against most of the epitopes on the native proteins because in many systems, most epitopes seem to be determined by the three-dimensional structure of the native molecule (15).

Another main problem has been the lack of suitable human myeloma lines to which normal antigen-stimulated human B cells could be fused (2,3,16). Naturally occurring human myelomas cannot readily be cultivated into long-term cell lines and synthesize the parent immunoglobulin chains *in vivo*. Epstein-Barr virus (EBV) immortalizes human B cells. EBV-transformed lines secreting specific human antibody to various antigens have been derived (17-20). One advantage of the EBV method is that the cultures are generally quite stable, while hybridoma lines are aneuploid and tend to loose chromosomes, often with the consequence that the hybridomas loose immunoglobulin (Ig) production and, therefore, need regular recloning. A disadvantage of the EBV methodology appears to be the relatively low secretion of Ig compared with that from hybridoma cell lines. Some investigators (21,22) have been successful in growing subcutaneous adapted human-human hybridomas in nude mice ascites. Truitt *et al.* (21) used pristane-primed, irradiated nude mice to grow human-human ascites. They obtained a 100 times greater antibody titer (100-300 μl/ml of specific antibody) than that of *in vitro* cultures. Although antibody production remained stable after several nude mice passages, genetic instability was found in the hybrids. Abrams *et al.* (22) have harvested milligram quantities of human monoclonal antibodies from NS1/human hybridomas grown in nude mouse ascites. Human hybridomas can also be produced by fusion of mouse myeloma cells with human lymphocytes (23,24). However, such hybrids have a high degree of instability, because human chromosomes are preferentially lost in such interspecific hybrids (25). Attempts to prevent the loss of human chromosomes have included irradiation of mouse fusion partners, and construction of so-called heteromyelomas (26). It remains to be demonstrated whether this cell line has any advantages compared with the other parental fusion partners.

I. HUMAN MONOCLONAL ANTIBODIES AS REAGENTS FOR THE IDENTIFICATION OF LEUKEMIA CELLS

MAbs reacting with various hematopoietic cells are now available, allow the distinction of various lymphoid and some myeloid cell populations (27), and have become important tools in diagnosis and study of normal hematopoiesis as well as leukemogenesis (28-33). Nearly all of the MAbs generated are of mouse origin. However, it is conceivable that the antigeneic spectrum recognized across an allogeneic barrier is more specific and identifies other antigens than is possible over a xenogeneic barrier (e.g., mouse-recognizing human antigens). The immune response of rodents against cellular components of human cells is primarily directed against those epitopes that are strongly immunogenic. Such epitopes may be specific for man (or primates), but not specific for a given individual and, at best, only specific for a human cell type. In the murine hybridoma system several different immunization procedures, such as inducing tolerance, have been developed in order to avoid an immune response against irrelevant antigens. Only a limited number of human MAbs with specificity for cell membrane antigens on human tumor cells has been reported (7,23,31-38). The importance of the human MAbs in cancer biology is based on the possibility that this technique may answer some of the main questions concerning human-associated antigens on leukemic cells and the possible immune response towards antigens on leukemic cells in the autochthonous host. Dissection of the antigeneic repertoire that the human immune system may react against on human cancer cells has been studied mainly by mixed hemadsorption and immune adherence assays using sera and cancer cells derived from the same patient. Three classes of surface antigens on malignant cells have been identified (39-43): (a) antigens strictly tumor-specific, in the sense that they show an absolute restriction to autologous tumor cells; (b) antigens shared by autologous and allogeneic tumors—recent evidence suggests that some of these antigens are differentiation antigens that may be detected on a restricted range of normal tissue (7,43); and (c) antigens expressed by an extensive range of normal and malignant cells. Antibodies to the latter class of antigens are relatively common, whereas antibodies to class (a) and class (b) are found only infrequently. Some of the most extensive studies have been reported by Shiku and Garrett and their associates (39,40), who used lymphocytes from draining lymph nodes of melanoma lesions as a source of anti-

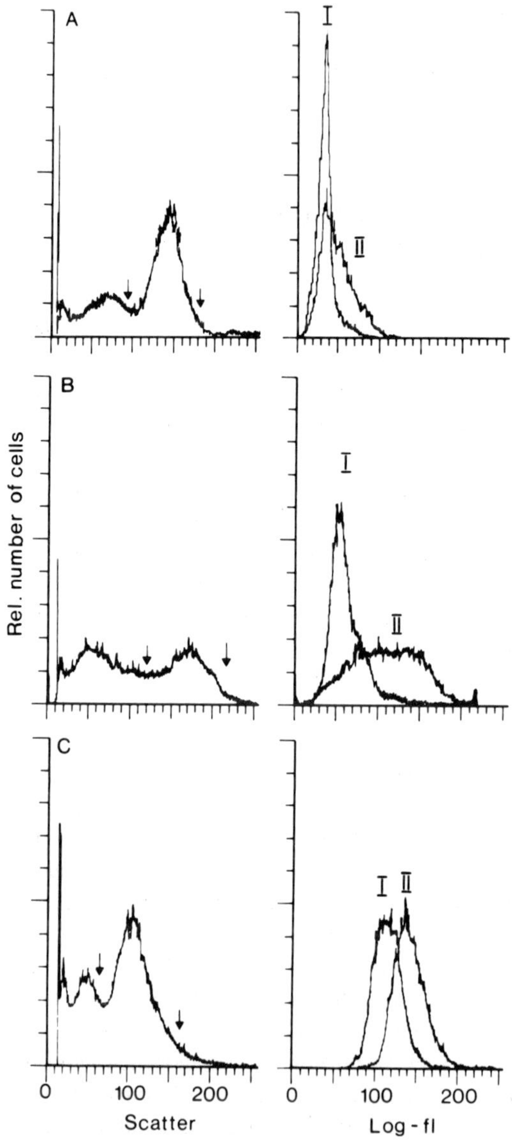

Figure 1 (A) FACS analysis of a sample of AML cells from Patient no. 18, from whom B lymphocytes were obtained to generate the AML-18 line. Left part of the histogram shows scatter signs. The gating is indicated by markers. Only cells within the markers were analyzed. Right part of the histogram shows fluorescence signal. I: negative control sample incubated with normal human Ig as first step.

gen-primed human B lymphocytes to generate human MAbs. Most of these human MAbs were found by immunofluorescence to react with intracellular structures that also were found in normal cells; only a few human MAbs bound to cell surface constituents. Only a few human MAbs have been produced that react with hematopoietic cells (7,44). In both cases, human-human hybridoma technology was used to immortalize human B lymphocytes from patients with acute myeloid leukemia (AML) and chronic myeloid leukemia (CML) to study the antigeneic repertoirs of the humoral immune response against the patient's own leukemic cells and against leukemic cells from other patients. This resulted primarily in generation of a human MAb (designated AML-18 [7]) with high specificity for human leukemia cells in contrast to the two human MAbs (designated AML-19 and CML-20 [44]) that seem to be specific for myeloid leukemia cells. The human MAbs obtained were bound to leukemic cells of the patients from which the B lymphocytes were obtained for fusion (Fig. 1). They also reacted to a different degree with AML cells of different subclasses (French-American-British classification [45]), with no correlation to any categories of the subclasses (Table 1). Moreover, a pronounced intratumoral antigenic heterogeneity in regard to reactivity with the MAbs was seen and indicates a high degree of diversity in the immunological phenotype within individual AML cell populations. Analysis of the MAbs binding to a panel of cells showed that the MAbs are highly specific for human leukemic cells (Table 2).

The AML-18, AML-19, and CML-20 hybridoma cells secreted Ig products (γ, κ) of the parental RH-L4 lymphoma and a new γ-chain and κ-light chain. The MAbs bind complement and can be used in a cytotoxicity assay. AML-18 hybridoma cells were injected subcutaneously into nude mice ($5\text{-}10 \times 10^6$ cells) mixed with 2×10^6 human foreskin fibroblasts. Six of 10 mice got subcutaneous tumors, of which four were successfully converted into ascites tumors upon two to five passages into other nude mice. However, ascites from three of these tumors did not have significantly increased antibody titer compared with culture

---

Figure 1 (continued)
II: AML-18 as first step reagent. Forty-five percent of the cells were stained (channel shift > 20 on a linear scale). (B) FACS analysis of AML-19-stained peripheral leukemic cells obtained from the patient from whom B lymphocytes were obtained to generate the AML-19 hybridoma line. The FACS settings and control samples were the same as for staining with AML-18. Fifty-five percent of the cells were positive. (C) FACS analysis of CML-20-stained peripheral leukemic cells, obtained from the patient from whom spleen cells were obtained and fused with RH-L4 cells, resulted in derivation of the CML-20 hybridoma cell line. The FACS setting and control samples were performed as described above. Twenty-seven percent of the cells were positive.

Table 1 Binding of the Human Monoclonal Antibodies (AML-18, AML-19, and CML-20) to a Panel of Leukemia Cell Samples

Type of leukemia	No. AML-18-positive samples / Total no. of samples	No. AML-19-positive samples / Total no. of samples[a]	No. CLM-20-positive samples / Total no. of samples[a]
AML-M1[b]	3/7	9/12	10/12
AML-M2	8/21	6/10	8/10
AML-M4	5/9	7/8	7/8
AML-M5	6/17	11/12	10/12
AML-M6	0/2	0/4	0/4
c-ALL	4/6	0/10	0/10
CML[c] (chronic phase)	0/2	4/4	3/4
CML (blast crisis)	1/2	4/4	3/4
CLL[c]	0/2	0/4	0/4

[a]The samples tested with AML-19 and CML-20 were not all identical, although the total numbers are.
[b]The acute leukemias were defined according to the FAB classification.
[c]CML and CLL were defined morphologically and clinically.

Table 2 Binding of Three Human Monoclonal Antibodies to Various Types of Malignant and Normal Cells as Analyzed by FACS and Dot-Blot/ELISA

Cell type/ line	Antibody[a]:	AML-18		AML-19		CML-20	
	Type of analysis[b]:	FACS	Dot-blot/ELISA	FACS	Dot-blot/ELISA	FACS	Dot-blot/ELISA
RH-L4		Neg	Neg	Neg	Neg	Neg	Neg
Daudi		Neg	Neg	Neg	Neg	Neg	Neg
U-266		Neg	Neg	Neg	ND[c]	Neg	ND
Molt-3		Neg	Neg	Neg	Neg	Neg	Neg
K562		+	+	++	+	++	+
HL60		++	++	++	++	++	++
U937		Neg	Neg	Neg	Neg	Neg	Neg
Fibroblast		Neg	Neg	Neg	Neg	Neg	Neg
Erythrocytes		Neg	Neg	Neg	Neg	Neg	Neg
Peripheral blood mononuclear cells		Neg	Neg	Neg	Neg	Neg	Neg
Granulocytes		Neg	+	Neg	ND	Neg	ND
Normal bone marrow		Neg	+	Neg	+	Neg	+
Thymocytes		Neg	Neg	Neg	ND	Neg	ND

[a]The antibodies were used in dilutions of 1:50-100, as obtained from supernatants of hybridoma cultures. In pilot experiments, these dilutions had proved to saturate the specific antigens on positive cells.
[b]FACS, dot-blot, and ELISA were performed as described in the text. FACS analysis was only performed on viable cells and therefore detects only cell surface antigens. Dot-blot was performed on triton-X100 cellular extracts, and ELISA was done on fixed cells. These two analyses detect both cytoplasmic and cell surface constituents.
[c]ND = not determined.

supernatants. The fourth tumor gave higher titers in some aspirates, but not in a predictable and reproducible way. Further attempts to grow AML-18 cells as ascites tumors were, therefore, abandoned. Attempts to grow AML-19 and CML-20 hybridoma cells in nude mice were unsuccessful. AML-19 and CML-20 hybridoma lines were aneuploid with modal chromosome numbers of 93 (AML-19) and 51 (CML-20) 4 months after fusion (Fig. 2). The hybrids were genetically unstable and 2 months later, both clones had lost chromosomes with modal chromosome numbers being 88 for AML-19 and 50 for CML-20. Immunoglobulin secretion was confined to cells with a hyperdiploid DNA content. The AML-19 and CML-20 MAbs reacted in immunoblotting with cell extracts from normal bone marrow (i.e., HL60 and K562 preparations). The cellular components blotted by the MAbs were different in normal bone marrow as compared with the components in the HL60 and K562 cell line. In normal bone marrow, an antigen with Mr ~ 20,000 d was identified, whereas two different cellular components with Mr ~ 14,000 d and Mr ~ 18,000 d were revealed in the HL60 and K562 extracts. The same bands were seen when nonreduced sample extracts were used. Microscopic immunofluorescence analysis showed that both human MAbs bound to intracytoplasmic and cell surface components on leukemia cells, but only to intracytoplasmatic structures on normal bone marrow cells. It is currently undetermined whether the two molecules found in leukemic cells are abnormally processed products of the compound in normal bone marrow cells or completely different molecules. Such antigenic structures found in and on the malignant cells, but not in the normal cells, may provide an insight into the mechanism of oncogenesis. Leukemic cells frequently reveal an antigenic pattern that they share with their normal counterparts during certain stages of development (i.e., so-called differentiation antigens). So far, a large number of such normal developmental antigens has been demonstrated on leukemic cells (46,47). It has not yet been possible to demonstrate a truly tumor-specific antigen.

The source of antigen-primed B lymphocytes has, in mouse hybridoma technology, clearly shown that the immunization schedule is crucial in obtaining high amounts of antibody-producing hybridomas. In our system, we have used peripheral blood lymphocytes from a patient with AML, and spleen cells from a patient with CML. It has previously been argued (4,5) that spleen lymphoid cells can be expected to be a superior source of antigen-primed cells compared with peripheral blood lymphocytes. We did not find any difference in the number of antibody secreting hybridomas between the two fusions. However, the patient with CML had received cytoreductive treatment prior to splenectomy and, in both cases, blood and spleen contained malignant cells. When using naturally antigen-primed B cells for fusion experiments from patients suffering from leukemia, one faces the problems that the lymphocyte source, whether it is peripheral blood, spleen, or bone marrow, often is infiltrated with leukemic cells and that sometimes the pa-

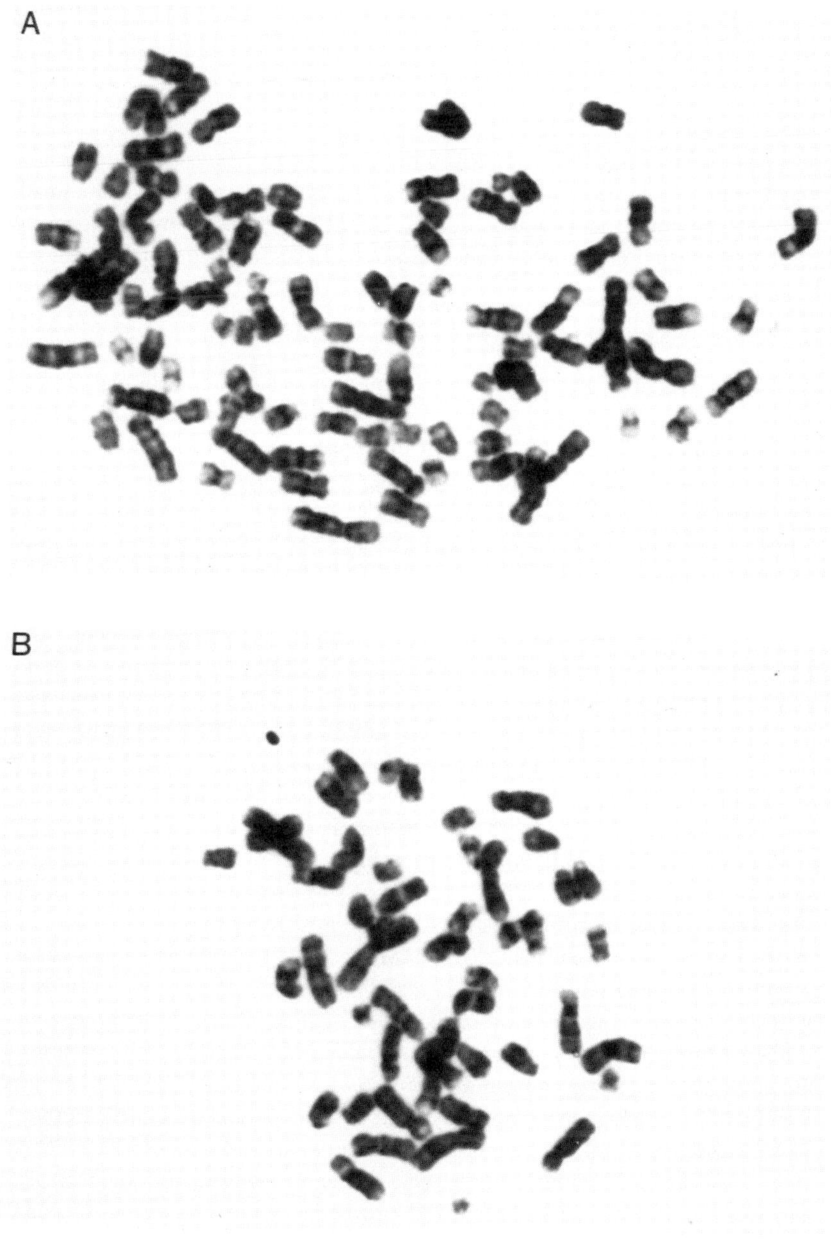

Figure 2 (A) Chromosomes from the AML-19 hybridoma line, 4 months after fusion. The line is aneuploid, with a modal chromosome number of 93. (B) Chromosomes from the CML-20 hybridoma line, 4 months after fusion. The line is aneuploid, with a modal chromosome number of 51.

tients have been in cytoreductive treatment, which may affect the antibody-producing lymphocytes as well as antigen expression on the leukemic cell. Another obstacle is that the amount of antigen-primed cells specific for the leukemic cells may be very small. Compared with the *in vitro* antigen-priming system, one has the advantage that the patients obviously have been exposed to the antigen for some time since it is possible to get IgG producing clones out of the fusions.

II. DIAGNOSTIC IMPLICATIONS: AML VERSUS ALL

Many attempts have been made by different groups to produce human leukemia-specific antibodies in animal species (for review, see 48,49). As with other human malignancies, it has been assumed that leukemic cells are likely to express unique antigens on their surface. However, when investigated closer, it has almost invariably been found that the supposed malignant cell characteristics are expressed on some normal cells at a particular stage of development or during a restricted phase of the cell cycle. The only leukemic-specific marker found to date is the Ph^1 translocation found in CML. Greaves et al. (50) and Billing *et al.* (51) have demonstrated the existence of an antigen associated with cells from many patients with ALL and some patients with CML in blast crisis. Antisera to this common ALL antigen (CALLA) was first produced in rabbits and required extensive absorption. Later, monoclonal antibodies specific for CALLA were produced by somatic cell hybridization (52-55) between a variant of P3/NS1/ 1-Ag4-1 as the parent myeloma cell line and spleen cells from BALB/c mice, which had been immunized with ALL cells emulsified in Freund's complete adjuvant. The produced MAb J-5 immuneprecipitates a single glycoprotein with Mr $\sim$ 95,000 d on cell membranes from LAZ 221, NALM-1, and CALLA-positive patients with ALL. The generated anti-CALLA-MAbs were positive with non-T cell ALL, distinguishing between T cell ALL, CLL, AML, and CML-stable phase, and were negative with the latter mentioned types of leukemias. The J-5 MAb also reacts with some cases of CML in blast crisis. The CALLA antigen is also present in nonhematopoietic tissues, such as renal tubular and glomerular cells from fetal and adult donors as well as from different kind of fetal tissue (56). It has not been possible to produce an antibody with any comparable reactivity to the CALLA antigen in AML leukemias. The diagnosis of AML cells has for a long time been done by negative criteria. One of the obstacles in immunophenotypic classification of AML has been that the knowledge about specialized subsets of myeloid cells has been insufficient and also because AML may involve a heterogenous cell population with respect to their stage of differentiation (57-60). One of the advantages of using human MAbs would presumably be that leukemic patients' immune response towards their own leukemic cells would be more selective and specific than it is possible to produce over a xenogeneic barrier, thereby avoiding reaction against irrelevant antigens, such as histocompatibility antigens. The leukemia-associated membrane antigens so far described appear to be predominantly normal differentiation antigens. These antigens are expressed by normal cells at an equivalent developmental level to the leukemic cell and are, therefore, not likely to be products of depressed ("oncofetal") genes. However, there is some evidence that these "normal" antigens on leukemic cells might, nevertheless, be immunogenic in some cases and elicit an antibody and/or cell-mediated response in the patient (61). This event may be one of the drawbacks of the rationale of immunotherapy in leukemia because the immune response might be effective against both tumor cells and their normal counterparts. This may not be tolerable in the case of acute leukemia. It has been argued that antigens other than differentiation antigens would occur on leukemic cells (48) These kinds of "leukemia antigens" may involve qualitatively new antigens associated with virus infection or genetic mutation. Such antigens would be immunogenic and, theoretically, could be used for active immunotherapy.

III. THERAPY

Previous studies (62,63) have demonstrated the efficiency of passive administration of antibodies in the treatment of selected animal tumors. In general, these studies made use of conventional heteroantisera specific for either virally induced surface antigens, normal differentiation antigens, or idiotypic tumor antigens. Some of the factors limiting serotherapy have been difficulty in producing antisera with desired specificity without extensive absorption, relatively low titer of these reagents, and inability to produce and administer the large quantities of specific antisera necessary for clinical use. With MAbs, many of these problems are circumvented because they have unique specificity; thus, the hybridomas proliferate continuously in culture and virtually unlimited amounts of antibody can be produced.

MAbs have been used in immunosuppressive therapy in cases of bone marrow transplantation as well as in preventing renal allograft rejection. In the case of renal allograft recipients, humans and monkeys have been treated with MAbs against the T cell population; humans have been given OKT-3 (IgG2a [64]), and cynomolgus monkeys have been treated with anti-Leu-2a MAb (IgG1 [65]). In both cases essentially complete clearing of the reactive cell population was observed along with significant prolongation of allograft survival. It is interesting that in the case of OKT-3 treatment, small numbers of T cells, which were nonreactive with OKT-3, but which expressed other T-cell markers, began to appear in the majority of patients 3 to 7 days after treatment. Since *in vitro* culture of these cells restored expression of OKT-3 reactivity, this was presumed to represent antigenic modulation. Nevertheless, the established rejection episode was promptly and decisively reversed without addition of any other therapy. Variable *in vivo* effects have been seen with the different MAbs used, and are presumably related to factors such as differences in antibody isotypes, target antigen affinity and density, and efficiency of cell-clearing mechanisms. In the majority of allograft recipients studied, the patients developed an immune response to the administered reagent. Both anti-idiotypic and anti-mouse immunoglubulin antibodies have been demonstrated (66).

The therapeutic value of many cytotoxic drugs is limited by their toxicity to hemopoietic stem cells in the bone marrow. Therefore, marrow can be harvested before administration of cytotoxic agents and reinfused after the drug has been excreted or metabolized (67). However, reinfusion of marrow may provide a source of future relapse if the marrow is infiltrated by malignant cells before treatment. Therefore, it would be of considerable value to "clean-up" the bone marrow in tumors where malignant-cell infiltration of bone marrow is common to eliminate malignant cells while sparing the bone marrow stem cells. In leukemias, such *in vitro* procedures have been performed using antisera (68) and monoclonal (69) antibodies in addition to heterologous complement and certain cytotoxic drugs (70). Treatment of marrow with monoclonal antibodies *in vitro* avoids some of the difficulties encountered when serotherapy/murine MAbs are administered directly to patients. Some of the advantages are that a large excess of antibody can be added to the system, and the marrow concentration can be varied. In the case of the anti-CALLA (J-5) MAb, *in vitro* treatment is particularly important since CALLA has been detected in normal adult kidneys (71). Modulation of certain tumor-associated antigens, such as CALLA, can occur *in vivo* as well as *in vitro*. The underlying mechanisms are virtually unknown, but probably comprise both shedding *and* internalization of the antigen-antibody complex in many antigen-antibody systems (72). Removal of the antibody from the cellular microenvironment leads, in most cases, to re-expression of the antigen. It remains to be examined whether prolonged exposure of cells to a specific MAb may result in suppression of expression of the corresponding gene. If so, the method will be suitable for analysis of the role of a given phenotypic feature for the malignant behavior and also for the induction of antigen-negative variant subclones that, together with antigen-positive subclones, seem highly suitable for determination of the gene(s) encoding for the antigenic molecule. However, more effective suppression of tumor growth *in vivo* may relate to destruction of antibody-coated tumor through antibody-dependent cell-mediated cytotoxicity or phagocytosis by cells of the transplant recipient (73,74).

In vivo monoclonal anti-idiotype antibody has been used in the treatment of B cell lymphoma (75), and polyclonal sheep anti-idiotype globulin has been used in treatment of a patient with chronic lymphocytic leukemia (CLL [76]). In the first case, the patient had progressive disease but entered complete remission after treatment. The patient did not generate an antibody reaction to the administered mouse anti-idiotype antibody and had no side-effects. In the latter case, the treatment produced a transient decrease in circulating leukemia cells, but was associated with considerable toxicity, including fever, rigors, and respiratory distress. The utilization of monoclonal murine antibodies in diagnosis and treatment of human leukemias and lymphomas for *in vivo* use has been reviewed previously (77). The hope is obviously that human MAbs will be far better tolerated upon injection and anaphylactoid side-effects avoided; however no data on the effects of injection of human MAbs into patients for diagnosis or treatment of specific diseases are yet available. It seems that the use of human MAbs for treatment is primarily relevant for eradication of micrometastases in patients who have achieved complete or significant partial remission with conventional therapy, although it can still be hoped that substances will be developed that, upon conjugation to MAbs, can result in eradication of larger tumor masses. Substances like α-particle-emitting radionucleides (e.g., ^{224}Ra, ^{211}At), chemotherapeutical drugs, the A-chains of toxins (e.g., ricin, diphtheria toxin), and tumor necrosis factor are among the most promising candidates, and may eventually reduce the otherwise very significant obstacles that intratumoral antigenic heterogeneity and antigenic modulation impose on the application of MAbs in tumor therapy. Although the generation of MAbs reactive with human tumor cells has circumvented many of the problems that followed the use of serotherapy, major limitations still exist. Some of the limiting factors that may still persist even with the advent of human MAbs are antigenic modulation as a consequence of binding of MAb to the cell surface *in vivo* (78,79), serum-blocking factors (80), the presence or release of circulating free antigen (81), impairment of the patients immunological response (80), and the implications of immunological enhancement for growth of autochthonous tumors (82).

IV. INTRATUMORAL PHENOTYPIC DIVERSITY AND CLONOGENICITY

Individual leukemic cell populations may be heterogenous with respect to many pheotypic features, such as growth characteristics, clonogenicity, sensitivity to drugs, antigenicity, and oncogene expression. This may have a negative impact on the use of MAbs in diagnosis and treatment. Leukemic progenitors are capable of both self-renewal and differentiation. *In vitro* studies of leukemic cell growth have demonstrated that only a minority of the leukemic blasts either fail to proliferate or undergo only one to five cycles of cell division. It would be of interest to identify an antigen associated with the clonogenic cell population in leukemias. The immunological phenotype of human leukemic cells as perceived by the human immune system may be substantially different from what can be revealed by mouse/rat antibodies. With the advent of reproducible and reliable *in vitro* antigen-priming systems, it might be possible to provoke a human immune response to weakly immunogenic antigens. Some of these aspects were recently demonstrated in murine tumors. The amount of tumor cells with metastatic capability is low in most tumor cell populations, including cell populations from metastatic foci. An antigen associated with the metastatic phenotype was recently described for a murine carcinoma (83). It was found that a detectable immune response against this antigen could be obtained across an allogenic immune barrier, but not over a xenogenic barrier. Identification of such an antigen has permitted a rational approach for analysis of genes that determine the metastatic process. On this level, the close association between hybridoma technology and DNA recombinant techniques will be developed.

V. CONCLUSION

Human MAbs can now be produced routinely. Production of human-human hybridomas seems, in most cases, superior to EBV transformation. Recently, however, construction by DNA recombinant technology of complete and specific antibodies was reported (84,85). Only low-level efficiency of assembly of the heavy and light chains were obtained by these procedures, indicating that these methods are not the methods of choice for production of specific MAbs. However, the synthesis and *in vivo* assembly of functional antibodies in yeast was recently reported (86), and it seems likely that further technological improvements in the production of MAbs by DNA recombinant technology eventually will make this technique superior to hybridoma methods. Besides the obvious areas of application for human MAbs in clinical oncology, human MAbs also have very important application in experimental cancer biology.

One of the fundamental questions in cancer immunology that remains, is whether human beings raise an immune response against autochthonous tumors. This question has not been addressed in several human tumor systems by the use of human MAbs and it seems, indeed, that human beings may react immunologically against their own tumor. The dissection of the antigenic repertoire that the human immune system may react against on human cancer cells is a major area of application of human monoclonal antibody technology.

We have used human-human hybridoma technology in an attempt to identify antigenic structures that may be specific for myeloid cells and/or their leukemic counterparts. This resulted primarily in generation of a human MAb (designated AML-18) with high specificity for human leukemia cells (7), but with a reactivity pattern that comprised both myeloid and lymphoid leukemia cells in contrast to the two human MAbs (AML-19 and CML-20) later generated that seemed specific for myeloid cells.

The staining pattern of different leukemic samples revealed, for a majority, a pronounced heterogeneity in intensity within each sample in line with previous reports on both experimental and human leukemias. Although, it cannot be excluded that a minor part of the antigen-negative cells are nonmalignant cells, the majority of the antigen-negative cells are leukemic cells. The lack of antigen on the leukemic cells, therefore, suggests that within each sample, these cells are diversified with respect to their stage of differentiation, concurring with a number of previous observations (57-60). The application of MAbs for the diagnosis of myeloid leukemic cells may, therefore, acquire the use of a panel of MAbs. Moreover, human MAbs are potentially very important experimental tools in studies of oncogenes and their products, and human MAbs against such products can be expected to be instrumental in studies on the importance of such genes for malignant transformation and behavior. Human MAbs can also be expected to be highly useful in studies on antigenic modulation, activation of the host immune response against tumor-associated antigens by immunization with anti-idiotypic antibodies, and the biological basis for metastasis. It can be expected that substantial new information relevant to both experimental and clinical cancer research will be based on the use of human monoclonal antibodies.

REFERENCES

1. G. Kohler and C. Milstein. Continuous cultures of fused cells secreting antibody of predefined specificity. *Nature, 246*:495 (1975).
2. C. M. Croce, A. Linnenbach, W. Hall, Z. Steplewski, and H. Koprowski. Production of human hybridomas secreting antibodies to measles virus. *Nature, 288*:488 (1980).
3. L. Olsson and H. S. Kaplan. Human-human hybridomas producing monoclonal antibodies of predefined antigenic specificity. *Proc. Natl. Acad. Sci. (USA)*, *77*:5429 (1980).
4. L. Olsson and H. S. Kaplan. Human-human hybridomas. Technical aspects. *Meth. Enzymol., 92*:3 (1983).
5. L. Olsson, H. Kronstrom, A. Cambon-de Mouzon, C. Honsik, T. Brodin, and B. Jacobsen. Antibody-producing human-human hybridomas I. Technical aspects. *J. Immunol. Meth. 61*:17 (1983).
6. J. L. Butler, H. C. Lande, and A. S. Fauci. Delineation of optimal conditions for producing mouse-human heterohybridomas from human peripheral blood B cells of immunized subjects. *J. Immunol. 133*:165 (1983).
7. L. Olsson, R. B. Andreasen, A. Ost, B. Christensen, and P. Biberfeld. Antibody producing human-human hybridomas. II. Derivation and characterization of an antibody specific for human leukemia cells. *J. Exp. Med., 159*:537 (1984).
8. P. A. W. Edwards, C. M. Smith, A. M. Neville, and M. J. O'Hare. A human-human hybridoma system based on a fast-growing mutant of the ARH-77 plasma cell leukemia derived line. *Eur. J. Immunol., 12*:641 (1982).

9. I. Kamo, S. Furukawa, A. Tada, Y. Mano, Y. Iwasaki, T. Ruruse, N. Ito, K. Hayashi, and E. Satoyoshi. Monoclonal antibody to acetylcholine receptor: cell line established from thymus of patient with myastenia gravis. *Science, 215*:995 (1982).
10. C. L. Reading. Theory and methods for immunization in culture and monoclonal antibody production. *J. Immunol. Meth., 53*:261 (1982).
11. L. Olsson and P. Brams. Human-human hybridoma technology. Five years of technical improvements, and its application in cancer biology. In E. G. Engelman, S. K. H. Foung, J. Larrick, and A. A. Raubitschek (eds.). *Human Hybridomas and Monoclonal Antibodies.* Plenum Press, New York (1985).
12. M. E. Kirch and U. Hammerring. Immunotherapy of murine leukemias by monoclonal antibodies. I. Effect of passively administered antibody or growth of transplanted tumor cells. *J. Immunol., 127*:805 (1981).
13. W. W. Young and S. I. Hakomori. Therapy of mouse lymphoma with monoclonal antibodies to glycolipid. Selection of low antigenic variants *in vivo. Science, 211*:487 (1981).
14. J. van Ness, U. K. Laemmli, and D. E. Pettijohn. Immunization *in vitro* and production of monoclonal antibodies specific to insoluble and weakly immunogenic proteins. *Proc. Natl. Acad. Sci.* (*USA*), *81*:7897 (1984).
15. D. Lane and H. Koprowski. Molecular recognition and the future of monoclonal antibodies. *Nature, 296*:200 (1982).
16. G. Kohler, Why hybridomas? *Hybridoma, 1*:1 (1981).
17. M. Steinetz and E. Klein. Human monoclonal antibodies produced by transformation with Epstein-Barr virus. *Immunol. Today, 2*:38 (1981).
18. E. Henderson, G. Miller, J. Robinson, and L. Heston. Efficiency of transformation of lymphocytes by Epstein-Barr virus. *Virology, 76*:152 (1977).
19. N. A. Brown and G. Miller. Immunoglobulin expression by human B-lymphocytes clonally transformed by Epstein-Barr virus. *J. Immunol., 128*:24 (1982).
20. N. Chiozacci, R. L. Wasserman, and H. G. Kunkel. Use of Epstein-Barr virus-transformed B cell lines for the generation of immunoglobulin-producing human B cell hybridomas. *J. Exp. Med., 156*:930 (1982).
21. K. E. Truitt, J. W. Larrick, A. A. Raubitschek, D. W. Buck, and S. W. Jacobson. Production of human monoclonal antibody in mouse ascites. *Hybridoma, 3*:195 (1984).
22. P. G. Abrams, J. A. Knost, G. Clarke, S. Wilburn, R. K. Oldham, and K. A. Foon. Determination of the optimal human cell lines for development of human hybridomas. *J. Immunol., 131*:1202 (1983).
23. J. Schlom, D. Wunderlich, and U. A. Tesramoto. Generation of human monoclonal antibodies reactive with human mammary carcinoma cells. *Proc. Natl. Acad. Sci.* (*USA*), *77*:6841 (1980).
24. R. Levy and J. Dilley. Rescue of immunoglobulin secretion from neoplastic lymphoid cells by somatic cell hybridization. *Proc. Natl. Acad. Sci.* (*USA*), *75*:2411 (1978).
25. N. R. Ringertz and R. E. Savage. *Cell Hybrids.* Academic Press, New York, San Francisco (1976).

26. N. N. H. Teng, K. S. Lam, F. C. Riera, and H. S. Kaplan. Construction and testing of mouse-human heteromyelomas for human monoclonal antibody production. *Proc. Natl. Acad. Sci. (USA)*, *80*:7308 (1983).
27. G. Janossy. Membrane markers in leukemia. In D. Catowsky (ed.). *The Leukemic Cell.* Churchill Livingstone, Edinburgh, London (1981).
28. E. S. Lennox. Monoclonal antibodies and tumor antigens-a perspective. In M. S. Mitchell and J. F. Oettgen (eds.). *Hybridomas in Cancer Diagnosis and Treatment.* Raven Press, New York (1982).
29. H. S. Kaplan, L. Olsson, and A. Raubitschek. Monoclonal human antibodies: a recent development with wide-ranging clinical potential. In A. J. McMichael and J. W. Fabre (eds.). *Monoclonal Antibodies in Clinical Medicine.* Academic Press, New York, London (1982).
30. R. W. Schroff, K. A. Foon, R. J. Billing, and J. L. Fahey. Immunologic classification of lymphocytic leukemias based on monoclonal antibody-defined cell surface antigens. *Blood, 59*:207 (1982).
31. M. F. Greaves, D. Delia, R. Newman, and L. Vodinelich. Analysis of leukemic cells with monoclonal antibodies. In A. J. McMichael and J. W. Fabre (eds.). *Monoclonal Antibodies in Clinical Medicine.* Academic Press, London, New York (1982).
32. M. Mitchell and J. F. Oettgen. Hybridomas in cancer diagnosis and treatment. In *Progress in Cancer Research and Therapy.* Raven Press, New York (1982).
33. R. H. Kennett, Z. L. Jonak, and K. B. Bechtol. Monoclonal antibodies against human tumor-associated antigens. In R. H. Kennett, T. J. McKearn, and B. Bechtol, (eds.). *Monoclonal Antibodies.* Plenum Press, New York (1980).
34. K. Sikora, J. Alderson, J. Philips, and J. V. Watson. Human hybridomas from malignant gliomas. *Lancet, i*:11 (1982).
35. A. N. Houghton, H. Brooks, R. J. Cote, M. C. Taormina, J. F. Oettgen, and L. J. Old. Detection of cell surface and intra cellular antigens by human monoclonal antibodies: hybrid cell lines derived from lymphocytes of patients with malignant melanomas. *J. Exp. Med., 158*:53 (1983).
36. M. C. Glassy, H. H. Handley, and H. Hagawara. UC 729-6, a human lymphoblastoid B-cell line useful for generating antibody-secreting human-human hybridomas. *Proc. Natl. Acad. Sci. (USA)*, *80*:6327 (1983).
37. R. J. Cote, D. M. Morrissey, A. N. Houghton, E. J. Beattie, H. F. Oettgen, and L. J. Old. Generation of human monoclonal antibodies reactive with cellular antigens. *Proc. Natl. Acad. Sci. (USA)*, *80*:2026 (1983).
38. M. Kararo and R. F. Irie. Human monoclonal antibody to tumor-associated ganglioside GD2: suppressed growth of human melanoma in nude mice. *Immunol. Letters, 8*:169 (1984).
39. H. Shiku, L. A. Takahashi, H. F. Oettgen, and L. J. Old. Cell surface antigens of human malignant melanoma. *J. Exp. Med., 145*:784 (1977).
40. T. J. Garrett, T. Takahashi, B. D. Clarkson, and L. J. Old. Detection of antibody to autologous human leukemia cells by immune adherence assays. *Proc. Natl. Acad. Sci. (USA)*, *74*:4587 (1977).
41. M. Pfreundschuh, H. Shiku, T. Takahashi, R. Ueda, J. Ronshoff, H. F. Oettgen,

and L. J. Old. Serological analysis of cell surface antigens of malignant human brain tumors. *Proc. Natl. Acad. Sci.* (*USA*), *75*:5122 (1978).
42. R. Ueda, J. Shiku, M. Pfreundschuh, T. Takahashi, L. T. C. Li, W. F. Whitmore, H. F. Oettgen, and L. J. Old. Cell surface antigens of human renal cancer defined by autologous typing. *J. Exp. Med.*, *150*:564 (1979).
43. T. Watnabe, C. S. Pukel, H. Takeyana, K. P. Lloyd, H. Shiku, L. T. C. Li, G. R. Travassos, H. F. Oettgen, and L. J. Old. Human melanoma antigen AH is an autoantigenic ganglioside related to G_{D2}. *J. Exp. Med.*, *156*:1884 (1982).
44. R. B. Andreasen and L. Olsson. Antibody producing human-human hybridomas III. Derivation and characterization of two antibodies with specificity for human myeloid cells. *J. Immunol.* (Submitted.)
45. J. M. Bennett, D. Carowsky, M-T. Daniel, G. Flandrin, D. A. G. Galton, H. R. Gralnick, and C. Sultan. Proposals for the classification of the acute leukemias. *Br. J. Haematol.*, *33*:451 (1976).
46. E. L. Reinheiz, P. C. Kung, G. Goldstein, and S. F. Schlossman. Discrete stages of human ultrathymic differentiation: analysis of normal thymocytes and leukemic lymphoblasts of T-cell lineage. *Proc. Natl. Acad. Sci.* (*USA*), *77*:1588 (1980).
47. E. L. Reinherz and S. F. Schlossman. The characterization and function of human immunoregulatory T lymphocyte subsets. *Pharmacol. Rev.*, *34*:17 (1982).
48. M. F. Greaves, G. Janossy, M. Roberts, et al. Membrane phenotyping: diagnosis monitoring and classification of acute "lymphoid" leukemias. In *Immunological Diagnosis of Leukemias and Lymphomas.* Springer Verlag, Berlin, New York (1977).
49. M. F. Greaves. Clinical applications of cell surface markers. *Prog. Haematol.*, *9*:255 (1975).
50. M. F. Greaves, G. Brown, N. Rapson, and N. T. Lister. Antisera to acute lymphoblastic leukemia cells. *Clin. Immunol. Immunopathol.*, *4*:67 (1975).
51. R. Billing, J. Minowada, M. Cline, B. Clark, and K. Lee. Acute lymphocytic leukemia-associated cell membrane antigen. *J. Natl. Cancer Inst.*, *61*: 423 (1978).
52. J. Ritz, J. M. Pesando, S. E. Sallan, L. A. Clavell, J. Notis-McConarty, P. Rosenthal, and S. F. Schlossman. Serotherapy of acute lymphoblastic leukemia with monoclonal antibody. *Blood*, *58*:361 (1981).
53. M. F. Greaves, W. Verbi, J. Kemshead, and R. Kennett. A monoclonal antibody identifying a cell surface antigen shared by common acute lymphoblastic leukemias and B lineage cells. *Blood*, *56*:1141 (1980).
54. M. Roberts, M. Greaves, G. Janossy, R. Sutherland, and C. Pain. Acute lymphoblastic leukemia (ALL) associated antigen. I. Expression in different hematopoietic malignancies. *Leuk. Res.*, *2*:105 (1978).
55. J. Ritz, J. M. Pesando, J. Notis-McConarty, H. Lazarns, and S. F. Schlossman. A monoclonal antibody to human acute lymphoblastic leukemia antigen. *Nature*, *283*:583 (1980).

56. R. S. Metzgar, M. J. Borowitz, M. H. Jones, and B. L. Dowell, Distribution of common acute lymphoblastic leukemia antigen in non-hematopoitic tissues. *J. Exp. Med., 154*:1249 (1981).
57. P. C. Nowell. The clonal evolution of tumor cell population. *Science, 194*: 23 (1976).
58. I. J. Fidler and I. Hart. Biological diversity in metastic neoplasms: origins and implications. *Science, 194*:23 (1981).
59. H. Rubin. Early origin and pervasiveness of cellular heterogeneity in some malignant transformations. *Proc. Natl. Acad. Sci. (USA), 81*:5121 (1984).
60. G. H. Heppner. Tumor heterogeneity. *Cancer Res., 44*:2259 (1984).
61. R. Harries. Leukaemia antigens and immunity in man. *Nature, 241*:95 (1973).
62. R. M. Ferguson, J. R. Schmidtke, and R. L. Simmons. Immunotherapy of experimental animals. In *Mechanisms of Tumor Immunity.* John Wiley & Sons, New York (1977).
63. L. L. Lanier, G. F. Babcock, R. B. Raybourne, L. W. Arnold, N. L. Warner, and G. Haughton. Mechanism of B cell lymphoma immunotherapy with passive xenogeneic anti-idiotype serum. *J. Immunol., 125*:1730 (1980).
64. A. B. Cosimi, R. C. Burton, R. B. Colbin, G. Goldstein, F. L. Delmonico, M. P. LaQuaglia, N. Tolkoff-Rubin, R. H. Rubin, J. T. Herrin, and P. S. Russell. Treatment of acute renal allograft rejection OKT 3 monoclonal antibody. *Transplantation, 32*:535 (1981).
65. H. Kreis, D. Norman, and P. Martin. Status of monoclonals used therapeutically in transplantation. *Transplant. Proc., 16*:1659 (1984).
66. G. J. Jaffers, R. B. Colvin, A. B. Cosimi, J. V. Giorgi, G. Goldstein, T. C. Fuller, J. T. Kurnick, C. Lillehei, and P. S. Russell. The human immune response to murine OKT-3 monoclonal antibody. *Transplant. Proc., 15*:646 (1983).
67. T. J. McElwain, D. W. Hedley, G. Burton, H. M. Clink, M. Y. Gordon, M. Jarman, C. A. Juttner, J. L. Millar, R. A. V. Milsted, G. Prentice, I. E. Smith, D. Spence, and M. Woods. Marrow autotransplantation accelerates haematological recovery in patients with malignant melanoma treated with high dose melphalan. *Br. J. Cancer, 40*:72 (1979).
68. B. Netzel, H. Ridt, R. J. Hass, H. J. Kolb, and S. Thierfelder. Immunological conditioning of bone marrow for autotransplantation in childhood acute lymphoblastic leukaemia. *Lancet, i*:1130 (1980).
69. J. Ritz, S. E. Sallan, R. C. Bast, L. A. Clavell, T. Hercend, J. J. Lipton, M. Feeney, D. G. Nathan, and S. F. Schlossman. Autologous bone-marrow transplantation in CALLA-positive acute lymphoblastic leukaemia after in vitro treatment with J5 monoclonal antibody and complement. *Lancet, ii*:60 (1982).
70. H. Kaizer, R. K. Stuart, D. J. Fuller, et al. Autologous bone marrow transplantation in acute leukaemia: progress report on a phase I study of 4-hydroperoxy-cyclophorphamide incubation of marrow prior to cryopreservation (abstr.). *Proc. Am. Soc. Oncol., 1* (1985).

71. R. S. Metzgar, M. J. Borowitz, N. H. Jones, and B. L. Sowell. The distribution of common acute lymphoblastic leukemia antigen (CALLA) in nonhematopoietic tissues. *J. Exp. Med., 54*:1249 (1981).
72. L. Chatenaud and J. F. Bach. Antigenic modulation—a major mechanism of antibody action. *Immunol. Today, 5*:20 (1984).
73. J. S. Economou, H. S. Shin, H. Kaizer, G. W. Santos, and D. S. Schron. Bone marrow transplantation in cancer therapy: inactivation by antibody and complement of tumor cells in mouse syngeneic marrow transplants. *Proc. Soc. Exp. Biol. Med., 158*:449 (1978).
74. M. Feeney, R. C. Knapp, J. F. Greenberger, and R. C. Bast, Jr. Elimination of leukemic cells from rat bone marrow using antibody and complement. *Cancer Res., 43*:3331 (1981).
75. R. A. Miller, D. G. Maloney, R. Warnke, and R. Levy. Treatment of B-cell lymphoma with monoclonal anti-idiotype antibody. *N. Engl. J. Med., 9*: 517 (1982).
76. T. J. Hamblin, A. K. Abdul-Ahad, J. Gordon, F. K. Stevenson, and G. T. Stevenson. Preliminary experience in treating lymphocytic leukaemia with antibody to immunoglobulin idiotypes on the cell surface. *Br. J. Cancer, 42*:495 (1980).
77. L. M. Nadler, R. Rtiz, and J. D. Griddin. Diagnosis and treatment of human leukemias and lymphomas utilizing monoclonal antibodies. In *Progress in Hematology*.
78. R. A. Miller and R. Levy. Response of cutaneous T cell lymphoma to therapy with hybridoma monoclonal antibody. *Lancet, ii*:226 (1981).
79. J. Ritz, J. M. Pesando, J. Notis-McConarty, and S. F. Schlossman. Modulation of human acute lymphoblastic leukemia antigen induced by monoclonal antibody in vitro. *J. Immunol., 125*:1506 (1980).
80. L. M. Nadler, P. Stashenko, R. Hardy, D. W. Kufe, K. H. Antman, and S. F. Schlossman. Serotherapy of a patient with monoclonal antibody directed against a human lymphoma-associated antigen. *Cancer Res., 40*:3147 (1980).
81. R. A. Miller, D. G. Maloney, J. McKillop, and R. Levy. *In vivo* effects of murine hybridoma monoclonal antibody in a patient with T cell leukemia. *Blood, 58*:78 (1981).
82. I. Hellstrom and K. E. Hellstrom. The role of immunological enhancement for the growth of autochthonous tumors. *Transplant. Proc., 3*:721 (1971).
83. L. Olsson and J. Forchammer. Induction of metastatic phenotype in a mouse tumor model by 5-azacytidine and characterization of an antigen associated with metastatic activity. *Proc. Natl. Acad. Sci.* (*USA*), *81*:3389 (1984).
84. S. Cabilly, A. D. Riggs, H. Pande, J. E. Shively, W. E. Holmes, M. Rey, L. J. Perry, R. Wetzel, and H. L. Heyneker. Generation of antibody activity from immunoglobulin polypeptide chains produced in *Escherichia coli. Proc. Natl. Acad. Sci.* (*USA*), *81*:8273 (1984).

85. M. A. Boss, J. H. Kenten, C. R. Wood, and J. S. Emtage. Assembly of functional antibodies from immunoglobulin heavy and light chains synthesized in *E. coli*. *Nucleic Acid Res.*, *12*:3791 (1984).
86. C. R. Wood, M. A. Boss, J. H. Kenten, J. E. Calvert, N. A. Roberts, and J. S. Emtage. The synthesis and *in vivo* assembly of functional antibodies in yeast. *Nature*, *314*:446 (1985).

11

Immortalization of the Human Immune Response to Human Cancers

MARK C GLASSY, SHAIK A. GAFFAR, ROBERT E. PETERS,* and IVOR ROYSTON

University of California-San Diego Cancer Center, San Diego, California

Rigorous and exacting manipulation of the human immune response may inspire new concepts not only in the diagnosis and treatment of human disease, but also in the understanding of the mechanisms of both the humoral and cellular arms of human immunology. To the tumor immunologist, the immortalization of the human immune response will allow investigators an opportunity to begin a systematic dissection of B and T cell functions and how they relate to the pathogenesis of cancer. Monoclonal antibody (MAb) technology, pioneered by Kohler and Milstein (1) and extended to humans (2,3), has provided a mechanism whereby individual windows within the human immune response may be critically analyzed. Since humans do make antibodies to their own tumor antigens (4,5), the immortalization of these Ig-secreting lymphocytes will provide a steady supply of the anti-cancer MAbs. In this report, we describe the results of a fusion of human parental UC 729-6 cells (6), with lymphocytes isolated from a regional draining lymph node of a cancer patient. The resulting human-human hybridomas secreted Ig reactive with human tumor antigens.

**Present affiliation*: Cytotech, Inc., San Diego, California

I. STRATEGY AND DESIGN OF TUMOR REACTIVE HUMAN MAbS

A. Source of Human Lymphocytes

At present, human MAbs to human tumors are produced from lymphocytes of cancer patients without prior intentional immunizations. The major sources of Ig-secreting lymphocytes within the body are peripheral blood, spleen, lymph nodes, tonsils, bone marrow, and cord blood. Schlom *et al.* (7) demonstrated and others confirmed (6,8,9) that B lymphocytes in regional draining lymph nodes of patients with cancer are primed to synthesize antibodies against tumor antigens. Additional evidence in support of this concept came in earlier studies from Old (5) by demonstrating that the sera of cancer patients do contain antibodies to their own tumors. Therefore, the immortalization of these lymph node lymphocytes through the now classical hybridoma technique will yield human MAbs reactive with human tumor antigens.

B. Human Fusion Partner

The production of human MAbs has been hampered somewhat by the difficulty encountered in reproducibly generating genetically stable Ig-secreting human-human hybridomas. This problem has been solved in our laboratory by developing and characterizing UC 729-6, a diploid 6-thioguanine-resistant human lymphoblastoid B cell line (6). A recent independent report (10) compared currently available human cell lines (both B cell and myeloma) for generating human hybridomas and concluded that UC 729-6 was the optimal cell line. The general characteristics of UC 729-6 (Table 1) have been reviewed elsewhere (11,12).

Table 1 General Characteristics of UC 729-6

1. Human lymphoblastoid B cell line derived from parental WIL-2 cells
2. 6-thioguanine-resistant and dies in HAT media within 10 days
3. Fc receptor-negative
4. HLA profile: HLA-A1, A2, B5, B17, DR4, DR7
5. Diploid with a $21p^+$ chromosome marker
6. Secretes $\leqslant$ 20-50 ng IgM/10^6 cells/ml day
7. Doubles every 17 hours

C. Case History

An 83-year-old white female, gravida 1, para 1, was admitted to UCSD University Hospital in July 1983 for a vulvar biopsy. Analysis showed a 5 × 6 cm left vulvar mass and a 2 × 3 cm fixed left inguinal node. A pathological examination showed the patient to have invasive squamous cell carcinoma of the vulva (T2N2M0). A radical vulvectomy and bilateral groin dissection were performed, including a node dissection of the left pelvic fossa, proctectomy, and transverse colostomy. Invasive epidermoid vulvar carcinoma with metastases to the left and right inguinal areas was also observed. Deep pelvic nodes were normal. Five of eight left groin nodes were positive, whereas two of nine right groin nodes were positive. Shown in Figure 1 is a hematoxylin-eosin (H and E) section of one of the patient's involved lymph nodes clearly demonstrating an invasive squamous cell carcinoma with an adjacent germinal center.

D. Fusion Summary

Details of the fusion and cloning of human-human hybridomas generated from UC 729-6 have been described previously (6). An involved lymph node from the patient described above was delivered to us within 3 hours of surgery. The nodal segments were immersed in serum-free RPMI-1640, trimmed free of extraneous tissue and capsular components, and teased with nugent forceps to make a single cell suspension. After large tissue aggregates settled, the cells in suspension were removed and washed twice, 500 *g* for 5 min/wash. All dissections and cell preparations were performed at room temperature. The isolated lymphocytes were resuspended at 5×10^6/ml in RPMI-1640 media supplemented with 10% fetal calf serum (FCS) and incubated overnight at 37°C in 5% CO^2 prior to fusion.

Using 35% polyethylene glycol 1500, 3.33×10^7 of the patient's lymphocytes were fused with 1.66×10^7 UC 729-6 cells according to previously described procedures (6). After the fusion, the cells were added to 96-well plates at 1.0×10^5 cells per well. The day after the fusion, the growth media was replaced by RPMI-1640 media supplemented with 10% FCS and glutamine, including hypoxanthine (1×10^{-4} M), amethopterin (2×10^{-7} M), and thymidine (1.6×10^{-5} M) (HAT media) (13). After 2-4 weeks in culture, hybrids visible to the eye were analyzed for human Ig secretion (see section II). Eighty hybrids resulted from 480 wells plated, 14 of which secreted IgG and four which secreted IgM.

II. PRODUCTION OF HUMAN-HUMAN HYBRIDOMAS

Supernatants from the hybridomas were screened for human Ig by an enzyme immunoassay (EIA) as described previously (14-17). Those found to secrete Ig were expanded and cloned by limiting dilution (1 cell/3 wells) without any feeder layer

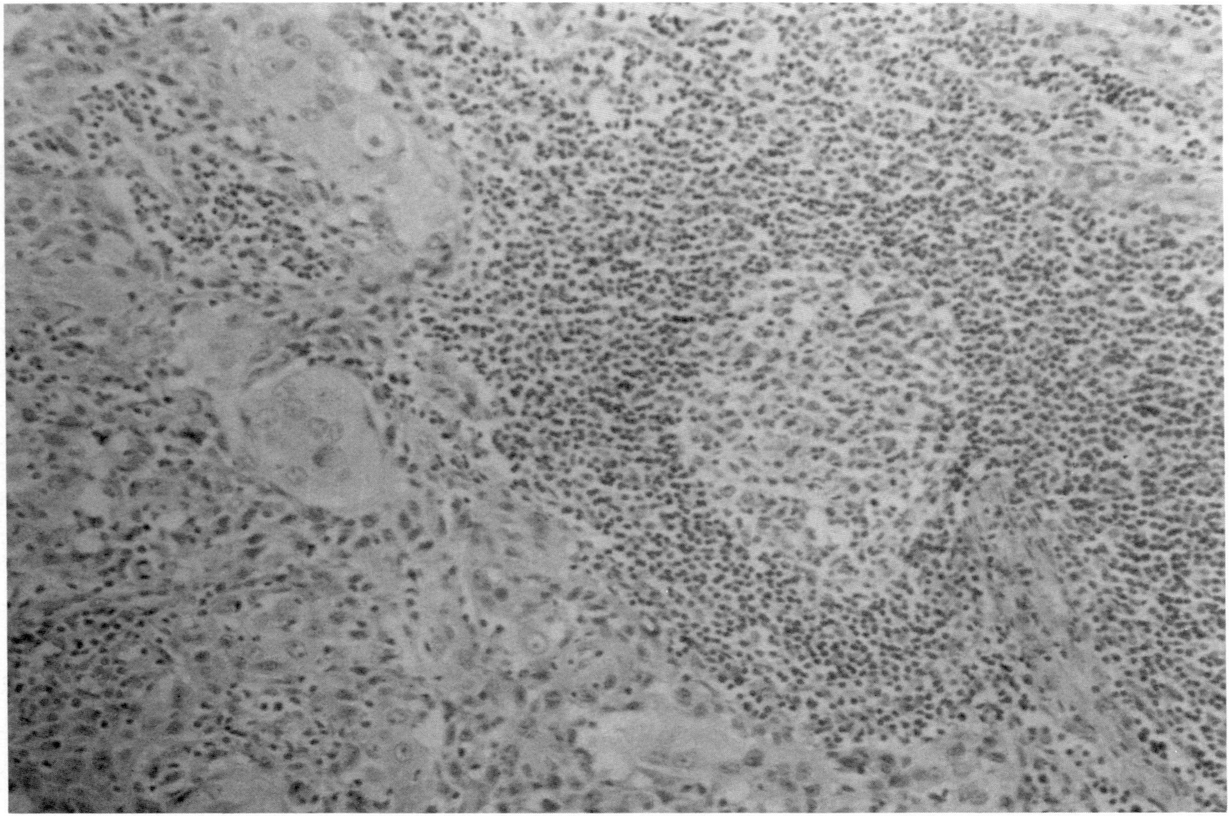

Figure 1 Hematoxylin-eosin section of a regional draining lymph node from the patient showing *in situ* vulvar carcinoma adjacent to a germina center (magnification ×400).

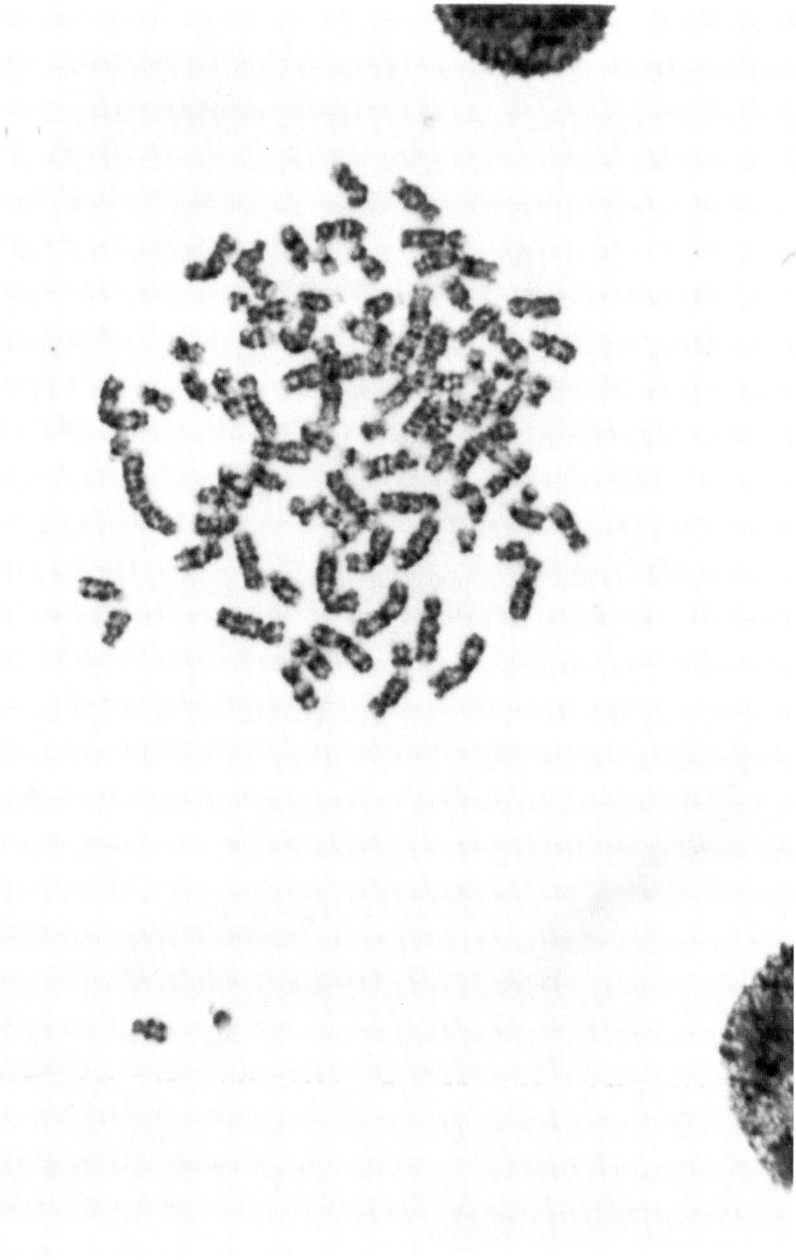

Figure 2 Karyotype of the VLN3G2 human-human hybridoma. A tetraploid modal chromosome number is apparent, and the $21p^+$ marker chromosome, indicative of parentage by UC 729-6, is present.

cells in RPMI media. Cryopreservation and thawing of these hybridomas has not resulted in any detectable adversity in stability and secretion.

The hybrids generated were tetraploid as judged by karyotypic (Fig. 2) and cytofluorographic analysis of their DNA content (Table 2). HLA phenotyping has also shown that these human hybridomas express antigens of both parental UC 729-6 and the patient's lymph node lymphocytes (Table 3).

Because large amounts of antibody would be required in a clinical setting, questions pertaining to the long-term stability of human Ig-secreting hybridomas are of paramount importance. The issue of long-term stability of these VLN hybrids was assessed over a 12-month period, during which we examined both DNA content (Table 2) and Ig secretion rate (Table 4). The generated data indicate that UC 729-6 is a genetically stable vector for the capture and immortalization of human B lymphocytes.

III. IMMUNOREACTIVITY

Of the 14 IgG-secreting hybrids, six passed initial reactivity screens against target cell bound antigens, whereas one of the four IgM-secreting hybrids passed. These seven hybridomas were cloned by limiting dilution (1 cell/3 wells) and expanded for further analysis. The reactivity of the six IgG human MAbs against a panel of normal and malignant cells is shown in Figure 3. The reactivity index (RI) was calculated from the following formula:

$$RI = \frac{O.D._{490} \text{ test MAb} - O.D._{490} \text{ background}}{O.D._{490} \text{ control} - O.D._{490} \text{ background}} .$$

The control consisted of an irrelevant human IgG used at the same concentration as the test human MAb.

As seen in Figure 3, these six IgG MAbs have broad reactivity profiles with human carcinoma cells, but do not react with hematopoietic or fibroblast cell lines and normal peripheral blood leukocytes. Of particular note, all six of the IgGs were very reactive with the A431 cell line, a carcinoma of the vulva, similar to the primary cancer of the patient used in these studies.

A titration of the VLN3G2 and VLN5C7 IgG MAbs against target cell-bound antigens is shown in Figure 4. Starting from an initial concentration of 450 ng/ml of VLN3G2 (Fig. 4A), we were able to obtain appreciable reactivity even at 450 pg/ml. There did not appear to be any major quantitative differences in the antigen expression by either the vulva, lung, or stomach cell lines since the reactivity of the MAbs was similar in each case.

Target A431 cells were analyzed by indirect immunofluorescence with VLN3G2 (Fig. 5). Cell surface and cytoplasmic staining patterns were evident.

Table 2 Cytofluorographic Analysis of Human Hybridoma DNA

	Relative DNA content[a]				
Cell type	2 months	4 months	8 months	12 months	24 months
UC 729-6	45 ± 2	44 ± 2	45 ± 4	45 ± 2	45 ± 2
VLN3G2	80 ± 2	81 ± 3	80 ± 4	80 ± 3	N.D.
VLN1H12	82 ± 3	81 ± 3	81 ± 3	80 ± 3	N.D.
CLNH5[b]	83 ± 3	82 ± 2	83 ± 3	83 ± 3	82 ± 3
MHG7[c]	74 ± 2	68 ± 3	55 ± 3	54 ± 3	51 ± 2

[a]Relative DNA content of UC 729-6 and the hybridomas was obtained by the propidium iodine method (6). At the indicated times after fusions, the DNA content of the cells was determined.
[b]CLNH5 is a human-human hybridoma described previously (6).
[c]MHG7 is a mouse-human hybridoma described previously (9).

Table 3 HLA Phenotype of UC 729-6 and VLN Hybrids

Cell line	HLA-A	HLA-B	HLA-DR
UC 729-6	A1, A2	B5, B17	DR4, DR7
VLN3G2	A1, A2	B5, B17 B27, BW44	DR4, DR7
VLN1H12	A1, A5	B5, B17 B27	DR4, DR7

Table 4 IgM Secretion (μg IgM/10^6 cells/ml/day) by Human Hybridomas over Time

Time (months)	VLN1H12	CLNH5	MHG7
1	1.58	2.36	2.84
2	ND	2.48	2.60
3	1.37	ND	1.92
4	ND	2.28	1.45[a]
5	ND	ND	2.11
6	1.25	2.43	1.87
7	ND	ND	1.49
8	1.29	2.36	ND
9	ND	ND	1.16[a]
10	1.31	2.43	2.48
11	ND	ND	2.27
12	1.28	2.24	2.06

At the indicated time points after the fusion, the amount of human IgM in the culture supernatant was determined by EIA. ND = not determined.

[a]MHG7, a mouse-human hybridoma, was subcloned by limiting dilution (1 cell/3 wells) at 4 and 9 months post-fusion to select for a higher secreting subclone.

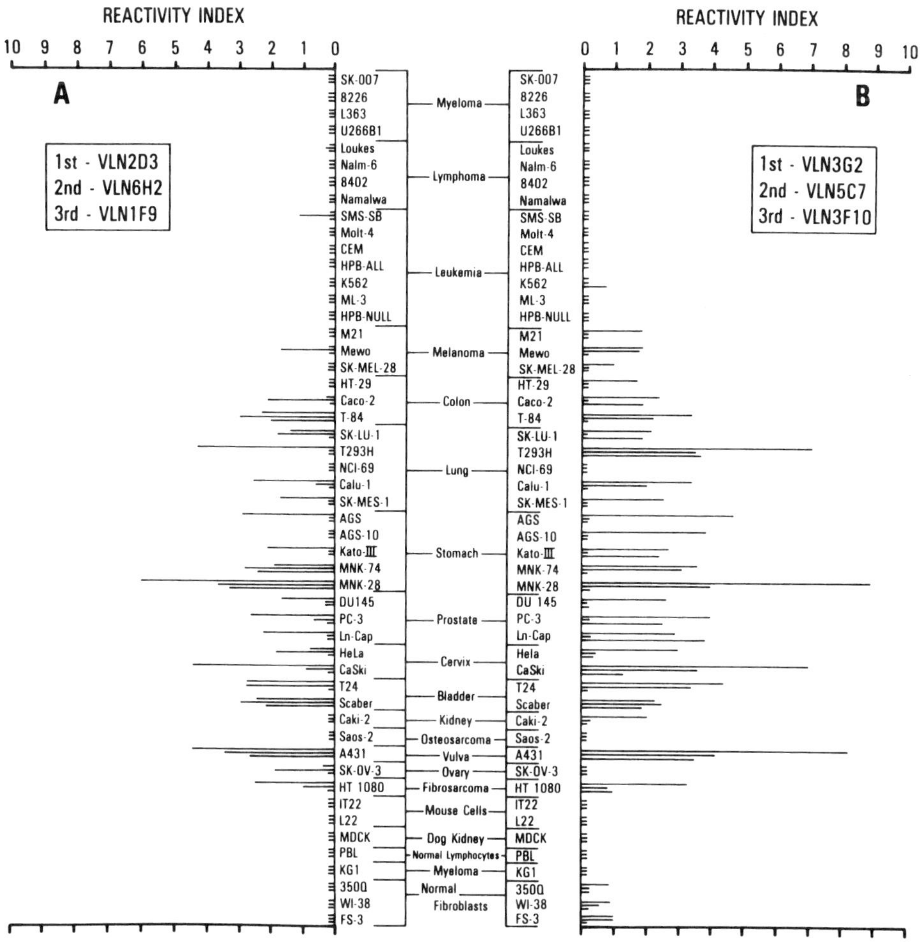

Figure 3 Enzyme immunoassay analysis of six human IgG MAbs from the VLN-UC 729-6 fusion against a panel of normal and malignant cells. The cells were prepared and tested for reactivity by the human MAbs as described previously (15). See text for an explanation of the reactivity index.

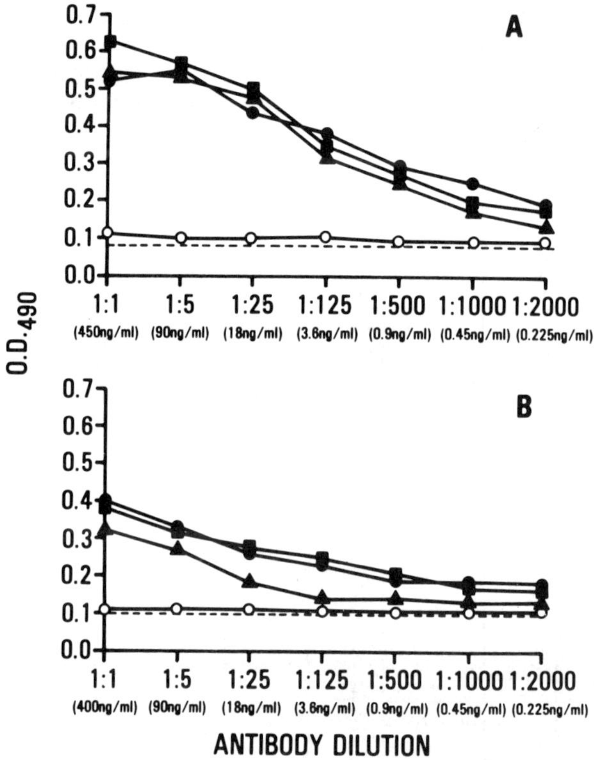

Figure 4 Titration of VLN3G2 (A) and VLN5C7 (B) human IgG MAbs against 2.0×10^5 target A431 cells(■), T293H cells (●), and MKN-28 cells (▲) by EIA. Controls consisted of an irrelevant human IgG and A431 cells (– – –) and the test human MAb and 8402 cells (○—○), an unreactive human T cell line.

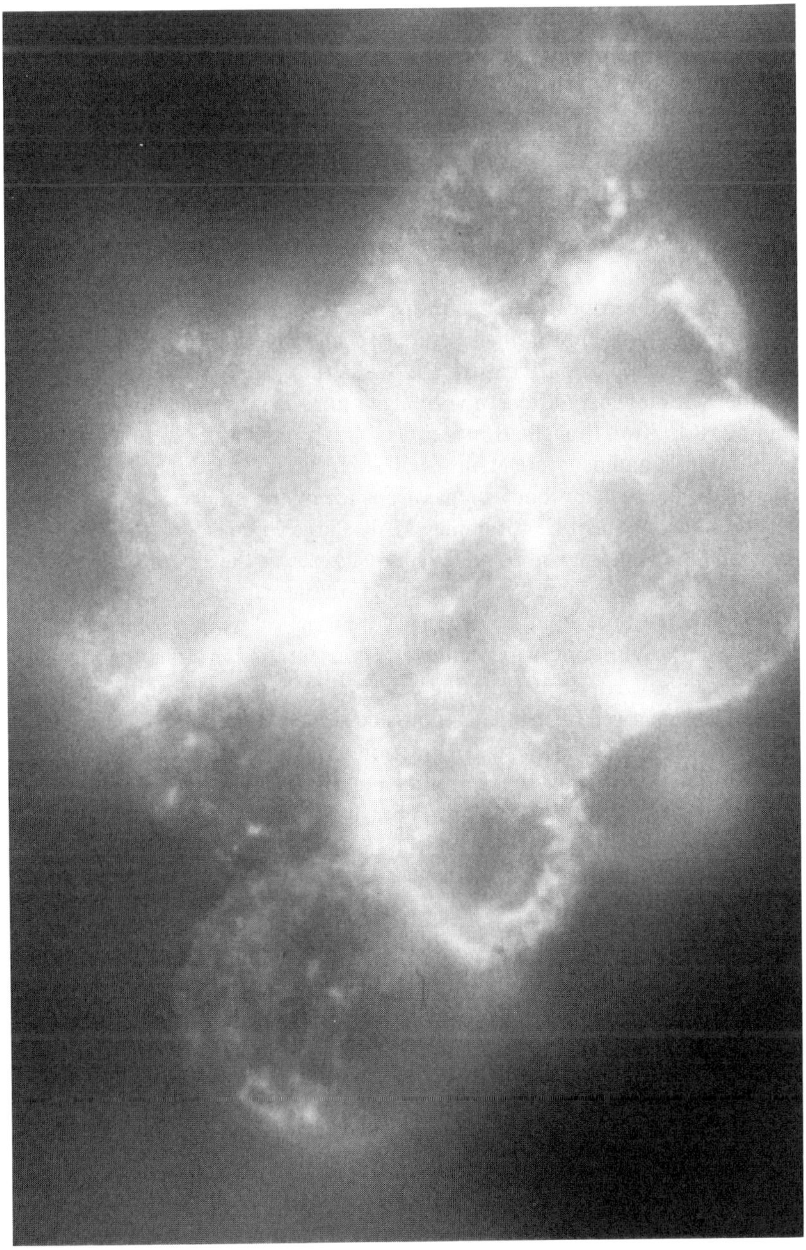

Figure 5 Immunofluorescence analysis of VLN3G2 and A431, a carcinoma of the vulvar cell line. A431 cells were incubated with purified VLN3G2 for 30 minutes at 4°C, washed, and then incubated with FITC-conjugated goat anti-human IgG for 30 minutes at 4°C.

IV. PURIFICATION

In our laboratory, human hybridomas were routinely grown in culture flasks containing RPMI-1640 medium supplemented with 10% FCS and glutamine (6). After 4 days of growth at 37°C in a 5% CO_2-humidified incubator, the cultures were harvested by centrifugation, and the supernates were collected. Starting with the hybridoma supernates, the strategies followed in the purification of the MAbs are outlined in Figure 6. According to this scheme, MAbs were isolated by standard biochemical procedures at physiological pH and by affinity procedures where antibodies were subjected to low acidic pH buffer. Even though the former method of purification is laborious and time-consuming, the antibodies are highly reactive and useful for *in vivo* studies, such as tumor imaging and therapy. In the later method of purification, the MAbs were eluted from the affinity columns either with low pH buffers or with high molar chaotropic agents like urea and guanidine HCl. Even though affinity procedures are rapid, these conditions are known to unfold and denature MAbs to different degrees, and many investigators prefer not to use such antibody preparations for *in vivo* studies.

To purify milligram quantities of human MAbs, large volumes of hybridoma supernates containing microgram to milligram quantities of the antibodies were pooled together. Handling large quantities of hybridoma supernates creates problems in research laboratories that are designed for analytical work. To decrease the starting volume, hybridoma supernates were concentrated in a dialysis bag surrounded by aquacide. After concentrating to a small volume, any insoluble precipitate formed was removed by centrifugation, and the clear supernatant was fractionated on a molecular sieving column. Fractions collected from the column were assayed for both antibody concentration and immunoreactivity against tumor antigens on target cells. Typical elution profiles of the growth media containing the MAbs of two of our human hybridomas, VLN3G2 and VLN1H12, are shown in Figure 7. Monoclonal IgG fractions (VLN3G2) separated from the IgM by the G-200 gel column were pooled, dialyzed, and chromatographed on a DE-52 ion-exchange column at pH 8.8. At this pH, human IgG elutes in the unbound fraction while nonimmunoglobulin proteins bind to the ion-exchange resin and require higher salt concentrations for elution. At this point, only the fetal calf serum immunoglobulins are the major contaminating proteins. These contaminants were removed from the human MAbs by passing the sample through a Sepharose-4B column conjugated with rabbit antibodies to fetal calf serum proteins.

Two major symmetrical protein peaks were observed in the G-200 runs (Fig. 7). Proteins in fractions 43-65 contained the IgG that reacted against a target A431 cell surface antigen(s). Higher molecular weight proteins in fractions 30-42 contained vestigial IgM that was not reactive with A431 cells. This IgM originated from parental UC 729-6, which secretes low levels of IgM. Both the immu-

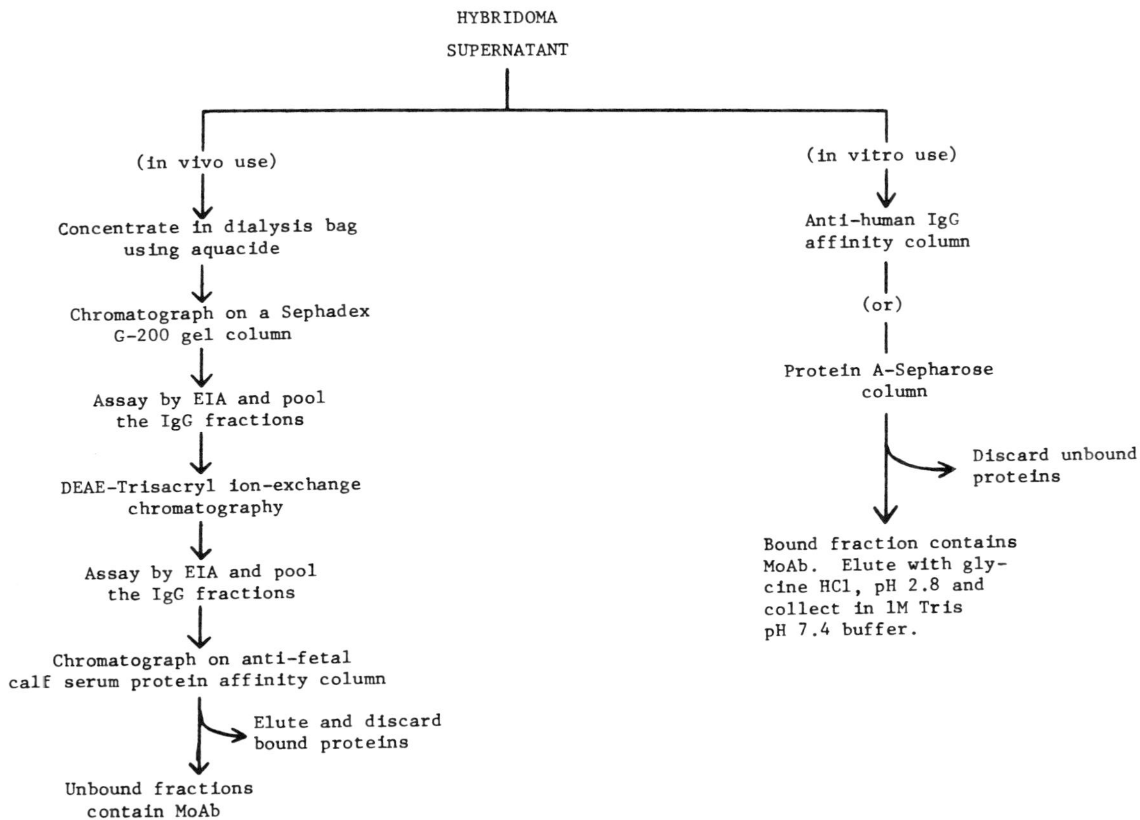

Figure 6 Flow diagram indicating our strategies for the purification of tumor-reactive human MAbs from hybridoma supernatant. For *in vivo* use, purification conditions are kept at physiological pH, though labor-intensive. For *in vitro* use, the antibodies are subject to potentially damaging extremes of pH by elution from affinity or protein-A columns.

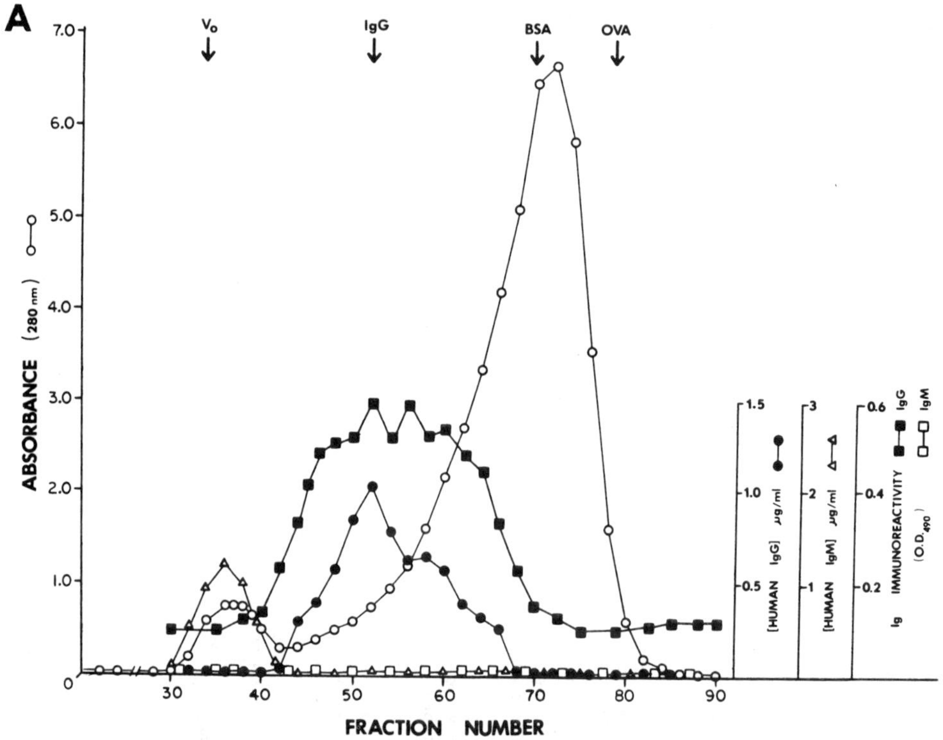

Figure 7 Sephadex G-200 chromatography of human hybridoma supernates grown in RPMI-1640 media supplemented with 10% FCS. (A) VLN3G2 culture supernatant (100 ml) was concentrated to 10 ml with aquacide, loaded onto a column (2.5 X 47 cm; void volume 73 ml), and eluted with PBS-collecting fractions of 2.35 ml at 4°C.

B

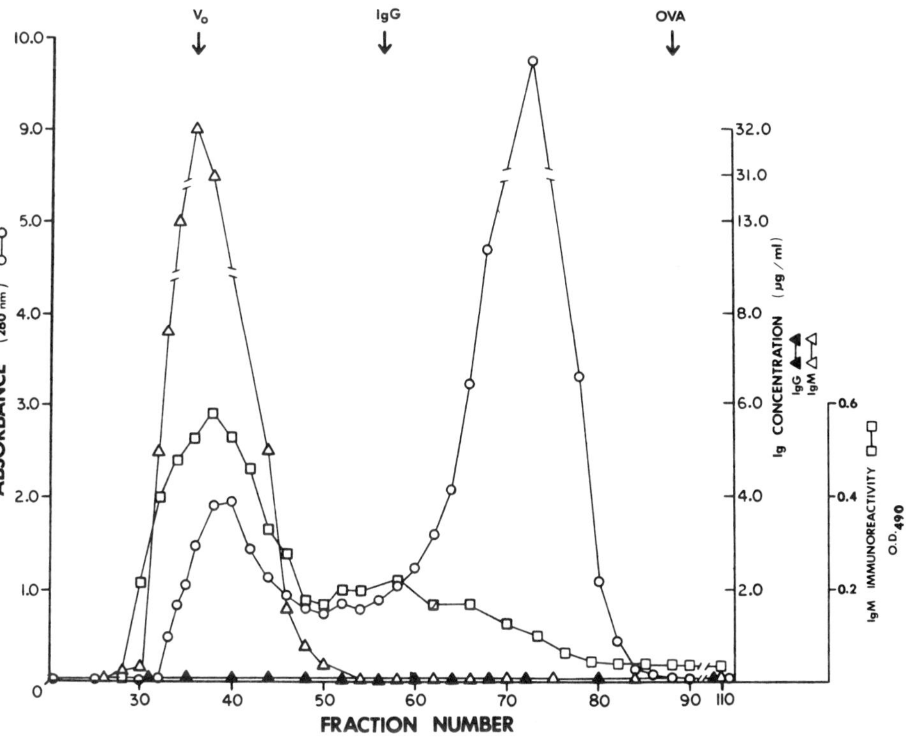

Figure 7 (continued) (B) VLN1H12 hybridoma supernatant (200 ml) was concentrated to 8 ml by aquacide and loaded onto the same column as described in Figure 6, and 2.0 ml fractions were collected at 4°C. All column fractions were read for absorbance at 280 nm and assayed by EIA to determine the concentrations of human IgG and IgM. To determine the immunoreactivity of the IgG and IgM in the column fractions, target A431 cells were used in a whole cell EIA described previously (15).

noreactivity and the IgG elution profile showed complete overlap in their G-200 fractions. Aggregates of IgG or monomers of IgM were not observed in any of the column fractions.

An alternative purification method for human MAbs is affinity chromatography, which is known to be direct and rapid, though it employs potentially very deleterious experimental conditions. Two of the most commonly employed reagents for this purpose are immobilized antibodies and protein A-Sepharose. Human IgG MAb preparations were passed through a column containing Sepharose-4B gel covalently conjugated to goat anti-human IgG antibodies. After washing the unbound proteins off the column with PBS, bound antibodies were eluted by passing glycine-HCl, pH 2.8, buffer through the gel. The acidic eluant containing the MAbs was then collected in 1 M, pH 7.4 tris buffer, to bring the pH of the solution to 7.4 immediately. Such antibody preparations are widely used in many *in vitro* studies.

Due to the low levels of proteins, human MAbs grown under serum-free conditions would be easier to purify. The growth of the VLN hybrids in commercially available serum-free media (Hana Biologics) was assessed (Fig. 8). Over a 6-day period, there was no significant change in the growth curves of the human hybridomas when cultured in RPMI-1640 media plus 10% FCS or in serum-free HB101 or HB102 (used according to manufacturer's instructions). There was an enhanced secretion of both IgG (Fig. 8A) and IgM (Fig. 8B) under serum-free conditions compared with serum-supplemented growth. Maximum IgG levels of VLN3G2 were observed during days 3-4 in HB102, whereas maximum IgM levels of VLN1H12 were observed on day 5 in HB102. Serum-free conditions may provide the appropriate milieu for the increased level of Ig secretion, in that there are no suppressor or inhibitory type factors which may be present in FCS that retard the rate of Ig secretion. The absence of these "factors" in serum-free media would allow Ig secretion to occur unimpeded.

V. ANTIGEN BIOCHEMISTRY

Approximately 5×10^6 mid-log phase A431 cells (a squamous cell carcinoma of the vulva) and T293H cells (an oat cell carcinoma of the lung) were intrinsically labeled with 100 μCi of ^{35}S-methionine (NEN) for 18 hours in methionine-free RPMI-1640 media supplemented with 10% FCS. Cells were scraped off with a rubber policeman, washed twice (500 *g* for 10 min/wash in RPMI-1640 media without serum), and lysed with NP-40 detergent (0.5% NP-40, 1 mM PMSF, 5 mM EDTA, 50 mM tris, pH 7.4) for 1 hour at 4°C. Extracted macromolecules were ultracentrifuged (100,000 *g* for 1 hour), precleared with affinity-purified irrelevant human IgG overnight at 4°C, and washed twice in a microfuge. To the cleared supernatant, 30 μg of affinity-purified VLN3G2 was added, incubated for 2

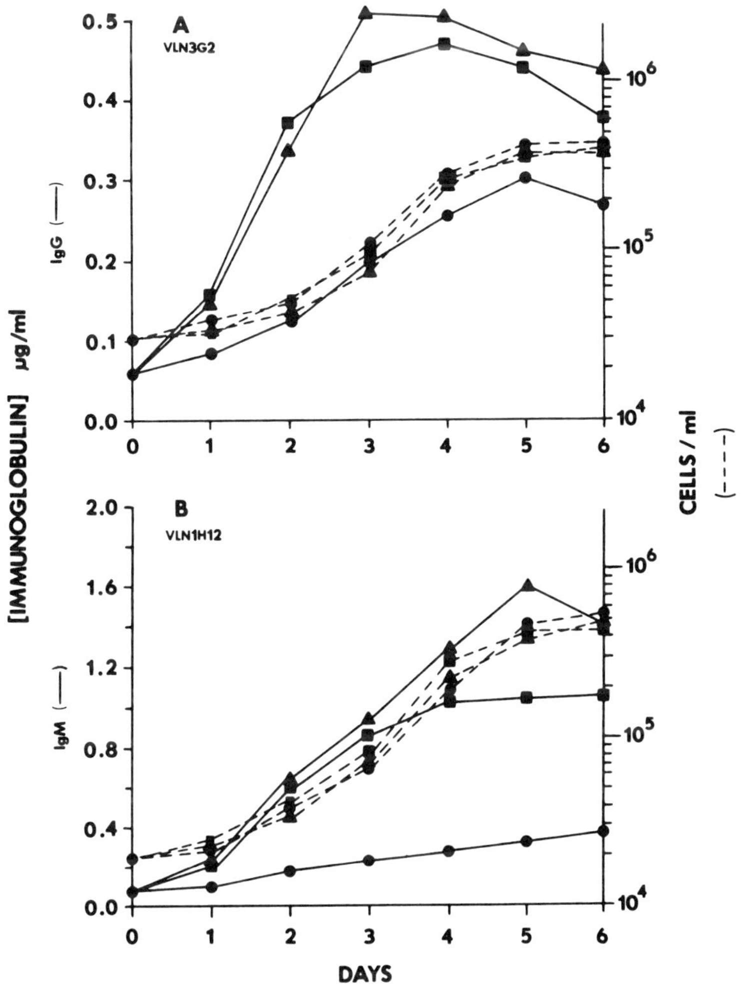

Figure 8 Growth of human-human hybridomas in serum-free media. Cells were washed three times in serum-free RPMI-1640 media and resuspended in HB101 (■), HB102 (▲) (Hana Biologics; cells were grown according to manufacturer's instructions), and RPMI-1640 (●) supplemented with 10% FCS and glutamine (6). At 24-hour intervals, both viable cell number (- - -) and Ig concentration (–) were determined. (A) VLN3G2-IgG. (B) VLN1H12-IgM.

Table 5 Molecular Parameters of Antigen(s) Recognized by VLN3G2

Experimental condition	A431 cell line	T293 cell line
Reducing[a]	48 K	48 K
Non-reducing[b]	48 K	48 K
Isoelectric point	5.85	5.0

[a]10% SDS-PAGE with B-mercaptoethanol
[b]10% PAGE.

hours at 4°C. After three washes, the samples were analyzed by SDS gel electrophoresis as described previously (18).

A summary of the data describing some of the general biochemical characteristics of the antigen(s) recognized by VLN3G2 is given in Table 5. Under nonreducing conditions, a single band was identified with an apparent molecular weight of 48,000 daltons (48 K) (pI of 5.8) from the A431 cell line that, under reducing conditions, resolved into a subunit with a molecular weight of 48,000 daltons. T293H cells also yielded a single band with an apparent molecular weight of 48,000 daltons (48 K; pI of 5.0), which resulted in one subunit with a molecular weight of 48 K under reducing conditions.

VI. CONCLUSIONS

The analysis of the human immune response to human tumor antigens (4,5) will hopefully generate a new understanding in the regulation of cancer, possibly leading to new therapeutic regimens. Our approach has been through the development of a human hybridoma system (6,11,14,16) by which we immortalized individual lymphocytes obtained from regional draining lymph nodes of cancer patients. The resulting hybridomas have secreted MAbs reactive with human tumor-associated antigens (6,9,11,19).

Because large amounts of human MAbs would be required for serotherapy, questions pertaining to the long-term stability of human Ig-secreting hybridomas are of significant importance. We have previously shown (20) that human-human hybridomas, with UC 729-6 as the fusion partner, were stable for up to 2 years (Tables 2 and 4). This was particularly evident when compared with mouse-human hybridomas (8,9,20), which nonrandomly loose human chromosomes

(21,22) and, therefore, have the potential to loose human Ig secretion, a problem encountered by others (8). The VLN human hybridomas described here were derived from UC 729-6 and have been genetically stable in culture for longer than 1 year, indicating that their long-term survival should not present any major difficulties.

The case presented here represents a model in understanding the human immune response to human tumor antigens. Antigens displayed by the malignant vulvar cells embedded within the lymph node stimulated an immune response, resulting in a proliferation of germinal centers (Fig. 1), areas known to be enriched in Ig-secreting B cells (23). These lymphocytes were collected and fused with UC 729-6, effectively immortalizing and, thereby, "freezing" a window of this immune response. The reactivity data obtained with the cells shown in Figure 3 suggest a restricted specificity of the recognized antigens to malignant adherent cell types. Whether this information will be supported using fresh frozen tissues is currently under evaluation. If these human MAbs react only with malignant cells in tissue sections or a subset of them, then these antibodies may have utility in the analysis and treatment of cancer.

The lymph nodes play a critical role in immune regulation, and their response to the antigenicity of tumor cells may trigger regional nodes to develop complex immune reactions (7). Regional lymph nodes draining tumors are routinely enlarged as a result of either immunoreactivity or metastasis, or both. In lymph node metastasis, the metastatic tumor cells first appear in the marginal sinus, from which they penetrate the medullary sinuses, the medulla, and the cortex, eventually resulting in total parenchymal replacement (24). In the case presented here, the patient was diagnosed as having metastatic squamous cell carcinoma of the vulva to regional lymph nodes (T2N2M0), one of which was used in this study. Based on our results, it appears that vulvar metastases embedded within regional lymph nodes, causing the patient to mount an immune response against her tumor antigens. If this is true, then questions are raised as to the apparent ineffectiveness of the antibodies in the course of her cancer. However, the prognostic value of germinal center hyperplasia in cancer patients, such as that observed in the case studied here, remains controversial (25,26), indicating the importance of other mechanisms in the disease.

VII. PERSPECTIVES

The role of the lymph node in tumor immunity has been inadequately studied and is poorly understood. The microenvironment within a regional draining lymph node is complex and regulated by a variety of host defense factors, such as genetics, age, hormonal milieu, variable metastasizing capabilities, the nature of the tumor antigens presented, and the different physiological responses of the patient. In the case presented here, we feel we have immortalized part of the immune response that the patient has mounted to her tumor antigens. This is partly based on the cell reactivity data of the human IgG MAbs generated from the fusion. The UC 729-6 cell line simply served as a genetically stable vector by which we immortalized the patient's human Ig-secreting lymphocytes.

One of the major goals in developing human hybridoma technology has been the analysis of man's immune response to his cells and tissues. In the future, this technology will provide a means whereby we can begin a systematic analysis of the human immune response to human cancers by immortalizing B cells from regional draining lymph nodes. It is hoped this will provide new information in developing better strategies and regimens for the war on cancer.

REFERENCES

1. G. Kohler and C. Milstein. Continuous cultures of fused cells secreting antibody of predefined specificity. *Nature, 256*:495 (1975).
2. L. Olssen and H. S. Kaplan. Human-human hybridomas producing monoclonal antibodies of predefined antigenic specificity. *Proc. Natl. Acad. Sci.* (*USA*), *77*:5429 (1980).
3. C. Croce, A. Linnebach, W. Hall, Z. Steplewski, and H. Koprowski. Production of human hybridomas secreting antibody to measles virus. *Nature, 288*: 488 (1980).
4. K. E. Hellstrom and J. P. Brown. Tumor antigens. In M. Sela (ed.). *The Antigens. Vol. 5.* Academic Press, New York (1979).
5. L. K. Old. Cancer immunology. The search for specificity. *Cancer Res., 41*: 361 (1980).
6. M. C. Glassy, H. H. Handley, H. Hagiwara, and I. Royston. UC 729-6, a human lymphoblastoid B cell line useful for generating antibody-secreting human-human hybridomas. *Proc. Natl. Acad. Sci.* (*USA*), *80*:6327 (1983).
7. J. Schlom, D. Wunderlich, and Y. A. Teramoto. Generation of human monoclonal antibodies reactive with human mammary carcinoma cells. *Proc. Natl. Acad. Sci.* (*USA*), *77*:6841 (1980).
8. K. Sikora and R. Wright. Human monoclonal antibodies to lung-cancer antigens. *Br. J. Cancer, 43*:696 (1981).
9. D. H. Lowe, H. H. Handley, J. Schmidt, I. Royston, and M. C. Glassy. A human monoclonal antibody reactive with human prostate. *J. Urol., 132*:780 (1984).
10. P. G. Abrams, J. A. Knost, G. Clarke, S. Wilburn, R. K. Oldham, and K. A. Foon. Determination of the optimal human cell lines for development of human hybridomas. *J. Immunol., 131*:1202 (1983).
11. M. C. Glassy, H. H. Handley, and I. Royston. Design and production of human monoclonal antibodies to human cancers. In E. G. Engleman, S. Foung, J. Larrick, and A. A. Rabbitschek (eds.). *Human Hybridomas and Monoclonal Antibodies.* Plenum Press, New York (1985).

12. M. C. Glassy, S. A. Gaffar, R. E. Peters, and I. Royston. Human monoclonal antibodies to human cancer cells. In R. A. Reisfeld and S. Sell (eds.). *Monoclonal Antibodies and Cancer Therapy, Vol. 27.* UCLA Symposia on Molecular and Cellular Biology; Alan R. Liss, New York (1986).
13. J. W. Littlefield. Selection of hybrids from matings of fibroblasts *in vitro* and their presumed recombinants. *Science, 145*:709 (1964).
14. M. C. Glassy and P. H. Cleveland. Use of mouse and human monoclonal antibodies in enzyme immunofiltration. In G. DiSabato, J. J. Langone, and H. Van Vunakis (eds.). *Immunochemical Techniques, Methods in Enzymology, Vol. 121.* Academic Press, New York (1986).
15. M. C. Glassy and C. D. Surh. Immunodetection of cell-bound antigens using both mouse and human monoclonal antibodies. *J. Immunol. Meth., 81*:115 (1985).
16. M. C. Glassy, H. H. Handley, P. H. Cleveland, and I. Royston. An enzyme immunofiltration assay useful for detecting human monoclonal antibody. *J. Immunol. Meth., 58*:119 (1983).
17. M. C. Glassy and H. H. Handley. Monoclonal antibodies and enzyme immunofiltration. In P. N. Cheremisinoff and R. P. Ouelette (eds.). *Biotechnology Handbook.* Technomic Publishing, Lancaster, Pennsylvania (1985).
18. B. J. Davis. Disk electrophoresis-II. Method and application to human serum proteins. *Ann. NY Acad. Sci., 121*:404 (1964).
19. H. Hagiwara and G. H. Sato. Human x human hybridoma producing monoclonal antibody against autologous cervical carcinoma. *Mol. Biol. Med., 1*: 245 (1983).
20. M. C. Glassy, H. H. Handley, C. Surh, and I. Royston. Genetically stable human hybridomas secreting tumor reactive human monoclonal IgM. *Cancer Invest.* (in press).
21. M. C. Glassy and S. Ferrone. Differential segregation patterns of human chromosomes in somatic cell hybrids constructed with human B lymphocytes and human melanoma cells. *Cancer Res., 42*:3971 (1982).
22. M. E. Kamarck, P. E. Barker, R. L. Miller, and F. H. Ruddle. Somatic hybrid mapping panels. *Exp. Cell Res., 152*:1 (1984).
23. P. Nieuwenhuis and D. Opstelten. Functional anatomy of germinal centers. *Am. J. Anat., 170*:421 (1984).
24. H. L. Ioachim. Metastatic tumors in lymph nodes. In *Lymph Node Biopsy.* J. B. Lippincott, Philadelphia, (1982).
25. M. Wernicke and A. Podesta. Host defense factors, tumor aggressiveness, and prognosis associated with carcinomas of the breast. *Hum. Pathol., 15*: 423 (1984).
26. I. Carr. Lymphatic metastasis. *Cancer Metast. Rev., 2*:307 (1983).

12

Construction of Stable Human Hybrid Clones Producing Antibody Reactive with Human Mammary Carcinoma

ANTHONY J. STRELKAUSKAS, CATHERINE L. TAYLOR, and PAUL H. ALDENDERFER
Medical University of South Carolina, Charleston, South Carolina

GLENN A. WARNER
Northwest Oncology Clinics, Seattle, Washington

In general, early human-human fusion experiments have followed in the footsteps of their mouse monoclonal predecessors, using human multiple myeloma cells as malignant partners instead of mouse plasmacytoma cells. These early attempts were almost always unsuccessful because most myeloma cells could not be adapted to long-term culture. However, there have been several cell lines developed for use as fusion partners, which have reportedly been successfully derived from human myelomas and adapted to culture. These include U266 (1), RPMI-8226 (2), KARPAS 707 (3), KMMI (4), HMy2 (5), IM9 (6), GM-1500 (7), and SK-007 (8).

The first report (8) of a successful human fusion utilized the IgE-secreting myeloma U266 to produce a hybrid cell-making antibody specific for dinitrophenol (DNP). At about the same time, Croce *et al.* (7) used an 8-azoguanine-resistant derivative of the lymphoblastoid line GM-1500 (called GM-1500 6TG-A11) as a fusion partner to describe the construction of clones producing antibodies that were positive in a measles virus system. This fusion partner and derivatives of it have been subsequently used by other investigators in attempts at cloning antibodies specific for DNA (9,10) or tetanus toxoid (11). Eisenbarth *et al.* (12) have also reported some success using a derivative of this line in experiments on type-1 diabetes mellitus.

Comparisons between different fusion partners (13,14) have shown that SKO-007 exhibits a lower fusion efficiency than LICR, while both are significantly less effective than mouse NS-1 cells (14). Separate human fusions have been done using a variety of methods to produce antibodies specific for tumors such as glioma (15), lung and cervical carcinoma (16,17), colon carcinoma (18), malignant melanoma (19), and even products of oncogenes. In addition, human clones are also being used in the area of human leukemias. The work of Larrick *et al.* (20) in the area of cloned antibody to tetanus toxoid is also of interest for demonstrating the utility of human hybridoma technology. In addition, the concept of using Epstein-Barr virus (EBV) infection as an initial step for the development of human antibody-producing clones has also been well-documented (21-23, and Part I, Chapter 1 of this book).

We present the description of a stable human clone that does not cross-react with normal breast tissue or malignant tissue. This clone was constructed using new techniques that do not require hypoxanthine/aminopterin/thymidine (HAT)-sensitive myeloma cells as fusion partners. It is a true genetic hybrid as evidenced by karyotypic analysis, and has been in continuous culture for over 3 years. In addition, we have been able to adapt this antibody to both a Latex agglutination assay and ELISA system, by which we can identify a serum antigen closely correlated to breast cancer. Using these MAb-derived systems, we can monitor and follow women who are in post-surgical stages of the disease and determine the extent of ongoing metastasis, in some cases as much as 10 months before it is clinically identifiable.

I. TECHNICAL INFORMATION

A. Binding Studies

In order to identify binding of molecules to tumor cell lines, two methods were employed.

1. Indirect Rosetting

Target cells at a concentration of 0.5×10^6 were incubated with a 1:5 dilution of patient serum for 1 hour at 4°C, washed, and rosetted with sheep red blood cells (SRBCs) coated with affinity-purified rabbit anti-human $F(ab')_2$ using methods described previously (24). One hundred cells were enumerated microscopically for positive binding of SRBCs, and expressed as a percentage of binding.

2. Indirect Immunofluorescence

Assays were accomplished using standard methods. Briefly, 100 μl of target cells at 5×10^6 cells/ml were pipetted into wells of 96-well plates, and centrifuged at 200 *g* for 5 minutes. A 1:5 dilution of each patient's serum was added to cell pellets, incubated for 1 hour at 4°C, and then washed three times. One hundred μl of FITC-conjugated to rabbit anti-human IgG was added to cell pellets and incubated for 30 minutes at 4°C. Cells were washed, pipetted onto slides, and microscopically examined for positive fluorescence.

B. Human-Human Fusion

Prior to any fusions, serum samples from potential donor patients were carefully screened for the presence of intrinsic anti-tumor antibodies using well-characterized tumor cell lines. Only those patients who exhibited obvious anti-tumor antibodies were used as peripheral blood lymphocyte donors. It is important to note that we had no success with patients undergoing standard protocols of chemotherapy and/or radiation, and had to utilize patients who had been receiving alternative forms of cancer therapy which were not immunologically destructive (see section II.A). Donor lymphocytes were fused with the malignant fusion partner cell line Ball-1 (a generous gift from Dr. Jun Minowada) as follows. Cells were washed and added together at a lymphocyte to malignant partner ratio of 2:1. The cell mixture was centrifuged at 100 *g* for 5 minutes, supernatant removed, and the pellet gently disrupted. Three hundred μl of a 30% polyethylene glycol (PEG) 4000 solution containing 7% DMSO in Hank's balanced salt solution (HBSS) was added and mixed for 30 seconds. Cells were then centrifuged at 70 *g* for a total of 6.5 minutes. Cells were washed with 5 ml of HBSS added immediately after centrifugation, resuspended in 5 ml of RPMI-1640 containing 10% fetal calf serum (FCS), incubated at room temperature (RT) for 1 minute, and then centrifuged at 100 *g* for 5 minutes. Supernatant was then removed and 5 ml of RPMI-1640 plus 10% FCS was added. After 5 minutes at RT, pelleted cells were gently resuspended and diluted to 5×10^6 cells/ml. These cells were sensitized with the appropriate HLA antisera (i.e., identifying antigens on the normal lymphocytes, but absent on the malignant fusion partner), incubated for 1 hour at 4°C, washed, and rosetted with sterile human red blood cells (RBCs) that had been coated with sterile rabbit anti-human Ig. Rosetted and nonrosetted cells were separated on a Ficoll/diatrizoate density gradient, and pelleted rosetted cells were collected, washed, and seeded into 24-well plates at a concentration of 2×10^6 cells/well. RPMI-1640 with 10% FCS was added to the wells and changed daily until the red cells had completely lysed.

C. Analysis of Immunoglobulin Production

Two hundred μl of affinity-purified anti-human IgG (mg/ml), diluted 1:20 using borate saline buffer (BSB), was added to each well of a 96-well EIA plate and incubated overnight at 4°C. Plates were washed three times with BSB, and excess binding sites were blocked using BSB containing 0.5% gelatin for 1 hour at RT. After three washes with BSB, 0.1 ml of fusion supernatant was added to wells in triplicate and incubated for 1 hour at RT and then washed three times with BSB. Peroxidase-labeled anti-human IgG (0.2 ml) was then added to each well and incubated for 1 hour at RT. After three washes with BSB, 200 μl of substrate solution containing 10 mg O-phenylenediamine, 6 μl of 30% hydrogen peroxide in 10 ml 0.1 M citrate buffer, pH 4.5, was added to each well. The color change was evaluated within 30 minutes.

D. Binding Analysis of Antibody from Putative Clones

The same method used for testing patient serum (Section I.A) was employed except that cell line targets were incubated with doubling dilutions of fusion supernatants concentrated 10-fold using Amicon Minicon concentrators.

E. Immunoperoxidase Staining of Human Tissue

Frozen tissue sections (7 μm), obtained from surgical material, were fixed in acetone for 10 minutes at RT, then washed in 0.05 M tris buffer for 20 minutes. Sections were incubated for 20 minutes with normal goat serum, blotted to remove excess serum, and incubated with affinity-purified anti-mammary carcinoma antibody (obtained from clones) or tris buffer overnight at 4°C in a humid atmosphere to prevent drying. The following day, sections were washed for 10 minutes in tris buffer, incubated for 30 minutes with biotintylated goat anti-human IgG (Vector), washed for 10 minutes in buffer, incubated for 45 minutes in Avidin solution (Vectastain ABC reagent), washed again for 10 minutes in buffer, and incubated for 5 minutes in peroxidase substrate solution (Vector). Sections were then washed with water, counterstained with hematoxylin, and examined microscopically.

F. Karyotypic Analysis

Cells to be karyotyped were washed with HBSS and adjusted in 15-ml tubes to 5×10^5/ml in 10 ml of RPMI-1640 containing 10% FCS. One hundred μl of colcemid (Gibco) was added for 10 minutes at 37°C. Cells were pelleted by centrifugation, and 0.075 M KCl was added dropwise to 1 ml. Cell suspensions were vortexed and an additional 9.0 ml of 0.075 M KCl was added for 30 minutes at RT. After pelleting, KCl solution was removed, and cells were acid-fixed using 3 parts methanol, 1 part glacial acetic acid, added dropwise to a volume of 1 ml. Pellets were vortexed and resuspended in an additional 10 ml of acid-fix-solution for 15-30 minutes at RT. After three washes using acid-fix, chromosomal preparations were made by dropping cell suspension onto slides from a distance of about 1 foot. Chromosome spreads were enumerated microscopically, photographs were taken, and karyotypic analysis was performed by the cytogenetics staff at the Medical University of South Carolina.

G. HLA Typing

HLA typing was done by the tissue typing laboratory at the Medical University of Sourh Carolina.

H. Latex Sensitization

An equal volume of unsensitized Latex, 0.81 μm (Difco, Detroit, MI) was added to purified antibody diluted in glycine-buffered saline (GBS). The solution was mixed and incubated for 1 hour at RT and then centrifuged at 5000 *g* for 10 minutes. The supernatant was decanted, and 2 ml of GBS containing 0.1% bovine serum albumin (BSA) was added. After a final centrifuge step as above, the mixture was resuspended in a volume of GBS with 1.5% BSA.

I. Serum Testing

Ten μl of sensitized Latex and 50 μl serum were added to one well of an agglutination slide. Serum and Latex were mixed at 130 rpm for 15 minutes and read for degree of agglutination.

II. FINDINGS

A. Selection of Patients for Fusion

In order to produce antibody reactive with mammary carcinoma cells, our laboratory chose to use lymphocytes from the peripheral blood of breast cancer patients in remission. Sera from women who were judged to be in remission were tested for the presence of antibodies by binding to a battery of mammary carcinoma cell lines consisting of SW527, MDBMA231, and CAMA. Additional cell lines such as SW620 (colon line), 8402, 8392, and HSB2 (lymphoid lines) were also used to obviate the initial possibility of selecting patients producing abnormally cross-reactive antibodies. For these studies, remission was defined by two criteria: (a) 3 or more years with no evidence of disease, and (b) a history of limited chemotherapy and/or radiation. The intent was to find women who had developed an active immune response against their tumor and whose immune system had not been adversely affected by long-term chemotherapy and/or radiation. Binding of serum antibodies to cell line targets was identified by either indirect immunofluorescence or indirect rosetting. Initial experiments were done using both test procedures, but since essentially parallel responses were observed, and the indirect rosetting procedure was simpler and less expensive, all subsequent screenings were done by indirect rosetting. An example of this rosetting is shown in Figure 1. These indirect rosettes are not subject to Fc receptor binding, and

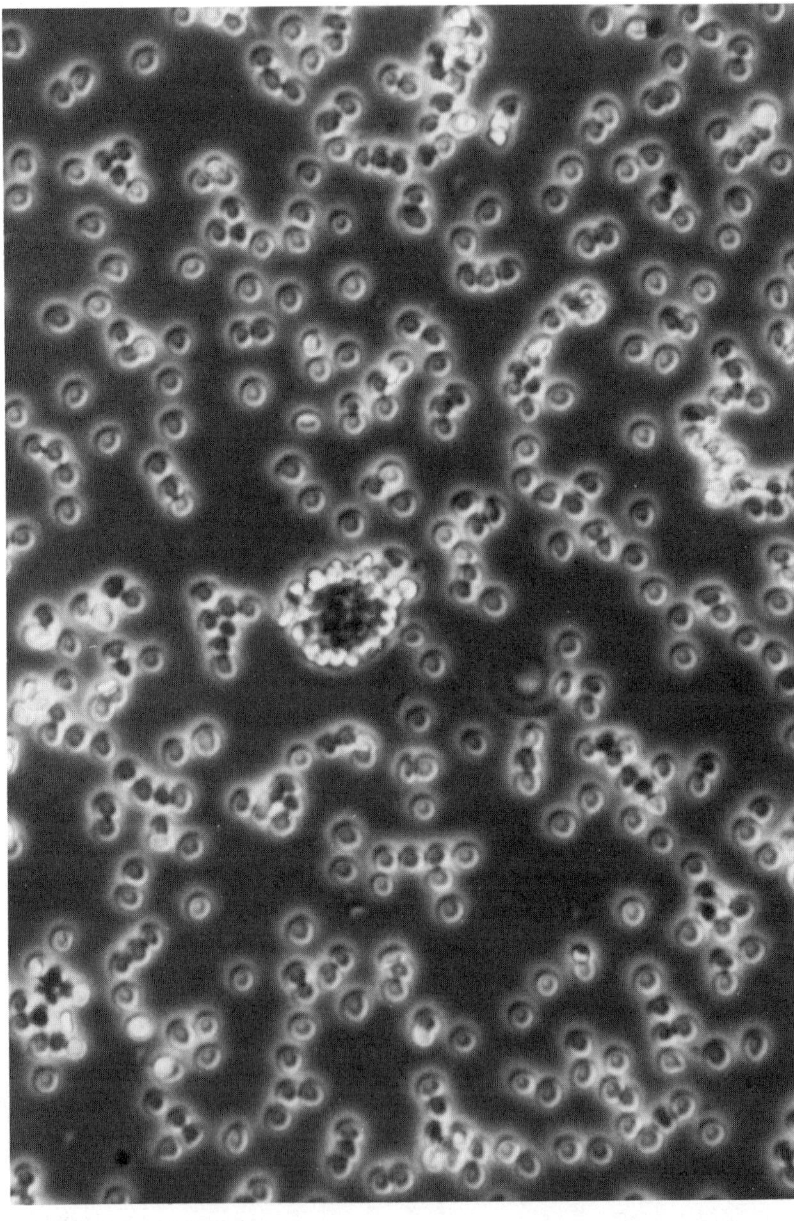

Figure 1 Indirect rosetting of SW527 cells after sensitization with serum from patient J.D. This patient met the criteria listed for fusion donors in that: (a) she was in remission for over 3 years, and (b) she had been exposed to limited chemotherapy or radiation during treatment.

Table 1 Evaluation of Serum Antibody in Recovered Breast Cancer Patients

	% Binding		
Serum dilution	Patient I.R.	Patient J.D.	Patient V.S.
1:2	86	82	76
1:5	87	62	24
1:10	66	31	36
1:50	70	26	38

controls for nonspecific rosetting using unsensitized tumor cells were run with each experiment. Unfortunately, of the 50 patients initially screened, only eight were satisfactory with respect to having apparently specific and potent antibody responses. Of these eight, we selected the three best responders for fusion. They were J.D., I.R., and V.S. (an example of the serum binding of these patients is shown in Table 1). Most of the women we screened were essentially immunodeficient in these binding assays, indicating the severity of deleterious effects resulting from commonly used chemotherapy and/or radiation protocols. It should be emphasized that we feel these preliminary screenings are essential for successful fusion.

B. Fusion

Our fusion procedure differs somewhat from mouse fusions as well as previously described human fusions in that no HAT selection is used. Instead, we developed a technique that takes advantage of "positive selection" of putative hybrid cells through the use of defined antibodies against surface markers associated with the lymphocytes of the patient, but absent on the malignant fusion partner (Fig. 2). This type of selection procedure allows for the use of a wide variety of possible malignant fusion partners. In our opinion, this is one of the most critical facets for the successful construction of human clones since it allows for the selection of a partner which will bring into the system those qualities necessary for effective and stable fusion. We chose Ball-1, a cell line, which was derived from a B cell lymphoma, for several reasons: (a) it contains but does not secrete intracytoplasmic mu and delta immunoglobulins, (b) it grows very well, and (c) it is Epstein-Barr nuclear antigen (EBNA)-negative. The fusion protocol used for lymphocytes from one patient (J.D.) is diagramatically illustrated in Figure 3. As shown, the construction of a stable clone secreting

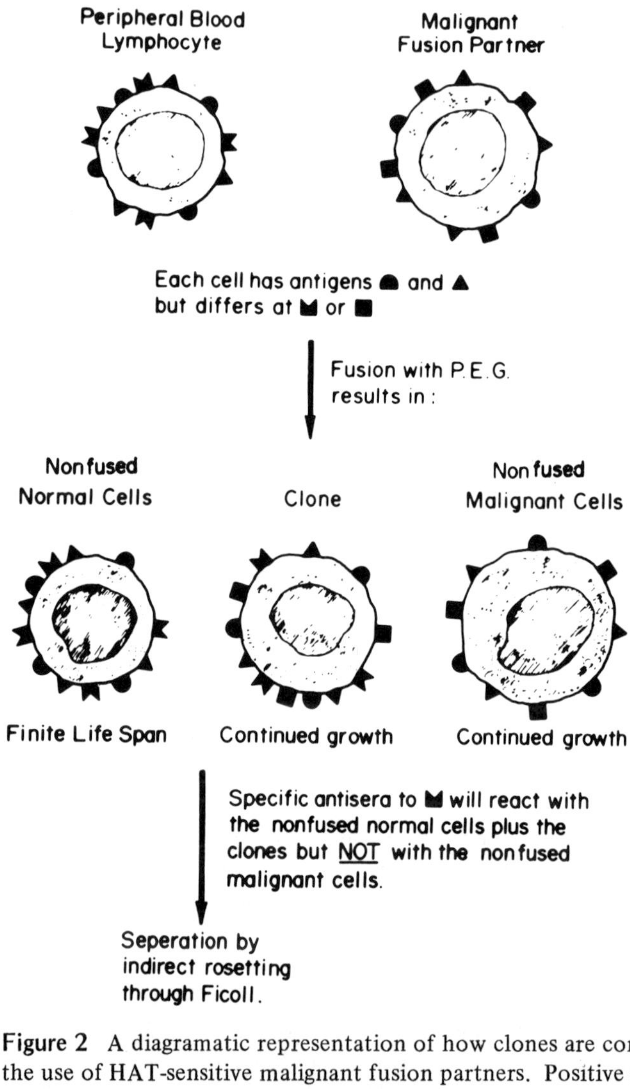

Figure 2 A diagramatic representation of how clones are constructed without the use of HAT-sensitive malignant fusion partners. Positive selection of clones takes advantage of defined antibodies (such as anti-HLA antibodies against surface markers associated with the lymphocytes, but absent on the malignant cells). After fusion, density gradient centrifugation is used to separate normal nonfused cells. Normal nonfused cells have finite life spans and will not survive in culture, thereby leading a purified population of clones.

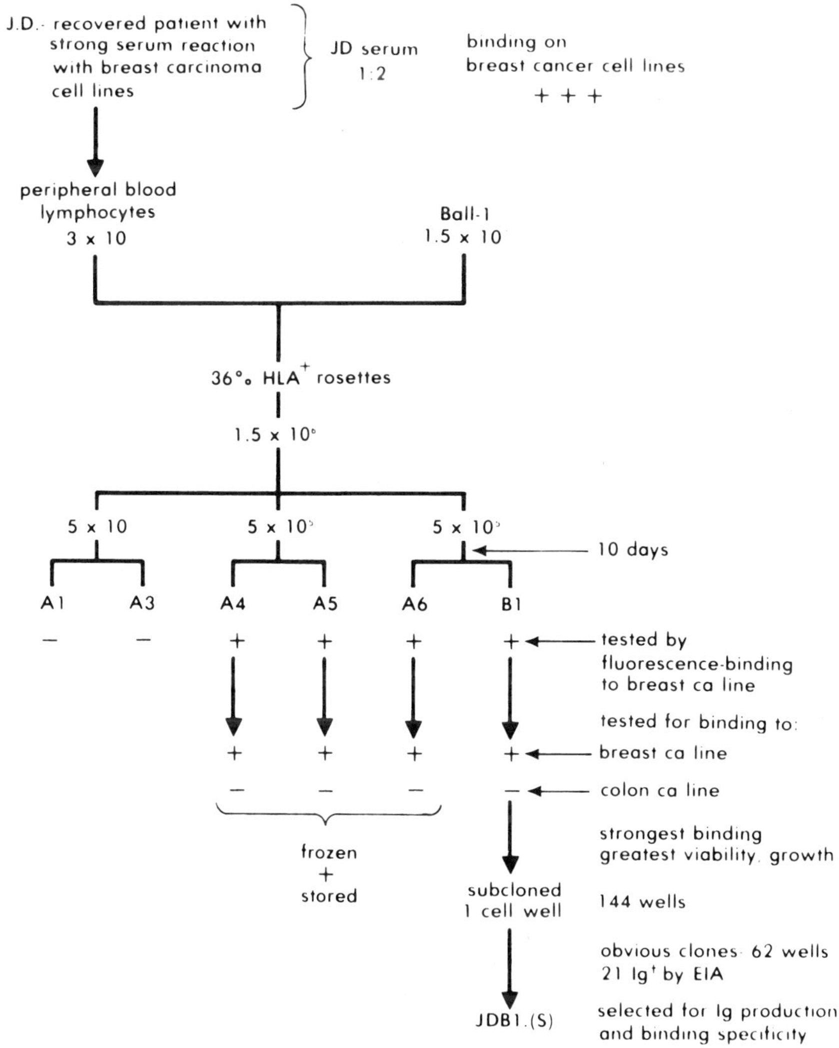

Figure 3 The fusion protocol used to construct JDB1 was followed by "positive selection" of putative clones. Separated clones were partially subcloned at first in order to enhance development of stable clones. This was followed by subcloning to one cell per well and testing for precise specificities.

antibody specific for mammary carcinoma cells involved only partial subclonings at first, in order to define the most vigorous growth before simultaneous testing for Ig production and specificity, again using cell lines. This intermittent and partial subcloning obviously changes the parameters usually used to calculate fusion efficiency. However, when cells from these partially subcloned, positive wells were further subcloned at 1 cell/well, with 144 wells seeded, 62 wells contained obvious clones while only 21 of these produced antibodies reactive with breast cancer cell lines.

C. Specificity JDB1 Antibody

As just noted, we combined identification of immunoglobulin synthesis and specificity of binding in all screening assays. This was extremely helpful in obviating the necessity to rescreen possible clones and limited the loss of time associated with more detailed examination of clones secreting antibody of undefined specificity. This screening was also enhanced by the rapidity of the indirect rosetting assay coupled with the use of cell lines to determine specific binding. The binding characteristics of subclone JDB1 and four other subclones are shown in Table 2. The subclone JDB1S is a subcloned variant of JDB1, which differs in that it grows more rapidly than JDB1 and shows a somewhat different pattern of binding-

Table 2 Reactivity of Human Anti-Mammary Carcinoma Antibody

Cell line	JD Serum	JDA4	JDA5	JDA6	JDB1	JDB1S
SW527 (breast)	2+	3+	3+	2+	2+	3+
MDMBA231 (breast)	1+	1+	–	–	1+	3+
CAMA (breast)	–	3+	1+	3+	3+	–
SW620 (colon)	–	–	–	–	–	–
CCL185 (lung)	–	–	–	–	–	–
HSB2 (lymph)	–	–	–	–	–	NT
8402 (lymph)	–	–	–	–	–	NT
SKW3 (lymph)	–	–	–	–	–	NT
JM (lymph)	–	–	–	–	–	–
L132 (normal fibroblast)	–	–	–	–	–	–
Normal E+	–	–	–	–	–	–

NT = not tested.
– = no binding.

ing. Typical tumor cell linc rosetting, using supernatants of JDB1, does not show contiguous binding of coated red cells as seen when using serum from patients such as J.D., but rather the binding of red cells in these studies can, in some cases, show a more patchlike pattern (Fig. 4). This may be because of continuously occurring modulation of surface antigens seen over time in culture with many cell lines. Support for this possibility comes from the fact that the percentage of positive cells will radically decrease in cases where target cell lines are not properly maintained and viability is allowed to decline.

Because binding to tumor cell lines cannot be relied upon to give unequivocal binding characteristics, JDB1 was also tested for binding to malignant or benigh breast tissue, using an immunoperoxidase staining procedure. JDB1 staining of tissue from a benign breast biopsy shows no staining of normal ductal structures or other areas, although a very slight artifactual background staining of connective tissue is apparent. In contrast, staining of malignant tissue sections with JDB1 shows a diffuse cytoplasmic staining of malignant cells. It should be noted that in some cases, this staining can take on patchlike particulate characteristics, depending on the fixation of tissue and the staining procedures used. Subsequent examination of tissue sections from other malignant breast tumors showed similar staining patterns, while two other normal breast biopsy sections as well as tissue sections from normal adrenal tissue and colorectal carcinoma were completely negative for immunoperoxidase staining with JDB1.

D. Genetic Characteristics of JDB1

The HLA types of the parental cells and the JDB1 hybrid are shown in Table 3. As can be seen, the clone, while conserving determinants of both of the parents (e.g., B35), also expresses some determinants not initially found on the parental cells as in the case of the A loci (A30/33). It should be pointed out that the undetermined X locus found in the J.D. parental type is most likely due to homozygosity at that locus, although a family study would be necessary to positively prove this. Also of interest is the fact that the malignant fusion partner Ball-1, which has been tested on several occasions over the past 3 years in culture, has expressed each of the three A loci antigens indicated in Table 3 at different times, suggesting a transient expression of surface antigens for this cell line.

Most importantly, karyotypic analysis of JDB1 and Ball-1 (Figs. 5a and b) strongly indicate that JDB1 is a hybrid of J.D. and Ball-1 for the following reasons: (a) no Y chromosome is seen in JDB1, even though Ball-1 is XY; (b) two X chromosomes are seen in JDB1 as would be expected since the parental cell J.D. was female; and (c) specific chromosomal differences between Ball-1 and JDB1 can be seen. For example, JDB1 appears to have translocations associated with chromosome number 4, and there are definite differences between the number 6 chromosomes in Ball-1 and those seen in JDB1. Interestingly, there is no clearcut explanation for the excision of some chromosomes and retention of others,

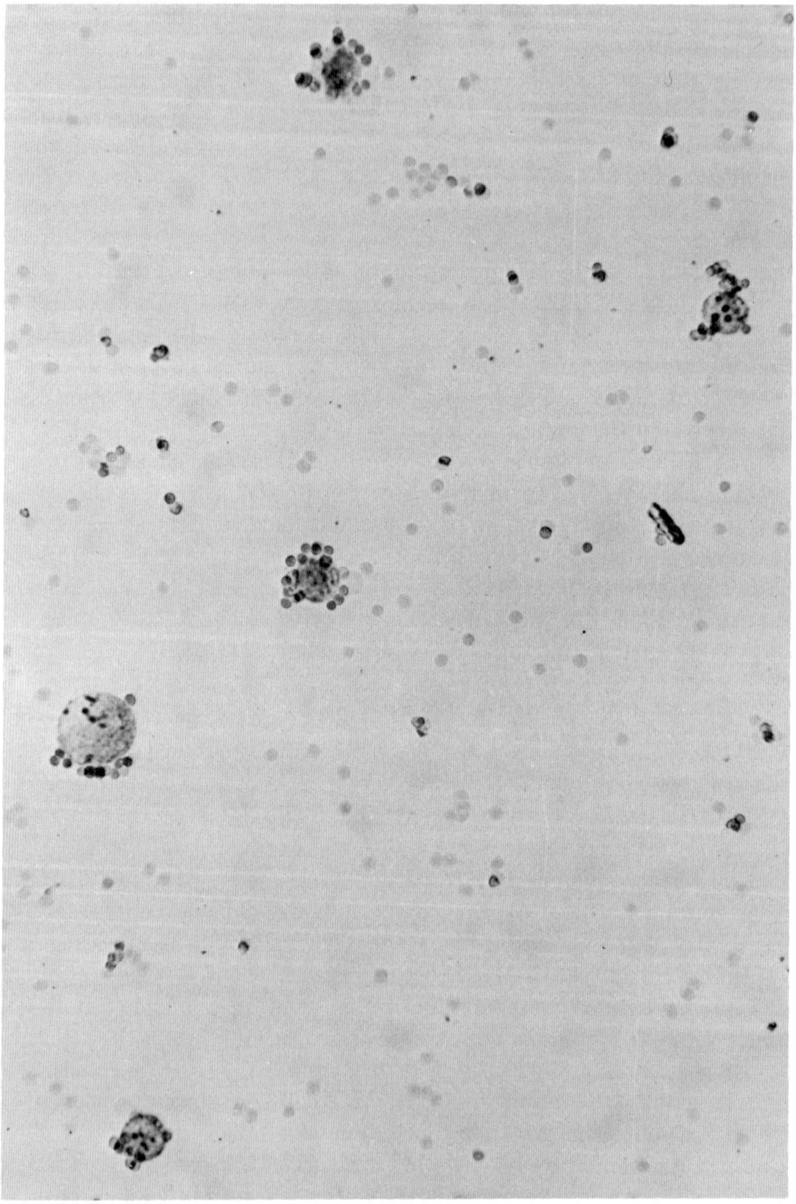

Figure 4 Indirect rosetting of breast carcinoma cells from the SW 527 line shows a patchlike pattern different than that observed when cells are sensitized with serum. SW527 cells were sensitized with supernatants of specific clones as described in Section I.A. Note that binding characteristics can diminish if cells are kept in culture for more than 3 days without transfer or are inadequately maintained.

Table 3 HLA Type of JDB1 and Parental Cells

	Loci			
	A	B	C	D[a]
JD breast cancer patient in remission	A1, X	BS, B35	CW_2CW4	–
Ball-1 (malignant fusion partner)	A3, A24, A31[b]	B51, B35	XXXX	–
JDB1 clone	A24, A30/33	B17/51, B35	XXXX	–

[a]HLA-D typing was not done.
[b]Ball-1 has been tested on several occasions over the past 3 years in culture, and has been positive for each of these loci at different times, indicating that there may be a transient expression of surface HLA antigens over time in culture.

but it is possible that this may be a totally random event. In addition, karyotypic analysis of JDB1, at regular intervals during the first 37 months in culture, has also shown a near normal diploid number of chromosomes in 98% of the cells examined. This number has continued to remain stable up until the present. We believe this chromosomal stability is the cause for the stability demonstrated by JDB1's continued growth in culture over the past 3½ years.

E. Antibody Production of JDB1

One of the more interesting aspects of JDB1 is its pattern of growth and immunoglobulin production. In short, for JDB1: (a) maximum antibody production appears to be correlated with keeping cell numbers at lower levels; (b) there appears to be a cyclical immunoglobulin production pattern, and (c) there are certain media restrictions required for adequate growth of JDB1. With regard to Ig production, when cells are kept at levels no higher than 1×10^6/ml, the average antibody detected by ELISA is approximately 1 μg/ml per 24 hr. The doubling time of JDB1 averages 20-24 hours. It should be pointed out that when cultures are followed daily over a period of several months, fluctuations in both of these parameters can be seen. At times, the cells appear to go into a resting stage where the viability remains constant, but the doubling time slows. These periods can last up to 2 days before rapid division resumes. There is no consistency seen in the pattern of these fluctuations, and their cause is still unclear.

The JDB1 clone produces an IgG/kappa molecule. Experiments using isoelectric focusing with immunoprint fixation have shown there is obvious microheterogeneity of this IgG when using anti-G_1, G_2, G_3, and G_4 antibodies (obtained from Miles Laboratories, Elkhart, IN) in that both IgG_1 and IgG_4 are ap-

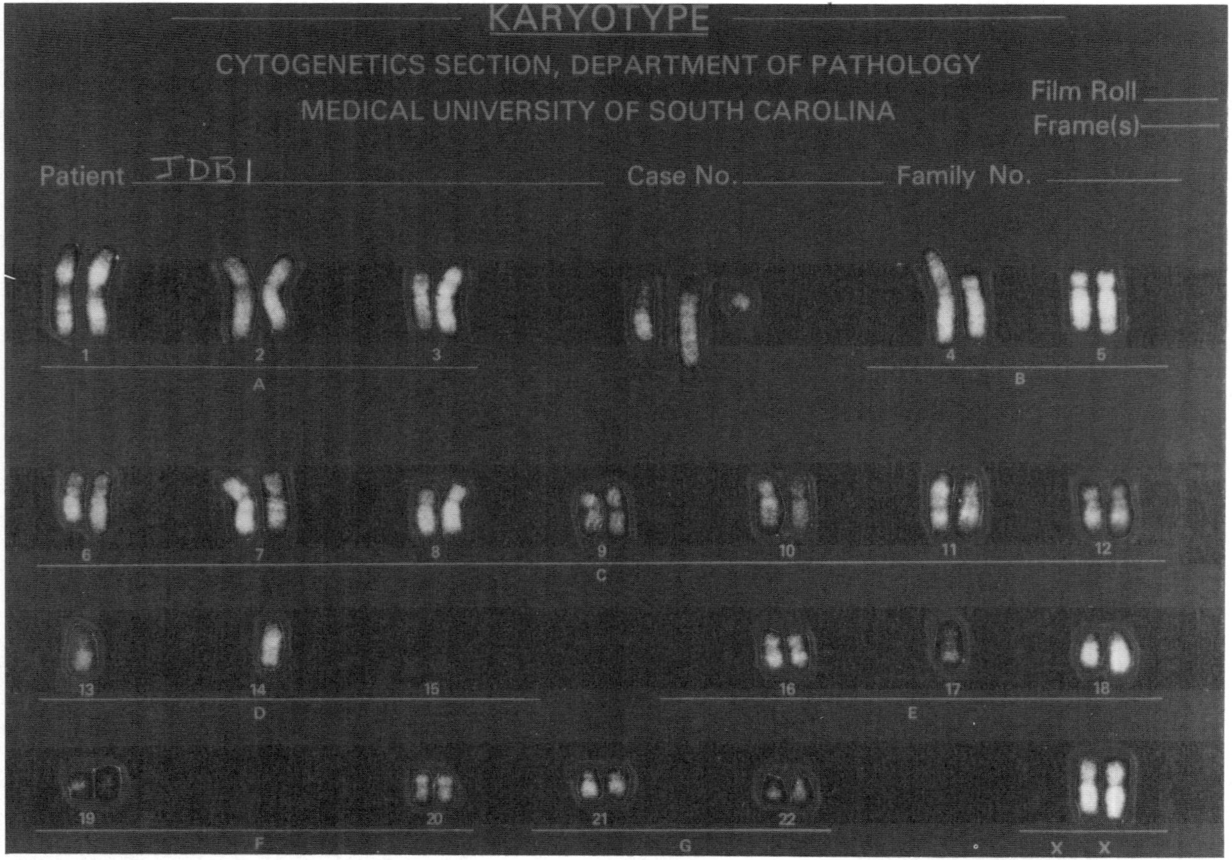

Figure 5 Karyotypic analysis of JDB1 and Ball-1. Cells were prepared after growth in colcemid and fixed as described in Section I.F. (a) Karyotype of JDB1 shows an XX genotype with three abnormal chromosomes that could not be positively identified. In addition, chromosome 15 appears to be missing.

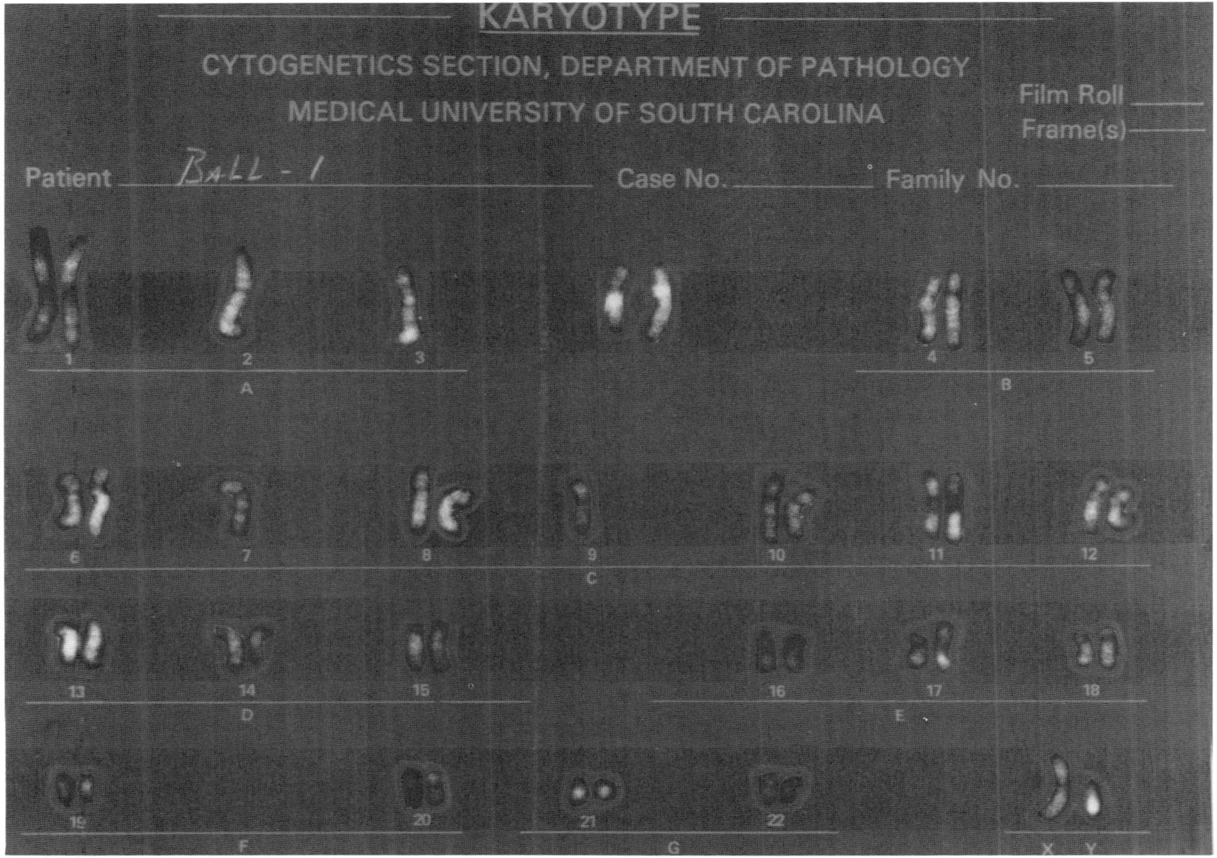

Figure 5 (continued) (b) The karyotype of Ball-1 shows an XY genotype with two unidentifiable chromosomal elements and normal number 15 chromosomes. It should be noted that in almost all JDB1 cells, there appear to be the three abnormal chromosomes, shown here, which probably have resulted from translocations.

parently produced. Interestingly, although Ball-1 is known to produce both mu and delta chains intracytoplasmically, we have been unable to detect secreted IgM in our assay. However, because of the common characteristic of mixed immunoglobulin types secreted by mouse-human clones, it would not be surprising to find a low level of mixed antibody molecules (i.e., part mu and part gamma).

F. Development and Clinical Significance of Breast Cancer-Associated Serum Antigen Testing

1. Serum Testing

Our previous work has shown us that some patients with breast cancer can develop an antibody response against breast cancer cell lines to their tumor, which we have been able to identify by either indirect rosetting or immunofluorescence. Since this binding assay is routinely used to check the specificity of putative anti-mammary carcinoma antibody-producing clones, we felt it would be worthwhile to determine if a serum antigen could also be identified in these patients. It is important to note that many previous attempts to define such an antigen have been only partially successful, and this has lead to the existing theories of complex antigenic heterogeneity believed to be associated with many types of cancer.

Our approach for identification of possible serum antigens was originally based on an inhibition of binding by cloned antibody (JDB1) to the mammary carcinoma cell line SW527. Analysis of serum was originally done to determine the levels of both intrinsic antibody and antigen. It was thought that those patients with high levels of antibody (as determined by the percentage of SW527 cells bound with serum antibody) would be clinically better than those without intrinsic antibody. Coupled with the level of serum antigen present, these data might lead to a more informative picture of the patient's situation and would be a useful monitoring system throughout the course of the patient's disease. As stated, the inhibition assay was based on the degree of inhibition of JDB1 binding to known breast cancer cell lines. Since JDB1 gives a constant and reproducible percentage of binding, the decrease in this percentage can be utilized on an arbitrary scale to identify the level of serum antigen present. This inhibition assay for antigen analysis, although reliable, was time-consuming and somewhat expensive. Consequently, we adapted the JDB1 antibody to a rapid Latex slide agglutination test for serum antigen. This new test system requires only 15 minutes to do and is easily read with the naked eye. It is also extremely inexpensive and requires only 50 μl of patients serum.

2. Blind Studies

Through the cooperation of the Northwest Oncology Clinic in Seattle, we have tested serum samples from patients with breast cancer, other forms of cancer, and normal controls for the presence of serum antigen. Each sample is tested in a blind fashion in which only the patient name appears on the sample. After determining the antigen and antibody levels, we examined the medical records of each patient tested to evaluate the clinical status at the time serum was taken. The physician is then called and given the results of these tests. In Table 4, we have summarized the findings of serum antigen analysis in 402 individuals. It can be seen that of the 215 breast cancer patients, 175 showed no clinical evidence of disease. Of these individuals, 9% were positive in our assay. In our experience, these individuals are good candidates for imminent relapse. Of the women who had clinically identifiable metastasis, 88% were positive by our assay. In addition, 18 of the 162 controls and patients with other forms of cancer were +/- to 1+ positive in our Latex test. Only one of these was a normal control woman, while two had mammary dysplasia secondary to melanoma. We have also found that our assay system can show positive results with a percentage of women who have severe fibrocystic disease (Table 4). This is certainly of interest because it has been postulated that this condition may be a predecessor to the onset of mammary carcinoma. Alternatively, any disease that disrupts the normal breast may expose antigens to which antibody may develop. In a second series of experiments, 91 blind samples were obtained from San Diego, California. Of these, 37 were controls (i.e., individuals without cancer or patients with other forms of cancer). It was found that three (8%) of the 37 controls were positive (though none were normal controls). The 54 samples from breast cancer patients were divided into four groups based only on the antigen levels seen. After testing, the clinical course of each of these 54 patients was determined (Table 5). This separate study also supported the possibility that we may be able to use this rapid assay as a valuable tool for monitoring patients over the course of their disease. This would be of great value to oncologists who until now have had little available to them in this regard. Our enthusiasm is greatly increased by the data illustrated in Table 6, which illustrates preliminary findings of longitudinal studies we have begun on six patients. Although many of these patients have maintained high levels of antigen, two have shown striking results. Patients M.B. and L.F. were found to be positive for antigen 10 and 5 months, respectively, prior to the identification of clinical disease activity. In addition, analysis of the serum antigen in patient L.L. closely followed the disease activity pattern, going from positive to negative as the patient went into apparent remission. The predictive and/or monitoring capability of this assay certainly can not be confirmed on the basis of the small number of longitudinal tests we have done so far. We are encouraged by these results and by the fact that our computerized data base now comprises nearly 500 patients, many of whom have been followed repeatedly.

III. CONCLUSIONS

The future utility of human monoclonal antibodies is hypothetically obvious. For the diagnosis of many diseases, human monoclonal antibodies may prove to be even

Table 4 Results of Blind Serum Antigen Assays

Serum samples from Seattle

Total	402
Breast cancer	215
Controls (nonbreast cancer)	162
Fibrocystic disease	25

Controls (total = 162)

144 negative (24 normal, 84 colon, 3 inflammatory breast cancer, 8 ovarian, 8 melanoma, 1 prostate, 2 thyroid, 7 endometrial, 3 testicular, 3 lung, 1 bile duct cancer)

18 positive (1 normal, 1 lung, 3 ovarian, 2 melanoma with mammary dysplasia, 1 thyroid, 10 colon)

Breast cancers

	(-)	(1+)	(2+)	(3+)
175 with no evidence of disease	159 (91%)	7	5	4 (9%)[a]
40 with mestatic disease	5 (12%)[b]	13	10	12 (88%)

Fibrocystics

16-negative

4-1+ agglutination

4-2+ agglutination

1-3+ agglutination

[a]9% putatively false-positive, but these patients may have active disease not yet identified.
[b]12% of patients in this group are false-negatives.

more sensitive than their murine counterparts, while therapeutic modalities using purified populations of these human molecules should theoretically have very few, if any, deleterious side-effects. Unfortunately, this utility has yet to be established. This is primarily due to the difficulties associated with constructing and maintaining stable human hybrids, and the disappointingly low levels of specific immunoglobulin many human clones produce in culture (24).

The experiments described here involve one of many hybrids we have produced using alternative methods for the construction of human clones. The JDB1 clone has been stable in continuous culture for approximately 3 years. It is a karyotypically identifiable genetic hybrid, producing approximately 1 μg/ml of

Table 5 Synopsis of Antigen Level and Clinical Course in Breast Cancer

Antigen levels (latex)	No. of patients	Clinical course
None (-)	20	19 apparently disease-free
		1 bone metastases
Low (+/-)	6	4 apparently disease-free
		1 bone metastases
		1 abnormal bone scan (possible disease)
Medium (1+ to 2+)	22	19 local recurrence or metastases
		3 no discernible metastases
High (3+)	6	6 extensive disease with metastases

antibody, which is very reactive with mammary carcinoma cells. This antibody is an IgG/kappa molecule which shows definite microheterogeneity by isoelectric focusing coupled with print fixation. In addition, in experiments not described here, we have found that this antibody will readily lend itself to the killing of mammary carcinoma cell line targets in ADCC assays using human peripheral blood lymphocytes as effector cells.

JDB1 antibody shows a definite and specific staining with malignant breast tissue, but no apparent cross-reactivity with benign breast tissue and no staining of other tumor or normal tissue. This is in partial contrast to the studies of others in the area of breast cancer. For instance, Schlom *et al.* (25) constructed a murine-human clone by fusion of NS-1 with lymphocytes from the draining lymph nodes of patients with breast cancer. However, in addition to an apparent cross-reactivity demonstrated by these antibodies, the clones were also highly unstable. In more recent work (26), this group has described a murine monoclonal which is apparently much more specific. In these recent studies, they showed that this monoclonal has little or no cross-reactivity with benign fibroid tissue. In studies using JDB1 to detect breast tumor serum antigens, we found that serum from women with severe fibrocystic disease but no clinically defined malignant disease can give us positive results. Studies are under way to determine the extent of this cross-reactivity with some fibroid tissue. Other investigators (14), using human-human fusion procedures, have also constructed clones producing antibodies reactive with breast cancer tissue using the fusion partners LICR-LON-HMy2 or SKO-007; however, these attempts were also unsuccessful with respect to specificity in that some of their clones were found to produce antibody which cross-reacted with human peripheral blood mononuclear cells. Interestingly, these

Table 6 Longitudinal Studies of Breast Cancer Patients

Patient	Group	Date	Ag	Ab (%)	Clinical data
M.B.	2	9/83	1+	13	NED
	12	6/84	2+	32	Relapse operative site
	17	7/84	-	38	After radiation
	23	10/84	2+	6	Advancing disease
B.T.	23	10/84	2+	22	Bone mets.
	25	11/84	1+	30	Bone mets.
	28	12/84	2++	72	Bone mets.
	30	1/85	2+	88	Bone mets.
	34	2/85	2+	8	Bone mets.
	36	3/85	2+	36	Bone mets.
	39	4/85	2+	28	Bone mets.
	43	5/85	1+	72	Bone and liver mets.
	44	5/85	3+	20	Expired due to liver failure
L.L.	20	9/84	1+	18	Bone mets.
	22	10/84	1+	14	Completion of radiation
	24	11/84	-	12	NED
	31	1/85	-	18	NED
	34	2/85	-	18	NED
	43	5/85	-	46	NED
M.S.	5	4/84	3+	40	Extensive bone mets.
	9	5/84	3+	20	Extensive bone mets.
	19	9/84	3++	42	Extensive bone mets.
	20	9/84	3++	38	Extensive bone mets.
	23	10/84	3++	66	Extensive bone mets.
	25	11/84	3++	18	Extensive bone mets.
	29	12/84	4++	N/A	Extensive bone mets.
		2/85	3++	52	More progressive bone mets.
	38	3/85	3+	50	Bone mets. and lymph node mets.
	38	4/85	3+	50	Bone mets. and lymph node mets.
	43	5/85	3+	42	Bone mets. and lymph node mets.

Table 6 (continued)

Patient	Group	Date	Ag	Ab (%)	Clinical data
R.P.	9	5/84	3++	38	NED
	10	6/84	2+	20	NED but pain
	13	6/84	1+	18	NED but pain
	15	8/84	1+	30	NED but pain
	19	9/84	2++	50	NED but pain
	21	10/84	1+	12	NED pain in thorax and scapula
	22	11/84	1+	16	CT scan shows brain mets.
	23	12/84	1+	16	Expired
A.F.	10	5/84	-	8	NED
	20	9/84	-	8	NED
	28	12/84	-	8	NED
	35	3/85	-	10	NED
	47	6/85	-	18	Remission NED

Mets. = metastases.
NED = no evidence of disease.

authors have apparently constructed what appear to be fairly stable clones, although they indicate that this stability may be predicated on vigorous and repeated subcloning. In other recent studies (27), mouse-human hybrids were constructed using lymphocytes from the lymph nodes of breast cancer patients and the murine myeloma cell line SP2/OAg. A total of 81 human Ig-producing clones were derived from 595 wells. Seventy-two clones produced IgG, and 15 of these were apparently operationally specific for breast carcinoma cells. There was also apparent variable reactivity with malignant epithelial cells from colon and stomach carcinoma patients. Perhaps most importantly, these clones have reportedly been in stable culture for 2 years. This long-term stability is in direct contrast to the majority of reports on cross-species hybrids. It will be important to determine possible differences in technology used by these investigators that may explain their enhanced stability. Unfortunately, no information as to the genetic characteristics of these stable mouse-human clones was given in this report.

The clone we have described here has been in stable culture for approximately 3 years. This stability may be due to the near diploid number of chromosomes found in over 98% of the cells. This chromosomal analysis also strongly suggests that these cells are hybrids of two parents since the nonmalignant parent is female, the malignant parent is male, and the clone is karyotypically XX. These chromosomal characteristics help to support the hybrid nature of this clone and, taken together with the fact that these clones exhibit diploid numbers of chromosomes, indicate that genetic rearrangements such as translocations have probably taken place. This type of rearrangement, although probably required for the establishment of stable long-term clones, must for now be considered to be a totally random event. Visual analysis of chromosomes during karyotyping of JDB1 suggests there may be minor difference in the length of the long arms of chromosome 14, but more precise analysis is necessary to be positive that this difference exists. A detailed genetic study of the chromosomes of JDB1 is currently under way.

During early attempts at construction of human clones, it was felt, and with good reason, that fusion using human peripheral blood lymphocytes would not be effective due to the low number of peripheral blood cells making the appropriate antibody. For this reason, some investigators (23-25) have chosen to use infection with EBV to increase the size of this antibody-secreting population and, therefore, more easily obtain clones of specific antibody secreting cells. Our data conflict with these observations in that we have used peripheral blood lymphocytes to produce many different types of clones with reasonable success. We feel the major reason for this difference is the stringent prefusion selection process we use. Because the serum of the recovered patient is thoroughly tested before their lymphocytes are used for fusion, we feel that we increase the chances of obtaining a successful clone. An additional asset is the use of our modified approach to clonal construction, which may allow vigorous and stable clones to be produced. This may be important because the inherent instability seen in many human clones may be the result of using malignant partners made more unstable through their mutation (i.e., to 8-azoguanine resistance or ouabain sensitivity). Lastly, the indirect rosetting procedure we have adopted may allow for more sensitive identification of antibody binding; consequently, these methodological differences may allow us to identify clones that might go unnoticed using standard procedures. Perhaps the major problem associated with JDB1 is that of the small amounts of antibody produced. Though the level of production has remained at approximately 1 μg/ml for several years, this is disappointingly low when compared with levels seen with murine systems. Attempts to increase these levels through serial transfection experiments have been initially successful and are being continued in our laboratory (see Part I, Chapter 7 of this volume).

Studies aimed at identification of the antigen recognized by JDB1 are also beginning in our laboratory, but as yet have given no clear-cut results. Interestingly, we have found that JDB1 will specifically identify a serum antigen in women with metastatic breast cancer, which can not be found in serum from most normal control women or women in remission with no evidence of disease. Clearly, one of the more important aspects of this work is the capability to monitor patients and, thus, predict the onset of relapse. We have tested more than 1200 samples, many of which have come from the same patients, and it has allowed us to build up a significant longitudinal study population. All of the clinical and experimental information has been placed on computer for easy access and more precise statistical evaluation. We feel confident that this test system is far superior to any test currently available for monitoring breast cancer patients. Another area of great interest is imaging and therapy, and we are currently engaged in a joint venture in which we are examining the utility of these antibodies for these purposes.

REFERENCES

1. K. Nilsson, H. Bennich, S. G. O. Johannsson, and J. Ponten. Established immunoglobulin producing myeloma (IgE). *Clin. Exp. Immunol., 7*:477 (1970).
2. Y. Matsuoka, G. E. Moore, Y. Uagi, and D. Pressman. Production of free light chains of immunoglobulin by a hematopoietic cell line derived from a patient with multiple myeloma. *Exp. Biol. NY, 125*:1246 (1967).
3. A. Karpas, P. Fischer, and D. Swirsky. Human myeloma cell line carrying a Philadelphia chromosome. *Science, 216*:997 (1982).
4. A. Togawa, N. Inoue, K. Myamoto, H. Hyodo, and M. Namba. Establishment and characterization of a human myeloma cell line. *Int. J. Cancer, 29*: 495 (1982).
5. P. A. W. Edwards, C. M. Smith, A. M. Neville, and M. J. O'Hare. A human/human hybridoma system based on a fast growing mutant of the ARH-77 plasma cell leukemia derived line. *Eur. J. Immunol., 12*:641 (1982).
6. L. K. Everson, B. M. Buell, and G. M. Rogentine. Separation of human lymphoid cells into G, S, and G cell cycle populations by use of velocity sedimentation techniques. *J. Exp. Med., 137*:343 (1973).
7. C. M. Croce, A. Linnenbach, W. Hall, Z. Steplewski, and H. Koprowski. Production of human hybridomas secreting antibodies to measles virus. *Nature, 288*:488 (1980).
8. L. Olsson and H. S. Kaplan. Human/human hybridomas producing monoclonal antibodies of predefined antigenic specificity. *Proc. Natl. Acad. Sci. (USA*), *77*:5129 (1980).
9. Y. Schoenfeld, S. Hsu-Lin, J. Gabriels, L. Silverstein, B. C. Furie, B. Furie, B. Stollar, and R. Schwartz. Production of autoantibodies by human/human hybridomas. *J. Clin. Invest., 70*:205 (1982).
10. Y. Schoenfeld, J. Rauch, H. Massicotte, S. Datta, J. Schwartz, D. Stollar, and R. S. Schwartz. Polyspecificity of monoclonal lupus autoantibodies produced by human/human hybridomas. *N. Engl. J. Med., 308*:414 (1983).

11. N. Chiorazzi, R. L. Wasserman, and H. G. Kunkel. Use of Epstein-Barr virus transformed B cell lines for the generation of immunoglobulin-producing human B cell hybridomas. *J. Exp. Med., 156*:930 (1982).
12. G. S. Eisenbarth, A. Linnenbach, R. Jackson, R. Scearce, and C. M. Croce. Human hybridomas secreting anti-islet antibodies. *Nature, 300*:264 (1982).
13. A. M. Houghton, H. Brooks, R. J. Cote, M. C. Taormina, H. F. Oettgen, and L. J. Old. Detection of cell surface of intracellular antigens by human monoclonal antibodies: hybrid cell lines derived from lymphocytes of patients with malignant melanoma. *J. Exp. Med., 158*:52 (1983).
14. R. J. Cote, D. M. Morrissey, A. M. Houghton, E. J. Beattie, Jr., H. F. Oettgen, and L. J. Old. Generation of human monoclonal antibodies reactive with cellular antigens. *Proc. Natl. Acad. Sci. (USA), 80*:2026 (1983).
15. K. Sikora, T. Alderton, J. Phillips and J. Waton. Human hybridomas from malignant gliomas. *Lancet i*:11 (1982).
16. H. Handley, I. Royston, and M. C. Glassy. The production of human monoclonal antibodies to human tumor associated antigens. In J. W. Parker and R. L. O'Brien (eds.). *Proceedings of the 15th International Leucocyte Conference.* John Wiley & Sons, New York (1983).
17. M. C. Glassy, H. W. Handley, I. Royston, and D. J. Lowe. Human monoclonal antibodies to human cancers. In B. D. Boss, R. Langman, I. S. Trowbridge, R. Dulbecco (eds.). *Proceedings of the 4th Armand Hammer Cancer Symposium.* Academic Press, New York (1983).
18. M. V. Haspel, R. P. McCabe, N. Pomato, M. J. Jenesch, J. V. Knowlton, L. C. Peters, H. Hoover, and M. G. Hanna. Generation of tumor cell reactive human monoclonal antibodies using peripheral blood lymphocytes from actively immunized colorectal carcinoma patients. *Cancer Res., 34*:3951 (1985).
19. R. F. Irie, L. L. Sze, and R. E. Saxton. Human antibody to OFA-7, a tumor antigen produced *in vitro* by Epstein-Barr virus-transformed human B-lymphoid cell lines. *Proc. Natl. Acad. Sci. (USA), 79*:5666 (1982).
20. J. W. Larrick, K. E. Truitt, A. A. Rabbitschek, G. S. Senyk, and J. C. N. Wang. Characterization of human hybridomas secreting antibody to tetanus toxoid. *Proc. Natl. Acad. Sci. (USA), 80*:6376 (1983).
21. D. Kozbor and J. Roder. Requirements for the establishment of high titered human monoclonal antibodies against tetanus toxoid using the Epstein-Barr virus technique. *J. Immunol., 127*:1275 (1981).
22. D. Kozbor, M. Steinitz, G. Klein, S. Koskimies, and O. Makela. Establishment of anti-TNP antibody-producing human lymphoid lines by preselection for hapten binding followed by EBV transformation. *Scand. J. Immunol., 10*: 187 (1979).
23. D. Kozbor, A. E. Lagarde, and J. C. Roder. Human hybridomas constructed with antigen-specific EBV transformed lines. *Proc. Natl. Acad. Sci. (USA), 79*:6651 (1982).
24. A. J. Strelkauskas and C. L. Taylor. Human hybridomas. The road to the future. In J. J. Marchalonis (ed.). *Lymphocyte Structure and Function.* Marcel Dekker, New York (1986).

25. J. Schlom, D. Wunderlich, and Y. A. Teramoto. Generation of monoclonal antibodies reactive with human mammary carcinoma cells. *Proc. Natl. Acad. Sci. (USA)*, *77*:6841 (1980).
26. D. Kufe, G. Inghirami, M. Abe, D. Hayes, H. Justi-Wheller, and J. Schlom. Differential reactivity of a novel monoclonal antibody (DF3) with human malignant versus benign breast tumors. *Hybridoma, 3*:223 (1984).
27. A. Imam, M. M. Drushella, C. R. Taylor, and Z. Tokes. Generation and immunohistological characterization of human monoclonal antibodies to mammary carcinoma cells. *Cancer Res.*, *45*:263 (1985).

13

Radiolabeled Human Antibodies That Localize Breast Cancer *In Vivo*

Selecting antibodies for clinical applications

KAREN G. BURNETT, JOAN M. HAYDEN, RACHEL HERNANDEZ, KATHLEEN M. WALDRON, NICKI J. McROBERTS, and ESTHER H. OH
Hybritech Incorporated, San Diego, California

Since the earliest reports on the production of human monoclonal antibodies (1,2), investigators have discussed the potential superiority of these reagents as *in vivo* pharmaceuticals. Several clinical investigators have confirmed that multiple administrations of a mouse monoclonal antibody will elicit a significant immune response in many human patients. This anti-mouse immunoglobulin (Ig) response reduces the efficacy of subsequent antibody treatment (3-5). It is reasonable to suggest that a human monoclonal antibody might be less immunogenic in humans. However, there are many technical limitations to the production of human antibodies. To our knowledge, only two groups have performed *in vivo* clinical studies with human monoclonal antibodies. In one report, Phillips *et al.* (6) demonstrated localization of an ^{131}iodine-labeled human IgG anti-glioma antibody in tumor cysts of a patient with recurrent glioma. More recently, one of us in association with investigators at the University of California at San Diego and at Davis (7,8) described *in vivo* biodistribution of three ^{111}indium-labeled human IgM anti-breast antibodies in mice and humans. Two of the three antibodies imaged tumor lesions in breast cancer patients.

Our laboratory has previously published descriptions of the anti-breast carcinoma antibodies used in the clinical studies at the University of California at Davis and at San Diego (9). In this chapter we provide a retrospective view of the production and characterization of these antibodies. In light of clinical experiences, we present a revised set of *in vitro* and *in vivo* criteria that should be used to select human antibodies for tumor localization studies in patients.

I. METHODS

A. Fusions

Antibodies were produced using lymphocytes obtained from regional axillary nodes of patients with breast carcinoma. Lymphocytes were teased from freshly resected lymph nodes obtained less than 24 hours after surgery, then frozen at -70°C in RPMI-1640 with 50% fetal calf serum (FCS) and 10% dimethyl sulfoxide (DMSO). Eighteen hours prior to fusion, lymphocytes were thawed and cultured in RPMI-1640 with 10% FCS.

The myeloma fusion partner was a subline of the mouse myeloma cell line P3x63Ag8.653 (10). In our experience this subline, designated P3/HT, is superior to most existing human and mouse lymphoid lines for routine production of clinically useful human monoclonal antibodies (11). P3/HT does not produce any detectable level of mouse Ig heavy or light chains. Also critical to production of clinical grade monoclonal antibodies, P3/HT is not infected with Epstein-Barr virus (EBV) or mycoplasma. Lymphocytes were thawed 18 hours before use and cultured in RPMI-1640 with 10% FCS.

P3/HT was fused to lymph node lymphocytes by the method of Gerhard (12) with fusion medium containing 35% polyethylene glycol (PEG) 1000 and 7.5% DMSO. Myeloma to lymphocyte ratios were varied from 6:1 to 1:1. After fusion, the cell mix was immediately resuspended in hypoxanthine/aminopterin/thymidine (HAT)-selective medium (13) and seeded at 10^5 cells/well into 96-well microtiter dishes. Culture medium routinely was supplemented with a feeder layer (10^4 cells/well) of mouse peritoneal macrophages or 10% conditioned medium. To develop conditioned medium, mouse peritoneal macrophages were stimulated *in vivo* with thioglycolate for 72 hours, then removed and cultured *in vitro* for 24 hours at 10^6 cells/ml. Spent culture supernatants were frozen at -20°C for future use.

B. Screens

1. Human Immunoglobulin

Three to 5 weeks after fusion, culture supernatants from growing hybrids were assayed for the presence of human IgG, IgM, and IgA. Goat anti-human Ig subclass-specific polyclonal antibody was dried onto Linbro plates overnight at 37°C. Test supernatants were incubated in coated wells for 1 hour, and bound antibody was detected by an enzyme-linked immunosorbent assay (ELISA) with horseradish peroxidase (HRP)-conjugated second antibody and orthophenylinediamine (OPD) substrate. Color development was measured by absorbance at 490 nm, and these values were plotted against a standard curve generated with purified polyclonal human Ig of the relevant subclass to quantitate antibody in the culture supernatants.

2. Cell Surface ELISA

Target cells were grown in stationary flasks, trypsinized and transferred to 96-well microtiter dishes. Seeded cells were allowed to adhere overnight under standard culture conditions, then fixed with 0.25% glutaraldehyde and stored at 4°C no longer than 2 months before use. Immediately prior to specific assay, target cells were washed with 5% horse serum in phosphate-buffered saline (PBS) and used in a standard ELISA.

3. Membrane and Cytosol ELISA

Membrane and cytosol fractions were isolated from human tumor cell lines grown in athymic mice or fresh frozen human tissues. Frozen tissue was grated into small pieces and then homogenized in 10 mM tris-HCl, pH 7.5; 2 mM $CaCl_2$; and 2 mM phenylmethylsulfonyl fluoride (PMSF). After a 1000 *g* low-speed spin, the crude tissue preparation was centrifuged 1 hour at 100,000 *g*. Supernatant was retained as the tissue cytosol fraction. The 100,000 *g* pellet was redissolved in homogenization buffer and layered over a 40%/20% discontinuous sucrose gradient.

After a 17 hour, 130,000 *g* spin, the 40%/20% interphase was removed, pelleted in homogenization buffer, and retained as the tissue membrane fraction. Selected human tissue cytosol preparations were depleted of endogenous Ig by passage over a column of goat anti-human Ig-coupled sepharose. Tissue fractions were frozen at -70°C until ready for use. For specific assay, membranes and cytosols were thawed, plated at 2 or 10 μg/well into Linbro dishes, and dried overnight at 37°C. Plates were then precoated with 10% horse serum in PBS and used in an ELISA. All specific binding assays on whole cells, membranes, or cytosols included both negative and positive controls. Positive controls were monitored to routinely give O.D. (490 nm) values of 1.0-2.0 as a basis on which to normalize among individual ELISAs.

II. RESULTS

A. Clone Production

Fusion frequency was closely tied to the viability and activation state of the lymph node lymphocytes at the time of fusion. Important parameters affecting viability and activation state were the extent of node schlerosis, age and immune status of the patient, and time since surgical removal of the node. As an extreme example, autopsy lymph nodes, however rapidly obtained, were poor lymphocyte sources. Therefore, clone production varied widely among different lymphocyte preparations. With 27 breast lymph nodes used in 63 identical fusion protocols, fusion frequency varied from 3.0×10^{-5} to less than 3.3×10^{-8}. However, 63% of the fusions yielded 1-10 hybridomas per million lymphocytes (fusion frequency 10^{-5}-10^{-6}).

B. Immunoglobulin Isotypes

Due to the large size and short serum half-life of IgM molecules, we wanted to obtain IgG human monoclonal antibodies for *in vivo* clinical applications. In 18 fusions with breast lymph nodes from 15 donors, a total of 628 hybridomas were screened for production of human IgG, IgM, and IgA. Forty-one percent of hybridomas secreted more than 0.1 μg/ml of human immunoglobulin. Relative frequencies of IgG-, IgM-, and IgA-secreting hybridomas were 31, 32, and 38%, respectively. This Ig distribution data indicated that hybridomas of P3/HT with human lymph node lymphocytes yielded large numbers of antibodies of all three isotypes to assess for anti-tumor reactivity.

C. Specific Reactivity

Lymph node lymphocytes of 59 breast cancer patients used in 104 fusions generated a total of 4642 hybridomas. Ig-secreting hybridomas were screened for reactivity against breast cancer in one of the following assays: (a) cell surface ELISA, (b) ELISA on membranes and cytosols of human tumor xenografts grown in athymic mice (here to be called nude mouse ELISA), and (c) ELISA on membranes and cytosols of human breast tumor tissues. In preliminary studies, we also examined the solid phase immunoisolation technique (14) and Cleveland assay (15) as alternatives to these ELISAs. However, in our experience, these two assays were unacceptable for routine screening procedures, as the latter frequently gave high background signals and the former was both relatively insensitive and limited to antigens that could be iodinated.

To assess specific reactivity with breast cancer, the hybridomas were initially assayed in one of the three screening formats just described. For cell surface ELISA, breast carcinoma targets were cell lines T47D, MCF-7, BT20, ZR75-1, and/or H925. For nude mouse tumor ELISA, the breast carcinoma targets were membranes and cytosols of Clouser, T417, and T386 breast cell lines. For human tissue ELISA, the breast carcinoma targets were membranes and cytosols from pools of three fresh frozen tumors. In the course of these studies, two separate pools were used. "Initial specific positives" were those hybridomas scoring greater than 20% of the standard positive control value in two assay runs on the same target tissue.

All three assay systems indicated that 1-3% of hybridomas produced with human draining lymph node lymphocytes secreted a human Ig which bound breast carcinoma (Table 1). Very few IgG antibodies were identified as initial specific positives. However, among the assays used in these studies, the membrane and cytosol ELISA on human tissues was least effective in identifying such IgG initial specific positive antibodies.

The initial specific positives identified from fusions with breast cancer lymph

Table 1 Identification of Human Antibodies Reactive with Breast Carcinoma

Assay system	Human breast cancer target tissue	Clones produced (no.)	Specific positives (no.)	Specific positives total clones (%)	IgG-specific positives[a] (no.)	IgG-specific positives[a] of total specific positives (%)
Cell surface ELISA	Cell lines T47D, ZR75-1, MCG-7, BT20, H925	1830	43	2.3	2	4.7
Membrane and cytosol ELISA	Nude mouse xenografts: Clouser, T386, T417	215	3	1.4	0	0
Membrane and cytosol ELISA	Pool of three human tumors	1237	20	1.6	0	0
Membrane and cytosol ELISA	IgM-nude mouse xenografts, IgG-, IgA-human tumors	998	31	3.1	2	6.5

[a]Specific positives = antibodies with ELISA reactivity greater than 20% of the positive control value on one or more target breast carcinoma tissues.

node lymphocytes bound a variety of target antigens, as suggested by the assay techniques used in screening. Cell surface ELISA specific positives were assumed to bind membrane antigen, although glutaraldehyde fixation may permeabilize cells and allow binding of antibody to intracellular components. However, among nude mouse and human tissue ELISA positives, 24% bound target cytosol alone, 22% bound membrane alone, and 54% bound antigen in both membrane and cytosol fractions. These results contrast markedly with those obtained by Houghton *et al.* (16), who found that 90% of human anti-melanoma monoclonal antibodies produced with lymphocytes from melanoma patients reacted with intracellular antigens.

Initial specific positives could be identified from virtually every lymph node donor whose lymphocytes yielded significant numbers of hybridomas. Only five of 59 lymph node lymphocyte pools yielded greater than 2% specific positive hybridomas. Notably, one preparation generated 17 positives from 198 hybridomas (8.5%). Only one of these positives, YBY088, showed selective binding in human tissue ELISA (see section II.D).

D. Cross-Reactivity

Each initial specific positive was tested in its respective assay system for cross-reactivity on other tissues. Antibodies showing the most selective binding were subsequently screened for reactivity with target breast cancer tissues in the other two assay systems.

The cell surface ELISA panel included colon, prostate, cervical, bladder, and lung carcinoma, melanoma, and normal fibroblast cell lines. None of the initial specific positives identified by cell surface ELISA bound exclusively to breast carcinoma. However, seven of the antibodies showed some selectivity on the cell line panel and did not bind normal fibroblasts 350Q or WIL. When assayed further in the nude mouse and human tissue ELISAs, only two of the seven antibodies, YBB190 and YBM209, bound membranes and/or cytosols of human breast tumors (Tables 2, 3, and 4).

Nude mouse and human tumor ELISA specific positives were screened against normal colon, lung, kidney, brain, prostate, liver, and normal breast membranes and cytosols. Approximately 48% of positives initially identified by tissue ELISA lost specific reactivity in this multiantigen screen without losing IgM production. Many of the initial specific positives may have resulted from IgM "stickiness," which is particularly problematic on solid phase immunoassay plates. Haskard *et al.* (17) have shown that in some instances, this "stickiness" is due to cross-reactivity of antibodies specific for epitopes on intermediate filaments. All but one of the antibodies which retained the ability to bind breast tumor membranes or cytosols also cross-reacted significantly with the normal tissue panel. One antibody showed selective reactivity by human tissue ELISA (YBY088) and also bound breast carcinoma lines by cell surface ELISA (Tables 2, 3, and 4).

Table 2 Reactivities of Three Human IgM Anti-Breast Carcinoma Antibodies in Cell Surface ELISA

	ELISA O.D. (490 nm)		
Cell type	YBB190	YBM209	YBY088
Breast			
T47D	>1.5	>1.5	0.72
MCF-7	>1.5	ND	ND
BT-20	1.02	1.5	0.15
ZR75-1	1.17	>1.5	0.72
Negative			
H907 (bladder ca)	0.00	0.61	0.00
350Q (fibroblast)	0.08	ND	ND
WIL (fibroblast)	0.00	0.36	0.00
Other tumor cell lines			
T-84 (colon)	1.45	ND	ND
SW480 (colon)	0.27	ND	ND
320DM (colon)	0.18	ND	ND
SW403 (colon)	ND	ND	0.05
SW620 (colon)	ND	ND	0.37
Colo205 (colon)	ND	ND	0.09
M103 (small cell lung)	>1.5	ND	ND
H2540 (large cell lung)	0.70	1.05	ND
A549 (lung adeno)	0.32	ND	ND
PC-3 (prostate)	0.40	0.33	1.13
DU145 (prostate)	0.10	0.27	ND
Panc-1 (pancreas)	0.71	0.70	ND
H907 (bladder)	0.29	0.38	0.16
SK-Mel (melanoma)	0.07	0.31	ND
Brown (melanoma)	0.00	0.07	ND
H998 (osteosarcoma)	0.12	ND	ND
SK-NSH (neuroblastoma)	0.05	ND	ND
Caski (cervix)	ND	ND	0.05

ND = not determined.
Source: Reference 9.

TABLE 3 Reactivities of Three Human IgM Anti-Breast Carcinoma Antibodies with Membrane and Cytosol Fractions of Human Tumor Xenografts

	ELISA O.D. (490 nm)		
Tumor	YBB190	YBM209	YBY088
Membrane			
T417 (breast ca)	1.27	0.13	1.29
T386 (breast ca)	0.38	0.19	0.84
Clouser (breast ca)	0.50	0.70	0.38
T84 (colon ca)	0.49	1.24	0.77
Brown (melanoma)	0.28	2.86	ND
Cytosols			
T417 (breast ca)	1.00	0.28	0.42
T386 (breast ca)	1.43	0.20	0.81
Clouser (breast ca)	0.48	0.45	0.46
T84(colon ca)	1.16	1.15	0.82
Brown (melanoma)	0.36	0.17	0.39

ND = not determined.
Source: Reference 9.

E. Antibody Selection

Our initial criteria for selecting antibodies to be used in clinical trials were simple. First, antibodies should be IgG. Second, they should react specifically with breast carcinoma and not cross-react significantly with normal human tissues. Third, the target antigen should be present in high density on breast tumor cell surfaces. Finally, the radiolabeled antibodies should localize to human breast tumor xenografts in athymic mice. However, none of our antibodies met these criteria. Therefore, we selected three antibodies with distinctively different *in vitro* binding patterns for *in vivo* studies. Cell surface nude mouse and human tissue ELISA data of the three antibodies selected for *in vivo* use are given in Tables 2, 3 and 4.

YBB190, an IgM antibody, showed selective reactivity with some breast carcinoma cell lines, little binding to normal fibroblast cell lines, and no binding to blood elements (monocytes, lymphocytes, granulocytes, and red blood cells) or bone marrow. By immunofluorescence assay YBB190 reacted with both the surface and the cytoskeleton of permeabilized breast cancer cell lines. However,

Table 4 Reactivities of Three Human IgM Anti-Breast Carcinoma Antibodies with Membranes and Cytosol Fractions of Human Tissues

	ELISA reactivity (as % maximum control)[a]					
	Membranes			Cytosols		
Tissue	YBB190	YBM209	YBY088	YBB190	YBM209	YBY088
Breast ca 1	0	90	0	2	159	2
Breast ca 2	0	295	170	40	116	2
Breast ca 3	0	121	83	36	277	0
Breast ca 4	0	47	66	0	237	1
Breast ca 5	0	22	0	0	40	50
Colon ca 1	0	ND	0	4	ND	24
Colon ca 2	0	ND	0	0	ND	0
Mucin colon ca	0	ND	8	69	ND	27
Benign breast 1	0	93	0	0	132	5
Benign breast 2	0	ND	10	0	ND	0
Benign colon	0	797	0	5	292	26
Benign kidney	0	178	0	0	394	22
Benign lung 1	0	273	0	0	324	2
Benign lung 2	0	56	0	0	64	55
Benign liver	0	270	0	0	424	31
Benign brain	0	22	0	87	80	26
Benign prostate	0	135	0	5	240	6
Benign pancreas	0	42	38	0	94	30
Benign bladder	0	139	0	26	155	0

[a]% maximum control = $\dfrac{\text{O.D.}_{490}\text{ nm test antibody}}{\text{O.D.}_{490}\text{ nm positive control antibody}} \times 100\%$.

ND = not determined.

Source: Reference 9.

immunohistochemical studies on cryostat sections suggested that YBB190 had a much more universal reactivity on normal tissues than indicated by the tissue ELISA. The tissue ELISA also suggested that the target antigen was predominantly intracellular. Subsequent studies have shown that YBB190 reacts with an epitope on three antigens (40-45 kd) associated with cytokeratin.

YBM209, also an IgM antibody, was identified initially by its selective reactivity in cell surface ELISA, suggesting that the target antigen was located on cell membranes. However, in tissue ELISA, the antibody bound to an antigen found in many tumor and normal tissue membranes and cytosols. The antibody did not bind blood elements or bone marrow. In immunofluorescence assays, YBM209 bound the cytoskeleton of breast tumor cell lines. We could not confirm that YBM209 target antigen was displayed selectively or to any extent on breast tumor cell surfaces, except by inference from the cell surface ELISA.

YBY088, another IgM antibody, was initially identified by specific ELISA reactivity on breast tumor membranes. Immunofluorescence assay confirmed that target antigen was located predominantly on cell surfaces and could not be detected on normal fibroblasts or blood elements. However, tissue ELISA showed that the antigen was present in cytosols and not in membranes of many normal tissues. Although this contradiction has not yet been resolved, a survey of several breast cancer tissues suggests that YBY088 antigen can be located within the cell or on the cell surface, perhaps expressed as a function of tumor progression or differentiation.

F. *In Vivo* Mouse and Human Studies

In studies described elsewhere (7,8), biodistributions and pharmacokinetics of the three human IgMs were assessed in mouse models. When purified and labeled with ^{111}indium, all three of these human antibodies cleared extremely rapidly from the serum of Balb/c or athymic mice, leaving less than 5% of the injected dose in the serum 24 hours after administration.

In human trials, each of the three ^{111}In-labeled antibodies exhibited unique pharmacokinetics when administered at identical 20 mg doses. YBB190 cleared extremely rapidly from patient serum, as it had in mice, with no uptake in tumor lesions. YBM209 and YBY088 cleared more slowly than YBB190 from patient serum. Both YBM209 and YBY088 antibodies showed approximately 20-30% dose uptake in liver; in addition, YBM was taken up to some extent in the gastrointestinal tract. At the 20 mg dose, YBM209 and YBY088 successfully imaged all confirmed breast tumor lesions in five of six patients tested. These clinical studies (8,9) indicated that successful imaging was correlated both with antibody dose and the presence of target antigen on tumors.

III. DISCUSSION

In revising our criteria to be used in selecting human antibodies for *in vivo* applications, we must now consider the following clinical observations. First, despite their large size and relatively short serum half-life, IgM antibodies effectively penetrated the tumor vasculature and accumulated in target tissue. Second, serum clearance rate was a critical component to imaging success, and the human antibodies showed distinctly different pharmacokinetics. Furthermore, mouse models could not predict the *in vivo* behavior of these antibodies in humans. Third, antibody localized to lesions in those patients whose tumors contained the target antigen. However, we could not confirm that target antigen was displayed predominantly on tumor cell surfaces. Fourth, the clinical human studies showed that *in vitro* cross-reactivity with normal intracellular components as detected in tissue ELISA did not interfere with *in vivo* specificity.

We had hoped that clinical studies might indicate that one *in vitro* assay system was most effective in predicting *in vivo* tumor specificity. At this time, we do not have sufficient data to draw such a conclusion. Our studies do point out the critical need for a model or assay system to predict pharmacokinetics of individual antibodies in humans. We are not aware of an animal model that meets this criterion. Alternatively, it may be possible to associate serum clearance rates with particular biochemical compositions (e.g., patterns of glycosylation). This must be an important focus for future investigations.

These studies have shown that it is possible to produce human monoclonal anti-breast carcinoma antibodies by hybridizing mouse myeloma cells with human breast lymph node lymphocytes. Although large numbers of IgG-, IgM-, and IgA-secreting hybridomas can be obtained from human lymph node lymphocytes, most of the antibodies that bind to breast cancer tissue are IgM. We have shown that the following considerations are important in selecting antibodies for clinical use.

1. One must have an assay that can assess the presence of target antigen on a patient's tumor in order to interpret clinical data.
2. Antibody specificity for the target tumor need not be absolute. Cross-reactivity with normal tissues, particularly with intracellular antigens, may not interfere with *in vivo* antibody localization.
3. An antibody whose target antigen is predominantly intracellular may be clinically useful. With *in vivo* studies of more human antibodies, it should be possible to define more precisely the extent of tumor specificity needed and the relative importance of cell surface versus intracellular location to make an antigen a good target for antibody-mediated diagnosis and therapy.

4. The antibody must have relatively slow clearance kinetics in humans to allow adequate tumor uptake. As discussed above, to our knowledge there is currently no assay system that can predict the biodistribution of a human antibody in a human.
5. Antibody subclass may not be a critical consideration for localization studies. After one has demonstrated that an antibody can localize to a target tissue, as we have shown for YBM209 and YBY088, biodistribution can be "fine-tuned" by making antibody fragments or altering the antibody delivery protocol.

In continuing studies with human monoclonal antibodies, our laboratory is now producing a bank of IgG anti-breast cancer antibodies. With these antibodies, we hope to clarify the importance of Ig subclass in tumor localization. In addition, we are using a new set of screening techniques to identify human antibodies to new cell surface and intracellular antigens. With such new antibodies, we will study the relative importance of antigen distribution to successful tumor localization. Certainly, it remains technically difficult to produce human antibodies of defined specificities. However, if these human antibodies can reduce the immunogenicity problem of mouse monoclonal antibodies, then our efforts are justified by the therapeutic potential of antibody-mediated cancer therapy.

REFERENCES

1. L. Olsson and H. S. Kaplan. Human-human hybridomas producing monoclonal antibodies of predefined antigenic specificity. *Proc. Natl. Acad. Sci. (USA)*, *77*:5429 (1980).
2. C. M. Croce, A. Linnenbach, W. Hall, Z. Steplewski, and H. Koprowski. Production of human hybridomas secreting antibodies to measles virus. *Nature*, *288*:488 (1980).
3. R. O. Dillman, D. L. Shawler, J. B. Dillman, M. Clutter, S. B. Wormsley, M. Markman, and D. Frisman. Monoclonal antibody therapy of cutaneous T-cell lymphoma (CTCL). *Blood*, *62*(suppl 1):212 (1983).
4. R. A. Miller, A. R. Oseroff, P. T. Stratte, and R. Levy. Monoclonal antibody therapeutic trials in seven patients with T-cell lymphoma. *Blood*, *62*:988 (1983).
5. R. W. Schroff, K. A. Foon, S. M. Beatty, R. K. Oldham, and A. C. Morgan. Human anti-murine immunoglobulin responses in patients receiving monoclonal antibody therapy. *Cancer Res.*, *45*:879 (1985).
6. J. Phillips, K. Sikora, and J. V. Watson. Localisation of glioma by human monoclonal antibody. *Lancet*, (Nov. 27):1214 (1982).
7. K. P. Ryan, R. O. Dillman, S. J. DeNardo, G. L. DeNardo, J. Beauregard, K. Burnett, C. Rulot, R. E. Sobel, D. J. Carlo, I. Royston, L. F. O'Grady, and

S. E. Halpern. Imaging of breast cancer metastases using ^{111}Indium radio-labelled human IgM monoclonal antibody. (Submitted for publication.)

8. K. G. Burnett, C. Birdwell, R. M. Bartholomew, D. J. Carlo, S. Halpern, R. O. Dillman, P. L. Hagan, K. P. Ryan, J. Beauregard, C. Rulot, R. E. Sobol, I. Royston, S. J. DeNardo, G. L. DeNardo, D. Macy, and L. F. O'Grady. Studies of ^{111}In-labelled human IgM monoclonal antibodies in mice and humans. (manuscript in preparation.)
9. K. G. Burnett, E. Oh, and J. Hayden. In R. L. Ceriani (ed.). *International Workshop on Monoclonal Antibodies and Breast Cancer.* Martinus Nijhoff Publishers, Boston (1985).
10. J. F. Kearney, A. Radbruch, B. Liesegang, and K. Rajewsky. A new mouse myeloma cell line that has lost immunoglobulin expression but permits the construction of antibody-secreting hybrid cell lines. *J. Immunol., 123*:1548 (1979).
11. K. G. Burnett, Y. Masuho, R. Hernandez, T. Maeda, M. P. King, and J. Martinis. In S. Chatterjee (ed.). *Monoclonal Antibodies: Diagnostic and Therapeutic Use in Tumor and Transplantation.* PSG Publications, Boston (1985).
12. W. Gerhard. Fusion of cells in suspension and outgrowth of hybrids in conditioned medium. In R. H. Kennett, T. J. McKearn, and K. B. Bechtol (eds.). *Monoclonal Antibodies.* Plenum Press, New York (1980).
13. J. W. Littlefield. Selection of hybrids from matings of fibroblasts *in vitro* and their presumed recombinants. *Science, 145*:709 (1964).
14. R. R. McKendall and W. Woo. Microtiter radioimmunoprecipitation assay of HSV-1 polypeptides with recovery and SDS-PAGE analysis of precipitated proteins. *J. Immun. Meth., 72*:461 (1984).
15. P. H. Cleveland, M. G. Wickharn, M. H. Goldbaurn, A. F. Ryan, and D. M. Worthern. Rapid and efficient immobilization of soluble and particulate antigens for solid phase radioimmunoassay. *J. Immunoassay, 2*:117 (1981).
16. A. N. Houghton, H. Brooks, R. J. Cote, M. C. Taormina, H. F. Oettgen, and L. J. Old. Detection of cell surface and intracellular antigens by human monoclonal antibodies. *J. Exp. Med., 158*:53 (1983).
17. D. O. Haskard, V. Gul, and J. R. Archer. Crossreactivity between solid-phase immunoassay plates and intermediate filaments demonstrated by human monoclonal antibodies. *J. Immun. Meth., 77*:291 (1985).

III

FINAL CONSIDERATIONS

14

Perspectives on Regulatory Considerations for Human Monoclonal Antibodies for Use in Man

VICTORIA SCHAUF*
Nassau County Medical Center, East Meadow, New York

This chapter is provided to outline some regulatory considerations that may be pertinent in the United States to the testing and licensure of human monoclonal antibody products. The Food and Drug Administration (FDA) is responsible for the regulation of monoclonal antibody products for human use if the products are to be shipped in interstate commerce. FDA activities have been discussed recently in *JAMA* Medical News (1). At this writing, most monoclonal products have been of murine origin. Murine monoclonal antibodies have been licensed for *in vitro* diagnostic use, and investigational use in man has been permitted; however, none have been licensed for human administration. Because knowledge is rapidly accumulating and the field is still evolving, it is too early to know what all the requirements for monoclonal products of human origin will be. However, some pertinent regulatory concerns are discussed with reference to some of the approaches outlined in the earlier chapters. The comments provided here are based on cited references and discussions with FDA staff, but do not constitute formal guidelines.

Previous affiliation: Food and Drug Administration, Bethesda, Maryland

I. THE BASIS FOR REGULATION

Monoclonal antibodies can be used therapeutically or diagnostically. Diagnostic applications could involve administration to man or use *in vitro*. The statutory authority for federal regulation of biological products for human administration and the producers of such products is the Public Health Service Act. The FDA Center for Drugs and Biologics, Office of Biologics Research and Review, is responsible for regulating biological products, including hybridoma products, for human administration, as well as for certain *in vitro* diagnostics that are used to test blood products that are to be used for human administration. Other *in vitro* diagnostics are regulated by the FDA Center for Devices and Radiologic Health under the Medical Device Amendments of the Food, Drug, and Cosmetic Act.

To implement these laws, the executive branch of the U.S. government publishes proposed rules in the *Federal Register.* After a period in which public comment is invited, the final rules are codified in the Code of Federal Regulations (CFR). Some existing regulations have been discussed in relation to their possible bearing on hybridoma products (2). The regulations describe what is required for a product to be investigated and marketed and have the force of law. Although at present there are no regulations that mention hybridoma products, the 21 CFR 200 and 21 CFR 600 series are pertinent.

The FDA may also publish Guidelines or Points to Consider. These may assist communication between product developers and regulators, but do not have the force of law. A notice regarding availability of "Points to Consider in the Manufacture of Monoclonal Antibody Products for Human Use" was published in the *Federal Register* (3) and discussed by Merchant (4) and by Hoffman *et al.* (5).

Products of human hybridomas, like all biological products that are intended for therapeutic use or *in vivo* diagnostic use in man, must be shown to be both safe and effective before they can be licensed in the United States for marketing. At the time of licensure, two licenses are issued to the manufacturer by the Office of Biologics Research and Review: a product license for the product and an establishment license for the manufacturing facility. Efficacy must be demonstrated by well-controlled trials before licensure.

The human safety and efficacy data which are part of the license application are collected by obtaining permission to test the biological product in man. Such testing of unlicensed biological products which move in interstate commerce requires submission to the FDA of a Notice of Claimed Investigational Exemption for a New Drug (IND). There must be sufficient preclinical animal and *in vitro* data described in the IND to warrant investigational use of the biological product in man. Namely, there has to be some reason to believe the product is more likely to do good than harm, or a favorable "risk-benefit" ratio.

Flexibility in safety criteria could be possible where the intended use is in a setting of life-threatening disease. However, patients in this category are often immunodeficient and have increased susceptibility to viral infection.

Information submitted to the FDA in an IND is considered confidential to protect the sponsor's trade secrets and is not available to the public under the provisions of the Freedom of Information Act (FOI). After licensure, some information concerning the biological product and the studies demonstrating safety of the product used in support of the license would become available to the public under the provisions of the FOI.

The Office of Biologics Research and Review will review INDs and licenses for all monoclonal products intended for *in vivo* human use, whether the monoclonal is used alone or coupled to a drug, toxin, or radioisotope. For monoclonal antibodies coupled to other agents, reviewers may receive input from other experts in the FDA regarding the coupled agent.

INDs have been submitted and studies are ongoing for *in vivo* human testing of monoclonals. No monoclonal antibody has yet been licensed for human use *in vivo*.

II. CONSIDERATIONS FOR HYBRIDOMA PRODUCTS FOR *IN VIVO* USE

FDA standards for monoclonal antibodies have not yet been fully established. The draft Points to Consider provides information that can be used in preparing and evaluating material to be submitted to the FDA concerning hybridoma products. Specific considerations will have to evolve with technological advances. In general, it appears that "the use of highly purified products with optimal specificity as established by rigorous and copious experimental data represents the best possibility of ensuring their safe and efficacious therapeutic use" (5).

A number of antibody-containing products, produced by techniques not involving hybridomas, are already commercially available. It would be desirable for similar products of hybridoma technology to offer the same or greater efficacy, safety, or availability. The specificity and potency of new monoclonal products should be compared to those of licensed polyclonal products for the same indication. Studies could also be designed to compare safety and efficacy.

For each hybridoma product, the origins of the product will need to be carefully considered in deciding on the product's potential risks. This will involve characterization of the fusion partners and their donors and tissues of origin; the immunogen; the immunization procedure; the screening procedure; the cloning procedure; and the seed lot system. The latter should be characterized as to identity, stability, and known microbial contaminants. If murine cells have been employed, testing of the manufacturer's working cell bank for potential human pathogens such as lymphocytic choriomeningitis virus (LCM), polyoma, reoviruses, or murine leukemia viruses is indicated. If human cells have been employed, tests for Epstein Barr virus (EBV), EBV genomes, cytomegalovirus, hepatitis B virus, and retroviruses, including human T-lymphotropic viruses, are advised. Cell lines that actively produce identifiable virus are discouraged as a source of monoclonal antibody. Even if virus is subsequently removed or inactivated, some pathogens, such as HTLV-III, might be unacceptable in certain situations. Testing for other viruses in human and simian cell lines and in the antibody-producing cell line itself is also indicated. Screening of human donors, whose cells are incorporated in the hybridoma, may also be appropriate.

Considerations related to identifying production systems include identification of tissue culture systems or animals, including harvest and passage of ascites, control measures for contamination during production, criteria for further use of cells, supernatants, or ascites, purification of final product, and system to fill final containers (21 CFR 211).

It will be necessary to show that hybridoma products are not changed in successive production lots by comparison to an initial, stable reference lot. It is recommended that each lot should meet criteria for specificity, quantity, stability, aggregation, denaturation, fragmentation, homogeneity, sterility (21 CFR 610.12), and *Mycoplasma* and polynucleotide contamination. Characterization by immunoglobulin class, subclass, and isoelectric focusing pattern is currently recommended. If additives are used to preserve sterility or physical properties of the antibody preparation, they should be described in the way they are used, and they should be proven safe.

Specific attention is required to exclude potential viral contamination. When mouse cells or mice are used, screening is indicated for LCM virus by animal or tissue culture inoculation. Mouse antibody production tests are used to detect LCM, reovirus type 3, polyoma, pneumonia virus of mice, mouse adenovirus, minute virus of mice, mouse hepatitis, K, ectromelia, Sendai, and GD VII. Appropriate assays to detect murine cytomegalovirus, EDIM, thymic, LDH viruses, or murine leukemia viruses are currently performed routinely. Serum additives to tissue cultures need to be shown free of adventitious agents.

Tests are also necessary on the monoclonal antibody preparation after it is dispensed into its final container, the "final-filled" product. These are likely to include: potency, electrophoretic migration on polyacrylamide gels, protein concentration, and identity (21 CFR 610.14), in addition to the final container tests standard for biological products, namely sterility (21 CFR 610.12), general safety (21 CFR 610.11), and pyrogenicity.

Other contaminating materials are of concern and may be required to be absent (e.g., pristane, penicillin) or in minimal concentrations (other antibiotics). Potentially harmful contaminants such as residual chromatography reagents or preservatives may need to be assayed. The stability of the product needs to be assessed to determine proper use under IND and to establish a valid dating period at licensure.

Preclinical evaluation in animals for toxicity and immunopharmacology is currently recommended, particularly for products intended to be administered therapeutically. If an animal model exists for testing efficacy, this testing could also be employed. Monoclonal antibody preparations should be screened for cross-reactivity with human tissues. Blood cells or cell lines might also be employed.

Additional considerations pertain to monoclonal antibody products coupled to toxins, drugs, or isotopes. If the complex is toxic, it is important that the targeting be of appropriate specificity, that the toxin and antibody be coupled as completely as possible, and that unbound toxin be quantitated and present only in tolerable amounts. Determination of the stability of the complex would be important, and the activity and specificity of the components need to be maintained in the complex.

Other FDA publications may be useful to developers of monoclonal antibodies. These include "Points to Consider in the Characterization of Cell Lines Used to Produce Biologicals" (6a) and "Licensing of a Biological Monoclonal Antibody Product Prepared by Hybridoma Technology" (6). Although not directly related, information to be found in Petricciani *et al.* (7) on manufacturing and safety concerns for other biological products, the interferons, may be of interest to the reader.

Although not mentioned in the draft "Points to Consider in the Manufacture of Monoclonal Antibody Products for Human Use," several recent scientific development may be of interest to developers of monoclonals. Methods for antibody production by human hybridomas have been described using serum-free medium (8). The advantages of serum-free media in large-scale production of therapeutic agents have been discussed by Fleischaker (9).

As previously unrecognized human blood-borne viral diseases are described, such as human parvovirus infection (10), further evaluation for contamination may be necessary. For further information on possible contamination of blood products, see *Infectious Complications of Blood Transfusion* (11). In the future, some contamination problems might be avoided by using the products of normal cells that have been transfected to produce antibody (see Chapter 7). Additionally, in the future recombinant DNA technology might provide products that supplant hybridoma products by overcoming several of the technical and regulatory problems with hybridoma products.

III. *IN VITRO* DIAGNOSTICS

FDA requirements for approval of products for marketing for *in vitro* diagnostic purposes differ from those for *in vivo* use. *In vitro* diagnostics are regulated by the Center for Drugs and Biologics if they are to be used to screen blood products for human use; otherwise, they are considered medical devices regulated by the Center for Devices and Radiological Health. In the latter case, products classified as being "substantially equivalent" to a product marketed prior to the Medical Device Amendments of 1976 can be submitted to FDA as a "510 (k)" notice, which requires a response within 90 days. This relatively rapid mechanism would not be applicable to a novel product not marketed prior to 1976. Hybridoma products could qualify for a 510 (k) status if polyclonal products of the same specificity were marketed before 1976. A number of murine monoclonal *in vitro* diagnostic products have already been marketed using this mechanism, including reagents to assay for IgE and human chorionic gonadotropin.

For novel products, a premarket approval application is required, and this may require extensive clinical evaluation of the product to establish its usefulness as a diagnostic reagent and to substantiate the manufacturer's claims. The evaluation is based on consideration of specificity, sensitivity, stability, reproducibility, and clinical correlations. The role of clinical factors, such as age, sex, genetics, nutrition, geography, and concomitant medications, is important to determine (12). Such characterization should help to establish the clinical usefulness of the product.

IV. PERSPECTIVES ON THE REGULATORY PROCESS

At the beginning of the century, children treated with diphtheria antitoxin prepared from a horse with tetanus died of tetanus. This unnecessary tragedy led to the recognition that the safety of biological products for human use and the producers of such products should be regulated by the federal government. Commercial distribution in the United States of human hybridoma products for diagnostic or therapeutic use in man will require prior approval from the FDA. Developers of such products may wish to consider this process in their planning. The regulatory requirements have scientific validity—data must be collected to show that the product is useful for its proposed indication and that it is reasonably safe. The regulatory process provides formalized documentation, based on in-depth peer review and inspection of data, product, and manufacturing plant, that the product and its manufacture have been properly evaluated. This evaluation of the product properly would be necessary for responsible businesses for reasons of safety and ethics, even if no regulatory requirements existed. These considerations permit a rational approach to developing applications to the FDA.

The cost of identifying drugs and biologics for possible human use, their preclinical development, formulation, and their pharmacological, toxicological, and clinical evaluation is generally quite high. Estimates of several millions of dollars per drug evaluated have been proposed. Moreover, evaluation does not always reveal a safe, effective, marketable product. The development process for novel human hybridoma products may be similarly difficult or more difficult if the hybridoma is unstable or if it is coupled to a toxic ligand. Even development of novel human hybridoma products for marketing for *in vitro* use may be quite involved.

Collecting, analyzing, verifying, and presenting the data needed to satisfy the regulatory requirements for approval or licensure of hybridoma products, like any other serious scientific endeavor, is complicated, time consuming, and has the potential for unexpected delays and disappointments. Individual investigators may have greater potential resources for initial discovery than for final application. It would not be surprising if novel human hybridoma products for *in vivo* use were brought to market by well-established firms with extensive experience and resources. The status and prospects of the monoclonal antibody industry as of 1986 have been reviewed (13).

FDA requirements are considered quite stringent compared to those of many other grovernments. Satisfying requirements in the United States may be accepted by other governments as sufficient for marketing in their countries. Some products may appear abroad before they are available in the United States. This lag has been criticized with the argument that the delay may have deprived consumers of valuable products for which no counterpart was available. The delay has protected consumers in the United States from dangerous products.

The regulatory process leading to licenses to market is an interactive one. The product's sponsor provides materials to FDA reviewers who render professional opinions as to safety and efficacy. The FDA then acts to issue a license, or the sponsor may be asked to correct problems that have precluded earlier licensure. Often there is considerable interaction between sponsors and the FDA. It is desirable for the sponsor of a product to contact the FDA early in the development-and-application phase to begin effective communication before investing time and money in evaluations that might not contribute to the product's ultimate approval for marketing. Ongoing dialogue can expedite the regulatory process. Sponsors who identify problems in meeting requirements may discuss with the FDA alternative approaches to meeting these requirements if appropriate.

V. PERSPECTIVES ON THE EVALUATION OF MONOCLONAL ANTIBODIES

Some reasonable assumptions about human hybridoma products need to be evaluated objectively. For example, human products should be better tolerated than mouse products because they are more closely related antigenically to the patient. However, this needs to be shown objectively. In fact, humans are usually not inbred, and this assumption may not be true. Another assumption is that antibodies specific for a tumor's antigens would be of therapeutic value. This too would need to be demonstrated objectively, for each tumor antigen, since it is also possible for such antibodies to do harm by "blocking" antigens that are the target of other, more protective immune responses.

In considering the recent technological advances in antibody production, it is wise to remember the long history of use of antibodies. From this perspective, specific antibodies have been useful in preventing only a few infectious diseases of well-characterized etiology and pathophysiology. Less often, serotherapy was somewhat useful in treating established infections, only to be supplanted by more effective specific chemotherapy directed toward the etiological agent. The simple notion of using antibodies to treat "cancer" has been disappointing, because it failed to recognize the diverse etiology and pathophysiology of a multitude of malignant processes. The new technology may be useful in delineating the latter and may lead to more rational approaches to treating malignant diseases.

It is important that the products for use in malignant diseases, as for other diseases, be evaluated objectively. Objective trials controlled to eliminate observer bias are important, and anecdotal observations that one or a few heterogeneous patients "did well" with a particular immunological treatment often fail to be confirmed. Small, open trials are appropriate to begin to test a product's safety, prior to beginning larger, controlled trials to evaluate efficacy. Objective evaluations based on scientifically rational approaches would be likely to contribute to the regulatory review.

ACKNOWLEDGMENTS

Giovanna Connor provided expert editorial assistance, and several other FDA personnel provided helpful advice; however, opinions expressed in this chapter are those of the author and not necessarily those of the Agency.

REFERENCES

1. Various authors, Medical News. *JAMA, 254*:2189 (1985).
2. Marc H. Bozeman, The regulation of hybridoma products. In *The Impact of Hybridoma Technology on the Medical Device and Diagnostic Product Industry* (Proceedings of the Educational Seminar, Arlington, VA, June 14-15, 1982), Health Industry Manufacturers Association Reports, Report No. 82-1, (1982), Chapter 9, pp. 63-82.
3. Federal Register, Docket No. 83N-0363, Biological Products; *in Vitro* or *in Vivo* Monoclonal Antibodies, . . . Availability of Draft Criteria for New Technologies; Request for Comments, Data, and Recommendations. Notice. *Fed. Register, 49*:1138, Jan. 9, 1984.

4. E. Bruce Merchant, Points to consider during monoclonal antibody production. In *The Impact of Hybridoma Technology on the Medical Device and Diagnostic Product Industry* (Proceedings of the Educational Seminar, Arlington, VA, June 14-15, 1982), Health Industry Manufacturers Association Reports, Report No. 82-1, (1982), Chapter 10, pp. 83-92.
5. T. Hoffman, J. Kenimer, and K. E. Stein. Regulatory issues surrounding therapeutic use of monoclonal antibodies: points to consider in the manufacture of injectable products intended for human use. In Ralph A. Reisfeld and Stewart Sell (eds.). *Monoclonal Antibodies and Cancer Therapy* (*UCLA Symposia on Molecular and Cellular Biology*), New Series, Vol. 27. Alan R. Liss, Inc., New York (1985), pp. 431-440.
6. Federal Register, Docket No. 83N-0070, Licensing of a Biological Monoclonal Antibody Product Prepared by Hybridoma Technology. *Fed. Register, 48*:50795, Nov. 3, 1983.

6a. Federal Register, Docket No. 84N-0154, Open Meeting; Public Workshop on Cell Substrates; Availability of Points to Consider; Request for Comments. *Fed. Register, 49*:23456, June 6, 1984.

7. J. C. Petricciani, E. C. Esber, H. E. Hopps, and A. Attallah. Manufacture and safety of interferons in clinical research. In P. E. Came and W. A. Carter (eds.). *Interferons and Their Applications.* Springer-Verlag, New York (1984), pp. 357-370.
8. S. P. C. Cole, E. H. Vreeken, and J. C. Roder. Antibody production by human X human hybridomas in serum-free medium. *J. Immunol. Meth., 78*: 271-278 (1985).
9. R. J. Fleischaker, Jr. Applying large-scale culture techniques to the *in vitro* production of monoclonal antibodies. *Pharmaceutical Manufacturing,* pp. 16-21 (January, 1986).
10. R. J. Whitley. Editorial, Parvovirus infection, *N. Engl. J. Med., 313*:111-112 (1985).
11. E. Tabor, *Infectious Complications of Blood Transfusion.* Academic Press, Inc., New York (1982).
12. Hipolito Nino. Bureau of Medical Devices position on approval of hybridoma-derived products. In *The Impact of Hybridoma Technology on the Medical Device and Diagnostic Product Industry* (Proceedings of the Educational Seminar, Arlington, VA, June 14-15, 1982). Health Industry Manufacturers Association Reports, Report No. 82-1, (1982), Chapter 11, pp. 93-104.
13. Jeffrey L. Fox. Monoclonal antibodies: a successful diagnosis, *ASM News, 52*:90-93 (1986).

15

Conclusions and Perspectives

ANTHONY J. STRELKAUSKAS
Medical University of South Carolina, Charleston, South Carolina

The chapters presented in this book represent the work of many, but obviously not all, the laboratories around the world doing research with human monoclonal antibodies. There are a number of other groups who are doing elegant studies in a variety of research efforts in which the construction and/or utilization of human monoclonal antibodies plays an integral role. Some of this work has recently been reviewed (1). Chapter 5, concerning human monoclonals specific for *Pseudomonas aeruginosa,* is an example of the utility of human monoclonals for infectious diseases. In the case of Pseudomonas infections, which cause severe problems especially in burn patients, passive immunotherapy through the administration of monoclonal antibody may be the most effective treatment available. Other infectious diseases may also be good candidates for this therapeutic approach.

A second clinical problem in which human monoclonals have applicability is that of autoimmune disease (2). The benefits of cloning the autoantibodies involved in these types of diseases are obvious. Purification and characterization of these pathological molecules could lead to the discovery or development of inhibitory molecules (either natural or synthetic), which might block the binding to and subsequent damage of tissue. In addition, these autoantibodies themselves, if modified to $F(ab')_2$ fragments, might also passively block these disease processes.

Human monoclonals may also play a role in the success of organ transplantation. Because the process of graft rejection is a cell-mediated phenomenon, current methods involve administration of drugs that inhibit immune responsiveness such that the organ survival can be prolonged. The clinical consequences of this approach are consistent with those seen in immunodeficient patients. In contrast to this generalized immunoincompetence, human monoclonal antibodies specific for the subset(s) of lymphocytes responsible for graft rejection would prolong graft survival without compromising the entire immune system. It should be pointed out that this type of approach has been utilized for several years in transplantation research; first through the use of anti-thymocyte globulin (ATG) mostly made in rabbits and horses, and later using murine monoclonals. Many of these systems have been reviewed by Janossy *et al.* (3). Two of the major problems associated with the use of heterologous antibodies are adverse side-effects and quantities required. There is some controversy concerning the frequency and severity of these side-effects, but everyone seems to agree that high doses of murine monoclonals (in some cases, gram amounts per dose) may be required to establish and maintain this type of supportive therapy. The economic consequences of these requirements are well known. Unfortunately, they become even greater in the case of human monoclonals.

Perhaps the greatest hopes for human monoclonals lay in cancer research and treatment. From the preceding chapters, it can be seen there are many varied approaches being used for the development of both diagnostic and therapeutic reagents in this field. Here again, there has been and continues to be extensive use of murine monoclonals, both diagnostically and therapeutically (4,5). Unfortunately, the results have not been as successful as hoped for. The reasons for this lack of success are, like many facets of the disease itself, simply not understood. One possible explanation may be the inability of a murine monoclonal to identify the probably subtle tumor-associated and/or tumor-specific antigens of human malignancies. If this is, indeed, the case, it would be assumed that even those subtle antigens might be more readily identified in a homologous as opposed to a heterologous system, making diagnostic assays using human antibodies the tests of choice. The same principle holds true for therapeutics with an added benefit that human molecules should have very limited side-effects. However, both diagnostic and therapeutic applications would require the production of large amounts of human antibody, which to date has been technically difficult and economically unfeasible. One other problem may be related to the therapeutic use of these molecules. In most cases, therapy has relied on the conjugation of toxic molecules, such as ricin or toxic drugs, to antibodies (for excellent reviews, see reference 3). Some of the questions that remain to be answered about this approach are: How many molecules are required to initiate a lethal event? How will toxic molecules be attached such that they still allow and, in some cases, facilitate the internalization necessary for function? Can toxic molecules be conjugated in such a way that they maintain lethal characteristics? Perhaps most importantly, does the conjugation of toxic molecules change the human antibody molecule enough so that it is then recognized as a "foreign" protein by the patient receiving the therapy? All of these questions are currently being addressed in laboratories worldwide, but to date there have been no concrete answers.

The utility of human monoclonal antibodies in clinical medicine is obvious. These antibodies have tremendous potential in practically all types of human disease, either as sensitive diagnostic tools or as passive immunotherapeutic modalities. This is the good news. The not so good news is that the field of human monoclonal antibodies still has many problems. Some of the most important of these are: 1) the difficulties associated with the construction of stable hybrids; 2) the specificity, or lack of it, seen with antibodies from some human clones; 3) the dreadfully low amount of antibody produced by the stable clones thus far established; and, as a result, 4) the terribly high cost required to produce the large amounts suitable for generalized use of these antibodies.

I feel that as these problems of stability and specificity are addressed and alleviated, human monoclonal antibodies in large quantity will be produced (probably by large pharmaceutical houses) through the aid of genetic engineering and will become the reagents of choice diagnostically and therapeutically in a variety of human diseases.

REFERENCES

1. E. G. Engleman, S. K. H. Foung, J. W. Larrick, and A. A. Raubitschek (eds.). *Human Hybridomas and Monoclonal Antibodies.* Plenum Press, New York (1985).
2. B. F. Haynes and G. S. Eisenbarth (eds.). *Monoclonal Antibodies: Probes for the Study of Autoimmunity and Immunodeficiency.* Academic Press, New York (1983).
3. G. Janossy, G. Goldstein, and A. B. Cosimi. Monoclonal anti-human lymphocyte antibodies: their potential in immunosuppression and bone marrow transplantation. In A. J. McMichael and J. W. Fabre (eds.). *Monoclonal Antibodies in Clinical Medicine.* Academic Press, New York (1983).
4. B. D. Ross, R. Langman, I. Trowbridge, and R. Dulbecco (eds.). *Monoclonal Antibodies and Cancer.* Academic Press, New York (1983).
5. A. J. McMichael and J. W. Fabre (eds.). *Monoclonal Antibodies in Clinical Medicine.* Academic Press, New York (1982).

Index

B

C

D

E

I